MINIMAL
Access
GYNAECOLOGY

Edited by Stephen Grochmal

Forewords by
Roger Baldwin and Charles Ellis Connant

RADCLIFFE MEDICAL PRESS, OXFORD AND NEW YORK

British Library Cataloguing in Publication Data

A cataloguing record for this book is available from the British Library.

ISBN 1 87090 573 3

Library of Congress Cataloging-in-Publication Data

Minimal access gynaecology / edited by Stephen Grochmal ; forewords by
  Roger Baldwin and Charles Ellis Connant.
      p.   cm.
    Includes bibliographical references and index.
    ISBN 1–870905–73–3 (hard) : $125.00
    1. Generative organs, Female- -Endoscopic surgery. 2. Laparoscopy.
  I Grochmal, Stephen.
    [DNLM: 1. Genital Diseases, Female- -surgery. 2. Endoscopy-
  -methods.   WP 660 M665 1994]
  RG104.7.M55   1994
618.1'45- -dc20
DNLM/DLC
for Library of Congress   94-37495
                                                                     CIP

Typeset by Bookman, Slough
Printed and bound in Spain

Publisher's Note

Gynecology or Gynaecology poses a dilemma for any publisher whose work is designed for an international readership. Radcliffe Medical Press has chosen to answer it on this occasion by providing the book, initially, in covers spelled Gynecology for North America and Gynaecology for the rest of the world. The text has been edited for English spelling with the exception of Charles Connant's foreword.

This solution will not satisfy the purists, to whom we can only offer our apologies.

Radcliffe Medical Press
August 1994

Dedication

Dedicated to the memory of my father, Stanley Peter Grochmal, my
mother Sophie, and to my son, Geoffrey Stephen, a source of
perpetual joy, and to Diane, whose undying love and encouragement
changed the course of my life.

Contents

Part I – Preparing for the Endoscopic Procedure

Part II – Non Gynaecological Associated Procedures

Part III – Laparoscopic Procedures

Part IV – Hysteroscopic Procedures

Part V – The Future of Endoscopic Surgery

List of Authors

Gregory T Absten, President, Advanced Laser Services Corporation, Columbus, Ohio, USA

Roger Baldwin, FRCOG, Chairman, Examination Committee, Royal College of Obstetrics and Gynaecology; Consultant Obstetrician and Gynaecologist, Medical Education Centre, Whipps Cross Hospital, London, UK

Jonathan S Berek, MD, Director, Vice Chairman of Department of Obstetrics and Gynecology, Santa Monica Hospital; Director, Division of Gynecologic Oncology, University of California, Los Angeles, California, USA

John R Brumsted, MD, Associate Professor, Division of Reproductive Endocrinology and Infertility, University of Vermont, Burlington, Vermont, USA

Vito Cardone, MD, Medical Director, Fertility Center of New England, Reading, Massachusetts, USA

Stephen Cohen, MD, Associate Professor, Associate Chairman and Director of Reproductive Surgery, University of Massachusetts Medical Center, Department of Obstetrics and Gynecology, Worcester, Massachusetts, USA

Charles E Connant, MD, FACS, FACOG, Assistant Clinical Professor, Department of Obstetrics and Gynecology, UMDNJ School of Medicine, Newark, New Jersey, USA

Martin Curlik, MD, Clinical Professor of Urology, Chief, Section of Laparoscopic Urological Surgery, New York University, New York, USA

Jean B Dubuisson, Professor, Clinique Universitaire, Port Royal, Paris, France

John Erian, FRCOG, Consultant Gynaecologist, Farnborough Hospital, Orpington, Kent, UK

Royice B Everett, MD, Medical Director, Baptist Laser Institute, Baptist Hospital; Associate Clinical Professor, Department of Obstetrics and Gynecology, University of Oklahoma, Oklahoma City, USA

Ray Garry, FRCOG, Director Minimal Access Gynaecological Surgery, St James University Hospital, Leeds; Consultant Gynaecologist and Medical Director, Women's Endoscopic Laser Foundation, South Cleveland Hospital, Middlesbrough, UK

Jacob L Glock, MD, Clinical Instructor and Fellow, Division of Reproductive Endocrinology and Infertility, University of Vermont, Burlington, Vermont, USA

Stephen A Grochmal, MD, Medical Director, New Jersey Laser Institute, Princeton, New Jersey, USA

Stephen G Harding, MRCOG, Research Fellow, Whipps Cross Hospital and St Bartholemew's Hospital, London, UK

Michael S Kavic, MD, FACS, Visiting Assistant Professor of Surgery, Northeastern Ohio Universities College of Medicine, McKees Rocks, Pennsylvania, USA

Fabrice Lecuru, MD, Clinique Universitaire, Port Royal, Paris, France

John M Leventhal, MD, Clinical Instructor in Obstetrics and Gynecology, Harvard Medical School, Boston, Massachusetts, USA

Jack M Lomano, MD, Director, South Florida Women's Center, Lee Memorial Hospital, Department of Obstetrics and Gynecology, Fort Myers, Florida, USA

Thomas Lyons, MD, Director of the Center for Advanced Videoscopic Surgery at West Paces Medical Center, Center for Women's Care and Reproductive Surgery, Atlanta, Georgia, USA

L Mandelbrot, MD, Clinique Universitaire, Port Royal, Paris, France

Bruce McLucas, MD, Assistant Clinical Professor, University of California, Los Angeles, California, USA

Lindsay McMillan, MRCOG, Director of Medical Education Centre, Consultant Obstetrician and Gynaecologist, Whipps Cross Hospital, London, UK

Ervin Moss, MD, Consultant, New Jersey State Society of Anesthesiologists, Board of Directors, Anesthesia Patient Safety Foundation, Verona, New Jersey, USA

Adam Ostrzenski, MD, PhD, Professor and Director of Operative Gynecology – Endoscopic Laser Surgery, Department of Obstetrics and Gynecology, Howard University College of Medicine, Washington DC, USA; Professor, Department of Operative Gynecology, Jagiellonian University School of Medicine, Kraków, Poland

William H Parker, MD, Chairman of Department of Obstetrics and Gynecology, Santa Monica Hospital, California; Clinical Professor, Department of Obstetrics and Gynecology, University of California, Los Angeles, USA

Andrew Pesce, FRACOG, Westmead Hospital, Sydney, New South Wales, Australia

Michael Slatkine, PhD, Director of Research and Development, Laser Industries, Tel Aviv, Israel

Martin Steel, MRCOG, Consultant in Obstetrics and Gynaecology, Victoria Hospital, Blackpool, UK

Carlos A Suarez, MD, Director, Institute of Minimal Access Surgery of South Florida; Associate Professor, Department of Surgery, University of Miami, School of Medicine, South Miami, Florida, USA

Chris Sutton, FRCOG, Consultant Obstetrician and Gynaecologist, Royal Surrey County Hospital, Guildford, UK

Samuel Tarantino, MD, Medical Director, The Florida Infertility and Endometriosis Center, Tampa, Florida, USA

Ernst Voss, MD, Research Fellow, Rush Green Hospital, Romford, Essex, UK

Anthony Weekes, FRCS, FRCOG, Director, European Endoscopic Training Centre; Consultant Gynaecologist, Rush Green Hospital, Romford, Essex, UK

Foreword

" . . . . . . ὠφελέειν εἰ μή βλάπτειν "

Hippocrates 460 BC

The old Hippocratic aphorism of 'Either do some good or do no harm' could never have been more appropriately applied than with the development of endoscopic surgery. This philosophy, which is to the great benefit of the patient, is all pervasive in today's surgical revolution.

When Robert A Kimbrough used to give his annual final lecture at the University of Pennsylvania Graduate School of Medicine (the famous 'pendulum' lecture, ie the swing back of medical thinking or medical procedures) he was attempting to portray these changes exactly as they are ironically applied to minimally invasive surgery (MIS) today.

After years of totally invasive procedures and techniques, the change has been in the progression to MIS (or techniques). This has now led to the formation at health care institutions of the Minimally Invasive Surgical Unit (MISU) concept.

Recent developments over the last two years, have led to an explosion of interest in operative endoscopy by other surgical fields. It is through the enthusiasm and assistance of the gynecologist, that the general surgeon began the laparoscopic cholecystectomy, and the urologist explored the abdominal cavity and used endoscopic methods to perform a lymphadenectomy.

Endoscopic procedures were in the minds of the earliest gynecologists and have been described in various medical writings, but from Pantaleone's original works on hysteroscopy the modality remained vaguely a diagnostic tool. It was not until recently, when advancements in optics and electronic enhancement of optical imagery along with the electronic uterine distension pump, made hysteroscopy a 'sine qua non' in gynecologic work, both in the office and hospital. As a result, this made many pronounce the demise of dilatation and curettage. In a similar fashion, laparoscopies were described, but were not applicable, until Kurt Semm was able to monitor the intra-abdominal pressure and this, along with the Roeder loop and intra- and extracorporeal knot tying, established what Semm called 'pelviscopy'.

The entry to the peritoneal cavity was entirely blind – as we know from paracentesis, with or without ascites – but became more certain with the application of the Verres needle or more recently the Adair-Verres needle and the Grochmal modification of it. Semm has also described a different entry into the abdomen, slightly more elaborate, yet quite safe after mastering it.

From this point on, with the explosion of electronic technology, hysteroscopic and laparoscopic surgical procedures have become universally known as minimally invasive surgery.

Following Goldrath's original report in 1981, the use of Nd:YAG laser technology has leaped forward. Over the last two years, optical catheters and laser fibers made an even further impact in the use of the laser. The free CO_2 laser beam was supplanted by the Nd:YAG sapphire tip, which very quickly gave way to the shaped laser fiber as the ultimate in convenience, safety and cost efficiency. Technological horizons are proceeding in the miniaturization of instruments and, as mentioned previously, procedures like microhysteroscopy, microlaparoscopy and falloposcopy are now a practical reality. Future developments will be in portable laser units for the physician's consulting rooms, and the introduction of three-dimensional visualization in all endoscopic arenas. This will make these techniques truly minimally invasive and in keeping with the premise at the outset of this Foreword.

At the 1991 Clinical Congress of the American College of Surgeons it was widely discussed and substantiated that MIS is now being explored in applications far exceeding its initial use to perform a cholecystectomy[1].

In gynecology, MIS procedures have replaced many laparotomies almost entirely. Consider two examples: the laparoscopic approach to ectopic pregnancy which is now well-established as the treatment method that confers comparable safety and efficacy to that of laparotomy and rare postoperative complications[6,7]. Or the transuterine tubal surgery which is now a non-invasive hysteroscopic procedure with results close to 90% tubal patency for proximal disease[2]. Is this not a revolution? Additionally, the new distal chip cameras, the 1.6 mm viewing 'eye' of the optical catheter and the arrival of digital computerization for virtual reality effects will push the techniques of endoscopy even further.

The assisted reproductive technologies now have various methods and techniques, with a dozen or so acronyms, each one denoting a new leap forward. To mention but one, the microsurgical fertilization with a 'window' in the zona pellucida. In genetics, there are other dramatic changes, such as the ability to biopsy preimplantation embryos, or to use the polar body for sex determination. However, some techniques have lost ground, for example, early second trimester amniocentesis has replaced chorionic villous sampling, which is in keeping with our Hippocratic premise[2].

Efficient endoscopy and MISU are dependent on good assistance and teamwork and perhaps, most of all, appropriately selected and properly functioning instrumentation which, if not chosen carefully, can make the procedure either impossible or unsafe. And finally, 'pari passu' with the mentioned equipment stringency, is the training of the gynecologist, which is sometimes rather complicated, as work is performed in two rather than three dimensions. This is definitely an acquired skill and requires progressive conditioning of one's proprioceptive centers – therefore a good 'anlage' is desirable.

Patient preparation is also more critical than before, because patients are not hospitalized as after conventional surgery. A good proportion of MIS is done for ovarian pathology and although ovarian cancer is not a common disease, it is not rare, and laboratory work should be directed to determine possible presence of malignancy and also to avoid confusion with endometriosis[4,5]. Perhaps future immunofluorescence techniques will allow us to differentially diagnose these disorders. In MIS there are no problems of critical care and metabolism, such as cytotoxicity, ischemia and reperfusion, inflammatory cytokines, or stress responses[3]. The only exception might be the monitoring of fluid overload during endometrial ablation.

Because of the very nature of MIS work affecting the reproductive processes, the issues related are necessarily societal issues. The ethical considerations have also not achieved consensus and this has led to moral uncertainty[9]. Similarly the new procedures are not complete, sometimes controversial and should not raise expectations too high, too fast[8,9]. And lastly, we should be concerned with the interference by third parties in the patient-physician relationship.

This book, however, is not about controversial points. It is instead concerned with the actual application of MIS, and is the outgrowth of the preceptorships given at the New Jersey Laser Institute – MIS with a great degree of safety.

How do patients feel about this new approach? I can illustrate this with the words of one of our patients after laparoscopic laser adhesiolysis and appendectomy: 'The first two weeks I was not so sure, but now I can tell you, I never felt better in my life'.

Charles Ellis Connant, MD, FACS, FACOG
Assistant Clinical Professor of Obstetrics and Gynecology,
University of Medicine and Dentistry, New Jersey

References

1   Anderson D (1992) Gastrointestinal and biliary conditions. *ACS, Bulletin.* **77**:27.

2   Gleicher N (1992) Gynecology and Obstetrics. *ACS, Bulletin.* **77**:32.

3   Maier RV (1992) Critical care and metabolism. *ACS, Bulletin.* **77**:22.

4   Syntex Annual Women's Healthcare Roundtable. Monograph 1991, (Women's Cancer Screening p. 77 Robert Bast, MD)

5   Menczer F *et al.* (1993) Cyst fluid Ca 125 levels in ovarian epithelial neoplasms. *Obstetrics and Gynecology.* **81**:25.

6   Barad D *et al.* (1990) Proceedings of the World Congress of Gynecologic Endoscopy AAEL 18th annual meeting Washington DC. *Endoscopy in Gynecology.* **1**:1.

7   Ory SJ (1990) Syllabus ACOG, PG120 Operative endoscopy: getting started and becoming proficient, 38th Annual Clinical Meeting, San Francisco, May 5–6.

8   Batt RE (1990) *Manual of endoscopy.* AAGL.

9   Jones HW (1992) Assisted reproduction. *Clinical Obstetrics and Gynecology.* **35**:749.

Foreword

The exciting revolutionary advent of endoscopic surgery, in which gynae-cology has led the field, does require adequate training and cannot be undertaken lightly. There must be adequate facilities for training, certification and examinations.

The role of the 'team' must not be overlooked in the training programme. Not all patients are suitable for the various gynaecological techniques and there is need for careful selection and preparation of patients.

Follow-up studies by way of a National Register in patient outcome is necessary to improve still further the great advantage of endoscopic surgery.

The role of the gynaecological surgeon is in the process of changing completely as techniques used successfully for many years are now out of date, and as minimal access techniques improve still further.

Roger Baldwin FRCOG
Consultant Obstetrician and Gynaecologist
Whipps Cross Hospital
Chairman, Examination Committee,
Royal College of Obstetrics and Gynaecology
London

Preface

The purpose of this book is to provide current information on endoscopic operative techniques for the gynaecological surgeon. It also presents new and perhaps rather futuristic concepts derived from technological developments.

If you absorb its material thoughtfully and practise its principles persistently, we hope that your endoscopic technique will improve and that you will not need to resort to a conventional surgical approach when it is not necessary. Ultimately, your patients will benefit from a shorter stay and recuperation time, with an equivalent if not a superior outcome.

As editor, I have had the pleasure of selecting contributors who have demonstrated significant expertise or who — through their research, invention, publication or development of techniques — are pioneers in endoscopic surgery. This book complements a larger series of texts dedicated to the various specialties which now employ the minimal access approach. I feel honoured to be contributing to such a wide-ranging project.

A large number of illustrations are provided to promote a better appreciation of the material. My goal was to present the information in a practical, concise and up-to-date way, and not cloud it with esoteric anecdotes or academic overtones.

The field of endoscopic surgery is evolving and in a continuous state of development. Interestingly, it has been the gynaecological surgeons in private practice, not the academic institutions of the world, who have led the way and brought minimal access procedures to their present level of development. I encourage you to use your imagination to take these procedures to even greater heights. As the century closes, we will undoubtedly see quantum leaps in new applications of minimal access surgery to gynaecology.

I wish to express sincere thanks to Andrew Bax and all the staff at Radcliffe Medical Press, for their splendid support in seeing this project to fruition. I must admit that at times I stretched their patience to the limit! Finally, my greatest appreciation goes to all the contributing authors for taking time from their schedules to share their experience in the brilliant chapters which have resulted.

Stephen A. Grochmal
August 1994

Part I: Preparing for the Endoscopic Procedure

Video Documentation: Are We Accountable?

Psychological Impact of Pelvic Surgery: A Comparison of Laparoscopy Versus Laparotomy

Basic Techniques and Practical Manoeuvres in Minimally Invasive Gynaecology

Laser vs Electrosurgery: An Overview

Enhanced Precision and Tissue Selectivity in Laparoscopic Microsurgical Procedures

Organization of the Minimally Invasive Surgery Unit and Trouble-Shooting for Operative Endoscopy

Video Documentation: Are We Accountable?

JOHN M. LEVENTHAL

'Does he write? he fain would paint a picture'

Robert Browning

Introduction

Documentation of any operative procedure, in one form or another, is accepted universally as one of the standards of medical care. As such its performance becomes a legally mandated step in the appropriate care of the patient undergoing surgery.

Although the dictated operative summary and written operative note remain the minimum accepted standard for documentation in most cases, rapidly evolving electronic documentation techniques – which by their nature are more objective – may very soon become the new standard to which the surgeon will be held responsible. In no area is this more likely to occur than in the field of endoscopic surgery, where the documentation equipment has become an integral part of the procedure instrumentation. The advent of electronic microcircuitry has enabled the rapid and accurate video imaging of almost every portion of any endoscopic operation, and has thus made the details of the operative procedure available to a wide variety of secondary observers.

What is video documentation?

Video documentation is the recording of observed phenomena by means of video imaging, in a format which will be available for secondary observers to study.

Is the videotape a document?

The American Heritage Dictionary defines a document as: '*1. A written or printed paper bearing the original, official, or legal form of something, and which can be used to furnish decisive evidence or information. 2. Anything serving as evidence or proof, as a material substance bearing a revealing symbol or mark.*' The video record certainly fulfils the second definition, and therefore we must accept (as the legal profession has done) that the videotape is a document[1].

Why document at all?

Video documentation of an endoscopic procedure serves a number of purposes, including:

- patient information and education
- health professional education and teaching
- review by the surgical team
- communication with referring physicians and others
- documentation for the patient record
- follow-up review
- possible medico-legal documentation.

The relative importance of these reasons depends upon who is using the document. The use of photographs or videotapes before the proposed surgery is an outstanding method of achieving truly informed consent, and serves to give the patient (and perhaps her family as well) a real basis for understanding the impending operation (Figure 1.1). After the procedure, the documentary material from the case itself can be shown to the patient and compared with the preoperative briefing material. A complete understanding of the problem on the part of the patient makes for both more effective treatment and often a better outcome. When the problem is infertility, this understanding is especially important.

Videotapes or videodiscs of endoscopic surgery are particularly valuable for teaching other physicians and members of the operating team. It is not necessary to utilize professional teaching videos for this purpose. The unedited tape, used with the written permission of the patient (with the patient identifying data removed) is often more valuable as a teaching aid than a more polished version, and is immediately available. The videotape is ideal for communicating the findings of a procedure to the referring physician as well.

All of these factors are important with regard to legal accountability. However, the legal status of videotaping of procedures is vague in almost all states and has seldom been addressed by legislative bodies charged with creating statutory law. Is the videotape an official part of the medical record? If so, whose record? Where should it be maintained, and for how long? Does the videotape belong to the patient, the doctor or the hospital? Can the tape be edited during or after the procedure? Can the surgeon videotape only those

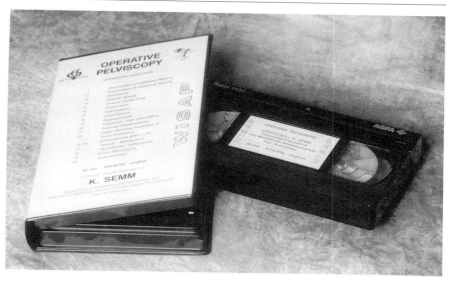

Figure 1.1: Teaching videotape used for preoperative counselling.

portions of the procedure believed to be significant? In 1986 a physician was supported by a court in New York in refusing to comply with a patient's demand for a videotape of a procedure, when the demand was made outside of the discovery procedures attendant to a malpractice action[2]. In Massachusetts in 1990, legal advice sought by a Boston hospital concerning the disposition of video documents held that the videotape was part of the hospital record and could be disclosed in any action brought against the hospital, which was responsible for its storage and preservation. It was therefore the opinion of the attorneys that any video recording made by a physician should belong to, and be kept by, the physician. They further advised that copies (never the original) of the videotape be given to the patient only if requested and signed for. The result of this course is to shift the responsibility and liability for that record to the physician and away from the hospital. In this latter instance, of course, the legal advice was sought by and rendered in the interest of the hospital, and perhaps it would have been somewhat different if an individual physician had been seeking similar information. These examples bring to light possible conflicts of interest between the physician and his or her hospital, and well demonstrate the dilemma which stems from the inability of lawmaking bodies to keep pace with rapid advancements in medical technology.

One area which has been addressed by many of the states is that of informed consent. It may well be that the consent laws offer a useful platform on which the patient and physician can reach agreement with respect to the various factors involved in videotaping[4]. It is perhaps from these various state laws that a method for defining the legal status of video documentation can be derived. If, as some experts contend, the informed patient is less likely to be a litigious patient, then perhaps videotapes of various endoscopic procedures are especially valuable sources of preoperative and postoperative information, and need to be regulated by the consent document itself. An understanding of the status of videotaping serves both the patient and the physician. While it should never be forgotten that the video record of the actual procedure can be helpful to a defendant physician involved in litigation, it must also be remembered that it is a potential source of trouble as well. If we are going to use the video document as the preferred medium for recording endoscopic procedures, the eventual legal decisions will have to take into account the protection and interests of both the patient and the physician.

Why video documentation?

Most forms of traditional documentation are subjective by their nature. They comprise the initial observer's concept of what was viewed at the time of the operative procedure, and therefore they often reflect the background and bias of the observer as much as they do the properties of the objects being observed. Therefore the written progress note or operative dictation is at best an interpretation, and (in modern parlance) not transportable as objectively representative of the original observations (Figure 1.2). In its attempt to record the findings of a surgical procedure accurately, even the most detailed operative dictation falls short of being truly objective. It can never be more than a document created out of the mind of the initial observer, and therefore a version of what was observed. The subsequent reader (the secondary

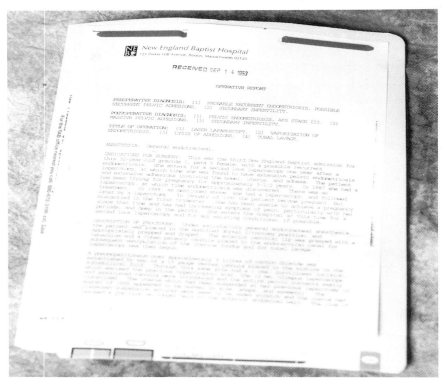

Figure 1.2: The operative dictation is at best a subjective interpretation of the endoscopic procedure.

observer) usually has no recourse to the original 'data', and must draw conclusions or base actions on the original observer's subjective documentation for better or worse. Modern video documentation, on the other hand, can provide every secondary observer with a fresh opportunity to draw conclusions from the original observations. Video documentation can enable a more accurate subsequent evaluation of the initial operative findings, and is by its very nature more informative than older methods of documentation. From the legal standpoint, however, this increased accuracy could serve to make the videotape the document of official reference, in the near future, with the physician accountable to it.

Technical requirements

Video imaging is a form of dynamic imaging, ie realtime motion is recorded. Static imaging is represented by the still photograph which captures a frozen moment of the procedure. Both dynamic and static imaging have important roles to play in the documentation of endoscopic procedures. In order to provide usable and accurate documentation, all visual recording systems, whether dynamic or static, depend upon sufficient illumination of the observed subject matter. This illumination in turn can be thought of as being dependent upon four variable factors: (1) the sensitivity of the recording system, (2) the transmission efficiency of the lens system used with the recording equipment, (3) the illuminating power of the light source, and (4) the size of the image to be recorded.

Sensitivity of the recording system

Photographic still imaging, which today usually means colour transparencies (35 mm slides), involves the use of colour slide film which is balanced for electronic flash illumination. Where the sensitivity of any silver-halide film varies with the chemical composition of the material, video sensitivity is a function of the electronics of the camera and recording system (*see* below).

Transmission efficiency of the lens system

Rigid endoscopes are made up of a series of lenses comprising a lens system. The design of the system is such as to provide for some calculated degree of magnification and optimal light transmission. Both are dependent on the design of the lens bundle, the diameter of the endoscope, the light transmitting properties of the lens material itself, and the distance over which the light must travel. Recently, with the advent of high-sensitivity, high-resolution microprocessor chips, the lens filled endoscope has begun to share the stage with a whole generation of entirely new instruments which employ a solid state microchip camera mounted at the distal end of a solid 'endoscope'. When conventional lenses are employed with these latter systems they are only for focus and magnification, and have little influence on the light transmission characteristics of the system.

The illuminating power of the light source

Since all photographic documentation requires the recording of material on or through light sensitive media, sufficient illumination is essential. The medium itself may be sensitive to light directly (eg silver-halide film), or indirectly, as transmitted through light sensitive electronic sensors (microprocessor chips). Electronic recording usually requires less light intensity than photographic imaging. This correctly implies that even very fast (high ASA) film is usually not as sensitive as the electronic light sensors of a microprocessor chip. The desired end-product of every recording is an image recognizable to the eye and accurately representative of the original object of observation. The illumination of the object must therefore be matched to the sensitivity of the primary recording medium.

Sufficient light depends on the source of illumination; the light generator (Figure 1.3). Virtually all light sources for endoscopy utilize a metallic arc bulb which produces light in the 'daylight film' range of 5 000° K to 6 000° K and is capable of producing brighter illumination (more lumens) than incandescent sources. Unlike an incandescent source, which can be varied throughout its entire range of illumination, the intensity of a metallic arc source can only be varied over a relatively small range. This is an important consideration in the design of video cameras requiring that the illumination

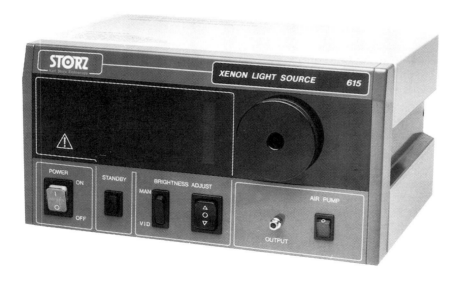

Figure 1.3: A typical metallic arc light source used for endoscopic procedures. (Courtesy of Karl Storz Endoscopy, America.)

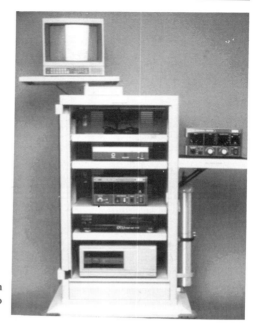

Figure 1.4: Endoscopic video recording system consisting of videocamera, monitor, and video cassette recorder (VCR).

intensity varies over a wide range of endoscopic applications. This requirement is generally addressed in the video camera by providing either an iris shutter driven by the light reflected from the field, or by dimming the illumination through the small range which is available with the metallic arc source.

The size of the recorded image

The amount of light necessary for successful imaging on film is inversely proportional to the size of the recorded image. More light is therefore needed for a 35 mm transparency image than for a 16 mm frame of a movie film. This principle is less important in the case of electronic imaging where the light gathering properties of the microprocessor chip are dependent upon the sensitivities of the individual units (pixels) and their density in the electronic chip array.

The video system

The typical video system consists of a video camera and monitor, videotape and video cassette recorder (VCR) (Figure 1.4). In the near future, optical laser discs and video-frame grabbers will become additional routine components to most systems in medical use. Not only is the video system the vehicle for recording endoscopic procedures, but it also serves as the means by which the surgeon visualizes the field. The arthroscopist has depended upon video monitor visualization for years, and the general surgeon, introduced to the laparoscopic approach more recently, has learned to be totally dependent

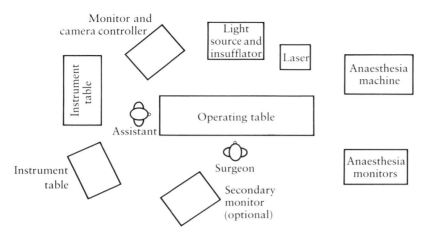

Figure 1.5: Diagram of operating room setup for operative laparoscopy utilizing two video monitors. Both the surgeon and the assistant have a clear view of the procedure.

upon it. The surgeon's eye in effect has been moved from the endoscopic eyepiece to the colour video monitor, thus bringing the previously concealed procedure into the immediate visual realm of the entire operating team as well. This has allowed for more efficient utilization of assistants and instrumentation and a significantly more comfortable position for the surgeon (Figure 1.5).

Video formats

Currently there is no worldwide agreement on the ideal electronic format for video-recording equipment. Although it has been the subject of numerous international meetings over many years, a universal format has unfortunately not emerged. In North America, parts of South America, Japan and parts of Asia, the National Television Standards Committee (NTSC) format is in general use. In most of Europe and Australia the Phase Alternation Line (PAL) format is the usual standard, although in France, the Séquence de Couleurs Avec Mémoire (SECAM) format is used. Other standards exist and newer ones arise at an alarming rate. Each format has its enthusiastic proponents and its own advantages and disadvantages with respect to image quality. From the practical standpoint, for the physician wishing to present his video material to larger audiences, this disparity causes considerable inconvenience when transporting videotapes overseas for lectures or meetings. Conversion facilities exist in most countries, but these add time and cost.

Equipment for video documentation

Microcircuitry and miniaturization have enabled the video camera to become an integral part of medical technique and documentation. In less than a

decade the operating room video camera has been transformed from a 1 kg
cylinder the size of a flashlight to a 50 g unit the size of the surgeon's finger.
While growing smaller and lighter, the resolution and sensitivity to light has
increased enormously. The improvement in camera resolution has been
accompanied by significant improvement in the quality of videotape material,
allowing for even smaller and less bulky VCR equipment.

The video documentation system can be considered to consist of five
essential components:

- video camera
- endoscope
- camera controller and video recorder (VCR)
- monitor
- light source.

The video camera

The vacuum-tube video camera, still used in most commercial television
studio work, continues to provide the highest-image resolution, but only by
the smallest of margins. Even this application is slowly giving way to the
three-chip camera with equivalent resolution. For medical and many other
applications, however, it has been replaced in almost all instances by the
solid-state microprocessor or single chip camera. Advances in solid-state
camera technology have been extremely rapid, and today these miniature
units are capable of resolutions and light sensitivities almost indistinguishable
from those of larger, bulky tube cameras.

There are currently two basic types of microprocessors used in solid-state
video cameras: (1) the charge-coupled device (CCD) chip, and (2) the metal-
oxide semiconductor (MOS) diode chip (Figure 1.6). The CCD chip generally
has greater light sensitivity but somewhat less resolution capability than the
MOS chip. Improvements in both types of chips, however, have been

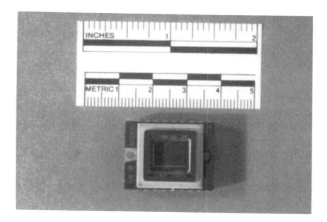

Figure 1.6: Charged coupled device microprocessor chip.

rapid. The addition of a negative charge to the MOS chip, creating the negative MOS diode chip, has resulted in a marked increase in light sensitivity for this device. In its present form the MOS or NMOS diode chip camera strikes a state-of-the-art compromise between sensitivity, dynamic range, noise, and what is termed 'lag' (the effect of light 'contaminating' the image before it can be moved from the collecting diode to the storage register). Even greater improvements in CCD technology, such as the hole accumulator diode (HAD) sensor and the frame interline transfer CCD (FIT CCD) by Sony, have given this technology some outstanding advantages over the older conventional CCD or MOS sensors.

Both the CCD and MOS microprocessors are integrated-circuit devices which utilize the principle of changes in electric resistance of metallic or silicon oxide in response to varying intensities of light striking its surface. The part of the chip facing the object being recorded is divided into an array of picture elements called pixels which are arranged along horizontal scanning lines. One of the major factors in determining the resolution of the chip is the number of horizontal lines: the greater the number of lines in a particular camera, the greater is its power of resolution. The NTSC format contains 700 pixels per line, whereas the PAL and SECAM formats contain 833 pixels per line. The latter formats therefore have inherently better resolution per line than the NTSC format used in the USA.

Although application requirements will vary from institution to institution, today's endoscopic video camera should have all or most of the following features:

- NTSC format (PAL or SECAM where appropriate)
- horizontal resolution of at least 400 lines – preferably more
- recorder on-off control or frame-grabber button at the camera head
- simple one-hand focusing at the camera head
- automatic and continuous white balancing
- automatic light intensity control or controllable from camera head.

Camera controller and recorder (VCR)

Light striking a pixel induces changes in resistance, which are stored in what is called the 'image register'. The electronic circuitry controlling the microprocessor chip allows for rapid sequential 'sweeping', or transfer, of the information stored in the image register to temporary storage in the 'storage register', thus freeing the image elements (pixels) for the next fragment of light stimulation. The rate at which this transfer occurs is known as the 'frame rate' and is measured in images per second. The frame rate varies with different electronic formats (see below). For NTSC format, used in the USA, the frame rate is 30 per second, while for PAL and SECAM the rate is 25 frames per second.

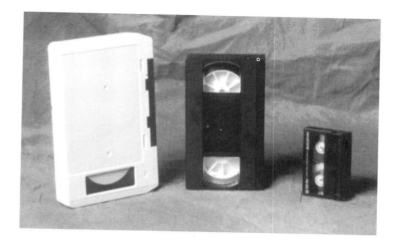

Figure 1.7: Videotapes in current use for recording endoscopic procedures (3/4 inch Umatic, 1/2 inch VHS and 8 mm).

The recording medium

Today, magnetic videotape remains the most widely used medium for recording, primarily because of its low cost and compatibility with most video systems. It is no longer necessary to employ 3/4 inch UMatic tapes for top-quality imaging. Half-inch VHS tapes (200 horizontal lines), Super VHS tapes (400 horizontal lines), and now 8 mm tapes of equal image quality are in common use, and are perfectly satisfactory (Figure 1.7). Video recording, however, has begun to move significantly into the digital age to accommodate the use of the computer. Laser optics or compact discs for archiving and fast retrieval of information are available and gaining in popularity. Videotape has the inherent disadvantages of physical bulk and inefficient access to specific images, while the CD can be instantly accessed, is small and rugged, and requires very little storage space. The optical disc (write once read many or WORM) is recorded by laser pitting of the media material, and is essentially not alterable. This characteristic of this media material may make it more acceptable than magnetic videotape as admissible evidence in litigation.

The monitor

Two types of monitor are available: analogue and digital. Most video monitors in current use in operating rooms are of the analogue type (similar to a home television set) and usually are capable of higher resolution than that of the camera employed. Because the original signal is customarily acquired as digital data, a digital–analogue converter is a common component of the camera controller. Digital monitors, which process the digital signal directly, are in increasing use and offer some advantages in clarity and resolution.

At least two monitors should be available in the operating room for easy vision of the surgeon and the assistant (*see* Figure 1.5).

The light source

A wide variety of light sources for endoscopy are available. For the surgeon desiring both photographic and video capability, the basic requirements are a metallic arc light with automatic light control and built-in synchronized electronic flash for still photography.

The endoscope

The smaller the diameter of the endoscope, the less the light transmissibility. It is therefore appropriate for good endoscopic documentation to use an endoscope with the largest size available for the particular requirements of the case. In the case of laparoscopy, this should be 10 mm for a diagnostic laparoscope and 12 mm for an operating scope with an instrument or CO_2 laser channel.

Frame-grabbing (still video)

In addition to the five components of the current-day video system listed above, the ability to obtain static (still) images by video is becoming increasingly desirable and available. The electronic approach to still images in endoscopic documentation is what is termed 'frame-grabbing'. The process involves the capture in digital form of a single frame of a videotape or real-time image and the subsequent printing out to hard copy material such as paper or transparency film. The process requires a computer for storage of the acquired frame and for output to a suitable printer to produce the hard copy, or picture. A number of colour printers are available in today's market. Depending on the system used, both prints and slides can be produced. The quality of the final image obtained, utilizing the newest equipment on the market, is little different from a still photograph. This approach to static images has proved to be valuable for capturing important parts of the operative procedure for insertion into the patient's hospital or office chart, but – although informative – it may raise some questions as to its admissibility in a court of law because it has been taken out of context with respect to the whole of the procedure. The process of frame-grabbing combined with the typed operative dictation is available commercially (Med Images, Inc©).

Archiving

Ideally, appropriate archiving of visual documentation material should require little space and should allow rapid and accurate retrieval of information. The endoscopic surgeon, with cabinets full of videotapes going back three years, may not agree that the ideal has been achieved. However, it is possible to transfer video images from videotape, or directly from the camera controller at the time of surgery, to optical laser discs which are similar to the compact music discs used in the home. These discs are capable of extremely large storage capacities, measured in gigabytes, and will allow almost instant retrieval of specific information. Interesting segments of a procedure may be coded digitally on the optical disc and retrieved in milliseconds by a bar-code reader or database search on a computer. Whole segments of video-imaging can be archived on a single disc; and, with the advent of advanced data compression techniques now in use, many videotape equivalents can be stored on a single disc. Colour transparencies can also be scanned, digitized and stored in their thousands on a single disc. Since this archived visual documentation data is stored in digital form, it can be transmitted over long distances by telephone or satellite, and thus can be available for viewing in widely separated geographic locations simultaneously and at any time. The legal question as to how long this material needs to be archived is, like other aspects of video documentation, an unanswered one. This author suggests that archived video records be kept the same length of time as the patient chart, and then destroyed.

The future

There are few fields of information management changing more rapidly than that of imaging technology. Endoscopic documentation is no exception. The optical lens endoscope will probably soon be replaced by the electronic endoscope, with the camera chip embedded into the distal end of the instrument, and looking through the endoscope will not be an option. The surgeon will be dependent upon the video system. With respect to image quality, high-resolution scanners (2 000 + lines) are even today capable of resolutions finer than the grain in conventional films, and camera resolution improves with each passing month.

Three-dimensional recording and viewing is in its infancy, but is already being applied to endoscopy in some crude ways. The whole world of virtual reality is just beginning to open up previously unimaginable possibilities. A virtual reality trainer for laparoscopic cholecystectomy, which allows the surgeon to manipulate the operative field in a way which is completely interactive and realistic, has already been introduced. The computer-generated organs displayed are still largely diagrammatic, but their replacement with video images of live structures is not far off.

In the short term, the increasing use of video documentation will un-doubtedly result in greater pressure on the legal system to address the questions raised by this technology. It remains to be seen whether the resulting decisions will apply in any universal sense, but local and institutional regulations are already in place in some areas. In the interim, informed consent may well be the best way to gain agreement between patient and physician[3]. With that in mind, a set of reasonable and practical guidelines for video documentation of endoscopic procedures is offered below.

Guidelines for video documentation

1. The consent form should be the defining document for all agreements between the patient and physician (and/or hospital) concerning the employment and disposition of the video record. To that end it should:

- state that a videotape of the procedure will be made, that the tape will be used to inform the patient of the operative findings, and perhaps (without identifying information) for instructional purposes as well
- clearly state that the physician may edit the tape or be selective in choosing which parts of the procedure to record
- confirm the patient's right to view the videotape postoperatively, to obtain a copy of the tape if desired, although the original videotape will remain the property of the physician (or hospital)
- contain a provision confirming the patient's understanding that the physician may choose *not* to record the procedure.

2. Every video document should be identified at the beginning and end with the patient's name, hospital or office record number, date of the surgery, and name of the surgeon.

3. The original recording, whether it be on videotape or compact disc, should be held in safe keeping by the physician or the hospital (if it is to be made a part of the official hospital record) for a period of time corresponding to the maximum statute of limitations applicable to the particular patient.

4. If the patient requests, an exact copy of the original may be given, the receipt of which should be acknowledged in writing and made a part of the patient record.

5. Under no circumstances should the surgeon erase or edit out a portion of a videotape which contains material depicting a surgical mishap. Such action could subject the surgeon to charges of records alteration in any subsequent litigation.

Conclusions

Are we accountable when we utilize the video camera to record our endoscopic procedures? It seems likely, with the rapid increase in the number of video imaged operations, that this technology will ultimately replace the written or dictated operative record, or at least be required to augment it. If that proves to be true, then the legal significance of the video record will parallel that of the written account. It is not likely that the techniques and legal requirements for video imaging in surgery will be standardized at any early date; however, as the use of the video document becomes more and more widespread in medical litigation, it becomes increasingly important for every endoscopist to adhere to a minimal set of guidelines with respect to the obtaining of informed consent from the patient, and the identification and recording of the endoscopic procedure.

The visual documentation of endoscopic procedures is currently the province of the video camera, and its many peripheral devices. There is little question that some measure of accountability for what happens on the video record will rest with the surgeon. From the legal viewpoint, in today's litigious atmosphere, the video document presents not only an objective picture of what was performed correctly, but also what may have gone wrong as well.

References

1   Miller RD (1991) The presentation of expert testimony via live audio-visual communication. *Bulletin of the American Academy of Psychiatry Law.* **19**:5–20.

2   *Hill v Springer* [1986] 132 NYS 2d 255.

3   Green HD, Jr (1991) Medical technology vs the law. *Professional Medical Monitor.* **1**:7–90.

Psychological Impact of Pelvic Surgery: A Comparison of Laparoscopy Versus Laparotomy

ADAM OSTRZENSKI

Introduction

As defined by the World Health Organization, health is not merely the absence of disease: it also encompasses an individual's physical, social and emotional well-being. Therefore the patient's emotional response to physical dysfunction and surgery must be considered as an integral part of any preoperative consultation.

Massler and Devanesan[1] suggested that any physical assault on the body (including surgery) is accompanied by an emotional reaction. Therefore the pelvic surgeon must be competent not only as a surgical technician: he must also be prepared to cope with the patient's feelings and anxieties.

According to Freeman[2], common emotional responses to surgery include:

- insecurity and vulnerability
- sense of being manipulated
- feelings of being attacked
- fear of dying (which may be expressed as fear of anaesthesia)
- fear of the unknown.

Other responses that he listed, however, may be offset by the use of endoscopy for gynaecological surgery, namely:

- anxiety
- fear of pain
- surrender of control
- fear of loss of identity (role, independence, attractiveness)
- depersonalization (by the hospital)
- helplessness

- emotional lability, sadness, tearfulness, inevitability
- regression and dependency
- feeling of illness — a state of non-health ('sick role')
- grief.

Emotional healing begins with grief, which is a natural and common response to gynaecological surgery. Denial, attempts to bargain with God, feelings of guilt, depression, anger and finally resolution/integration are well defined stages of grief that ultimately enable the sufferer to cope.

Psychological and physical importance of the uterus

Gynaecological diseases are unique in their nature, since they affect not only a woman's emotional well-being through their association with her sexual identity, body image, and self-esteem, but also her physical and social life — in particular her sex life. The genital organs are the most important factors in one's sexual identity. The emotional significance of the genital organs must, therefore, be kept in mind when contemplating gynaecological surgery. To help a patient through the grieving process, physicians must understand the symbolic value of their patients' genital organs. For most women, the uterus is associated with menstruation. Menarche is a symbolic rite of passage from childhood to feminine adulthood. The monthly rhythm of the menstrual cycle provides a sense of routine, regularity and predictability that bolsters a woman's emotional stability. For this reason, the uterus plays a significant symbolic role in a woman's emotional life[3,4].

For most women, regardless of their level of education, the uterus is a symbol of sexual repose and sexual gratification, as well as a symbol of the ability to bear children. The uterus, breasts, external and internal genitalia also are associated with a woman's feelings of attractiveness, sexual desirability and self-identity. To preserve this self-image, maintaining the health of the patient's reproductive organs is essential. Surgical removal of any of the genital organs, particularly the uterus, can negatively influence the patient's self-concept of femininity[5].

In the USA, hysterectomy is one of the most common surgeries performed during the child-bearing years. Dicker et al.[6] reported that from 1970 to 1978 more than 3.5 million women ranging in age from 15 to 44 underwent hysterectomies in the USA, 72% abdominally and 28% vaginally. The less well prepared the patient is for such a drastic surgical intervention, the more emotionally disturbing the surgery may be[7].

In 1962, Melody published his observations on the depressive reaction following hysterectomy[8], and stated: 'The social roles available to an individual, as well as one's body image, self-concept, and self-evaluation, are to a large degree determined by the social contact organs and their symbolic meaning to the individual'.

Hampton and Tarnasky[9] compared the emotional reactions of women who underwent hysterectomies with those of women who underwent tubal ligation and concluded that the depression that follows a hysterectomy is associated with more than losing the ability to conceive children.

Moore and Tolly[10] concluded that the majority of first depressions in hysterectomy patients actually developed before the surgery took place. It is important for pelvic surgeons to be aware of this psychological effect in order to support their patients effectively[8,11,12].

After a hysterectomy a woman may feel sexually dysfunctional, as if she has lost her attractiveness and sexual desirability. This constitutes a feeling of de-sexing and the destruction of her identity as a female. The loss of the ability to conceive may also lead the patient to believe she has lost her femininity. Hysterectomy can be psychologically disturbing and leave a woman feeling as if she has a hole in her body[13].

Barnes and Tinkham[14] explored the surgeon's influence on the patient's emotional responses to surgery and concluded:

> 'Surgeons tend to be activists rather than empathetic listeners and many of them need to distance themselves from the patient's feelings and fears as a kind of protective insulation against the things they see every day. Some do not hear the patient and instead relate to her as a uterus, breast or an appendix, not a human being in distress. At times one observes a kind of "cut-and-run" syndrome in some surgeon–patient relationships. There are also doctors with a tendency to react to their patient's problems in terms of their own personal and moral value system.'

Counselling

These findings indicate that a surgeon who takes the time to listen to and counsel his patient can have a positive influence on the patient's emotional response to the surgery. The surgeon himself must properly prepare the patient for surgery, an important task that should never be delegated to a physician's assistant, a resident or a nurse. Information about the surgical procedure, reassurance and emotional support will help modify the patient's negative feelings. Providing the patient with a thorough understanding of the surgical process will result in a positive attitude that will be reflected in the postoperative course. Instead of feeling like a powerless victim, she now becomes an important, decision-making partner.

The physician also should enlist the help of the patient's family and close friends who can serve as important allies in the patient's emotional support structure before and after surgery, particularly following hysterectomy, after which depression is a common emotion[15–17].

Surgeons should be aware of the sexual partner's role in the pre- and post-hysterectomy patient's emotions. If the sex partner is distant or detached, or if he sees the patient as less sexually attractive after hysterectomy, she is more likely to become depressed than if he has been emotionally supportive. Therefore counselling not just the patient but the partner is essential.

The need to perform hysterectomy

Knowing hysterectomy's devastating psychological effect, gynaecologists must take great care not to perform such surgery unless it is medically necessary. We must first consider why hysterectomies are performed. The most common indication for hysterectomy is fibroma of the uterus[18]. The fibroid uterus as a medical entity is considered benign, with very little tendency to become malignant. As such, the fibroid tumour can be removed and the organ preserved by performing myomectomy. Consequently, myomectomy and not hysterectomy should be the procedure of first choice for the patient with a fibroid uterus.

However, hysterectomies continue to outnumber myomectomies as the surgical procedure chosen for the fibroid uterus. Traditionally, myomectomy has been reserved for patients who are of reproductive age and whose fibroids are symptomatic (symptoms can include pelvic pain, pelvic pressure and/or abnormal uterine bleeding, anaemia, dyspareunia and compression of pelvic-abdominal structures). It is generally accepted that if the size of the uterus exceeds that of a 12-week gestation, hysterectomy should be performed, since uterine size alone may compress the ureters against the pelvic bone and cause complications in kidney function. However, with the varied and sophisticated technologies currently available (including ultrasound, magnetic resonance imaging, laser and operative pelviscopy), advanced surgical techniques and advances in anaesthesia, hysterectomy should be an occasional rather than a routine surgical choice for patients with fibroids.

Problems which laparoscopy can minimize

Surgeons can also minimize the gynaecological patient's emotional distress by performing laparoscopic surgery, rather than traditional laparotomy. As listed previously, there are 15 common emotional responses to surgery, the following 10 of which can be minimized when the laparoscopic procedure is applied instead of traditional laparotomy.

Surrender of control

Although surrender of control cannot be eliminated completely by endoscopy, it will be greatly minimized. During any hospital stay, the patient must surrender herself to the physician or physician-consultant(s) and hospital medical personnel in charge, and the longer the patient stays in the hospital, the longer she feels controlled by and at the mercy of the medical and hospital personnel. Laparoscopic procedures require only a short hospital stay. Most patients will be discharged on the day of surgery or the next day, unlike with the same uncomplicated procedure performed by laparotomy, in which the average length of hospitalization in the USA is four to five days.

Depersonalization

The patient, who already may be experiencing negative emotional feelings about surrender of control, must undress and put on a hospital gown. In most instances, she then is placed in a room with an unknown roommate whose selection is beyond her control. Unfamiliar hospital routines can be unnerving, and the patient is confronted continually with strangers, such as physician assistants, nurses, assistants to the nurses and, in teaching institutions, students, residents and technical personnel. Again, because laparoscopy shortens the patient's hospital stay, her feelings of depersonalization will not last as long. The patient's feelings of depersonalization can be further decreased if the laparoscopic procedure is performed in a free-standing surgical centre instead of a hospital. In such a centre, well-trained laparoscopists are able to perform even complicated types of surgery and their patients can go home on the same day or on the morning after surgery. It is the author's experience that even after a video laparoscopic panhysterectomy, the patient may go home on the day of surgery.

Helplessness

When patients are told they need surgery, the accompanying feelings of helplessness can be significant. The promise of endoscopy can dispel the patient's concerns about large incisions associated with laparotomy, because endoscopy requires only a 5–15 mm abdominal incision, compared with a 10 cm minimal incision for laparotomy. Even when the pelvic mass is large (fibroid, cyst, endometrioma, ectopic pregnancy, pelvic abscess etc), the knowledge that she will go home on the day of surgery and will have a very small abdominal incision tends to minimize the patient's feelings of helplessness.

Anxiety

Anxiety associated with being isolated from family and/or friends, being cut, undergoing the surgical process, being anaesthetized, suffering pain etc can be minimized by endoscopic surgery. This procedure will not eliminate anxiety, but it will substantially reduce it, particularly when the surgery is performed outside of a standard hospital facility.

Fear of pain

Fear of pain can be controlled when the patient is adequately prepared emotionally before the surgical procedure is performed. The patient's fear of pain is drastically reduced when the surgical procedure is explained and a comparison is made between laparotomy incisions and endoscopic abdominal incisions. Unfortunately, these issues frequently are either not addressed at all or are addressed inadequately before surgery. One way to lessen a patient's fears of surgery is to allow her to view, in a physician's office, a videotape of a similar procedure. Operative laparoscopic incisions are far less dramatic than skin laparotomy incisions. Because the patient's fear of pain dramatically increases with the size of the incision, the smaller the incision, the less the fear of pain.

Fear of loss of identity

The genital organs are the most important organs in the sexual identity of humans, and any surgery, particularly organ removal, will lead to the fear of losing that identity. New endoscopic techniques such as hysteropexy[19], in cases where the uterus is prolapsing or where the uterus is malpositioned, pelvic herniorrhaphy[3] and colpopexy[4] are only a few examples of how endoscopy can cope successfully with organ preservation.

Emotional lability, sadness, tearfulness, inevitability

These feelings will effectively be reduced by using endoscopy, because of the short stay in the hospital, small incisions, much faster healing, and a shorter recuperation period than with laparotomy. Since the postoperative recovery time is much shorter, the patient can return to her daily routine within a few days of endoscopic surgery. This is an especially valuable factor in view of the fact that the female workforce has grown considerably in the last decades; women will want to minimize the time taken off for surgery and recuperation.

Regression and dependency

Postsurgical dependency is directly associated with the pace of recovery; endoscopy substantially minimizes the patient's postoperative dependency. The minimal discomfort and lower complication rate of the endoscopic procedure tend to increase the patient's activity and to speed the process of regaining independence.

Feeling of illness

Most patients perceive the ambulatory type of surgery that endoscopy offers as a less serious medical procedure than one requiring a hospital stay. If the same surgery is offered via laparotomy, which automatically confines the patient to a hospital bed for several days, the patient will see it as a more serious medical problem. On the other hand, coming home the same day following an endoscopic surgery practically obliterates the patient's feeling of illness. 'It must not be so bad with me if you can do this surgery through a very small hole and I can be home the same day' — so said one patient after the presurgical consultation for a salpingo-oophorectomy.

Grief

When the endoscopic approach is offered, feelings of grief can be significantly diminished, particularly if the endoscopic surgeon can avoid removing the organ. In a case of uterine prolapse, for example, in most instances the surgeon can suspend the healthy uterus and repair the diseased structure[19], rather than performing a total hysterectomy.

Conclusion

It is only a matter of time before 95–97% of all gynaecological surgery will be performed via the laparoscope. However, progress is slow in gynaecological surgery, and only a few pelvic surgeons are prepared to perform this advanced endoscopic technique. General surgeons are performing a growing number of surgical procedures with the endoscope: cholecystectomy, appendectomy, herniorrhaphy, posterior cul-de-sac of Douglas herniorrhaphy[3] and bladder repair[20]. Acceptance of this new technique by the medical community can provide enormous benefit for the patient.

References

1   Massler DJ and Devomesan MM (1978) Sexual consequences of gynecological operation. In: Comfort A (ed). *Sexual Consequences of Disability*. Philadelphia, G. Stickley.

2   Freeman MG (1985) Psychological aspect of pelvic surgery. In: Telinde (ed). *Operative Gynecology*, 4th edition. Philadelphia, Lipton Co.

3   Ostrzenski A (1992) Endoscopic pelvic herniorrhaphy with CO_2 laser. *Gynecologic Endoscopy*. **2**: 136.

4   Ostrzenski A (1992) Laser video laparoscopic colpopexy. *Gin Pol*. **63**(7): 317.

5   Wolf SP (1970) Emotional reactions to hysterectomy. *Postgraduate Medicine*. **47**: 156.

6   Dicker RC *et al*. (1982) Hysterectomy among women of reproductive age. *Journal of American Medical Association*. **248**: 323.

7   Benedict R (1938) *Psychiatry*. **1**: 161.

8   Melody GF (1962) Depressive reactions following hysterectomy. *American Journal of Obstetrics and Gynecology*. **83**: 410.

9   Hampton PT, Tarasky WG (1974) Hysterectomy and tubal ligation: A comparison to the aftermath. *American Journal of Obstetrics and Gynecology.* **119**: 949.

10 Moore JT, Tolley DH (1976) Depression following hysterectomy. *Psychosomatic Medicine.* **17**: 86.

11 Dennerstein L *et al.* (1962) Sexual response following hysterectomy oophorectomy. *Obstetrics and Gynecology.* **83**: 401.

12 D'Escopo DA (1962) Hysterectomy when the uterus is grossly normal. *American Journal of Obstetrics and Gynecology.* **88**: 115.

13 Birns MT (1989) Inadvertent instrumental perforation of the colon during laparoscopy: nonsurgical repair. *Gastrointestinal Endoscopy.* **35(1)**: 54.

14 Baines AB, Tinkham CB (1978) Surgical Gynecology. In: Notma Norman MT, Nadelsson CC (eds). *The woman patient: medical and psychological interface.* Plenum Press, New York.

15 Baker MG (1968) Psychiatric illness after hysterectomy. *British Medical Journal.* **2**: 91.

16 Bragg RL (1965) Risk of admission to mental hospital following hysterectomy or cholecystectomy. *American Journal of Public Health.* **55**: 1403.

17 Richards DH (1973) Depression after hysterectomy. *Lancet.* **2**: 430.

18 Dicker RC *et al.* (1982) Complications of abdominal and vaginal hysterectomy among women of reproductive age in the United States. *American Journal of Obstetrics and Gynecology.* **144**: 841.

19 Ostrzenski A (1992) A new video laparoscopic laser hysteropexy in infertility treatment. *XIV World Congress on Infertility and Sterility Abstracts.* **209**: 94.

20 Ostrzenski A (1992) Psychological advantages of advanced endoscopy vs. laparotomy in gynecologic surgery. In: Klimek R (ed). *Pre-peri-natal psycho-medicine.* DWN Dream, Kraków.

3

Basic Techniques and Practical Manoeuvres in Minimally Invasive Gynaecology

LINDSAY McMILLAN, STEPHEN G. HARDING and ANDREW PESCE

Introduction

Advances in the development of endoscopic equipment and techniques over the last five years have brought about profound changes in the way gynaecological surgery is practised.

The incorporation of recent developments into clinical practice has been fuelled not only by the individual's desire to acquire new skills, but also by an increased tendency of our patients to seek out new treatments publicized in the lay media. This presents a predicament to gynaecologists, because most of them have only recently (if at all) taken up operative endoscopic procedures. They are largely self taught, although they are likely to have received initial guidance on one or several of the regular courses in Europe, the United States and other countries. Despite this, patients requesting endoscopic surgical procedures invariably have a high expectation of the results of such surgery: so how is it possible for the gynaecologist to incorporate endoscopic techniques, using new instruments and unfamiliar technologies such as laser and electrosurgery, into a busy hospital or private practice?

Patient expectations

The main advantages of endoscopic surgery over laparotomy are the lower patient morbidity and faster recovery time. However, the patient is more likely to consider the surgery to be 'minor' and is therefore less tolerant of complications. Similarly, if a laparotomy is later found to be necessary, this causes more distress than if it had been performed initially.

Patient expectation of the outcomes may be completely unrealistic. This is best demonstrated by the patient who believes her endometriosis will finally be cured by the 'new laser operation'.

The gynaecologist must ensure that the patient understands the nature and potential results of the procedure. This is no less important an issue than obtained real consent for other procedures, but potentially more of a problem because of high patient expectations. It would be prudent if, at least in the learning phase of endoscopic surgery, the gynaecologist only operates endoscopically on patients who would otherwise require conventional surgery, and ensures that the patient is aware of this. In this case, proceeding to an unexpected laparotomy is less likely to be seen as an indication of failure of care.

Laparoscopic operations

Changes in laparoscopic surgery have been greater in the last five years than any that have taken place in the past 50 years. Technological developments in endoscopy with the advances and refinements in the use of ultrasound equipment, MRI and CAT scanners, new imaging techniques and the use of fibreoptics and lasers, gynaecologists now have a formidable diagnostic and therapeutic arsenal.

The video camera has been the catalyst for these epic changes in endoscopic surgery. It has allowed us to enhance and magnify the image that we see through the endoscope, so that precision is increased and tissue damage reduced. Assistants now play a greater part in endoscopic surgery, as they are able to view the operation on the monitor along with the surgeon. Continued development of camera technology has led to the manufacture of microscopic videochip cameras, the smallest of which can be inserted directly into the patient. It is now possible for at least 90% of all gynaecological operations to be done endoscopically.

Unfortunately, with this rapid development of endoscopic surgical techniques, problems have arisen that need to be recognized and overcome.

When setting out to perform laparoscopic surgery it is essential to acquire as much information as possible about the condition to be treated, because it will dictate primarily whether the surgeon is sufficiently skilled and trained to perform the operation, and secondly the likely length of the procedure. Ultrasound scans, particularly transvaginal scans, are extremely useful in the diagnosis of ovarian cysts and tumours, benign and malignant tumours and uterine abnormalities. For instance they can demonstrate not only the presence of fibroids, but also their exact size, number and location.

Establishing a pneumoperitoneum

The majority of complications in laparoscopic surgery occur at the time of abdominal entry. Surgeons performing laparoscopic techniques should be able to recognize and deal with any complications that may arise. All patients should be assessed before surgery; any potential problems with the establishment of a pneumoperitoneum should be predicted and consideration given to how these may be avoided.

Incision

Initially the patency and spring mechanism of the Verres needle should be checked.

The site of the Verres needle insertion is dictated by the individual patient, not necessarily by the surgeon's preference for a particular site. Scars from previous abdominal surgery may make the use of the traditional intraumbilical insertion point hazardous, and alternative sites of entry may need to be used (Figure 3.1).

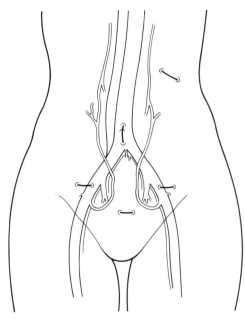

Figure 3.1: Sites of entry for the Verres needle. (Illustration courtesy of the Department of Medical Illustration, St. Bartholemew's Hospital, London)

One of the sites associated with the lowest incidence of morbidity is the suprapubic site. The Verres needle is inserted vertically in the midline and passed through the deep fascia and the peritoneum until it touches the uterus, which is manipulated vaginally. This method is considered to be suitable for those who are commencing their training in laporoscopy, as the complication rate is low. The main contraindication to this method is pregnancy, as the fundus of the soft pregnant uterus is difficult to palpate with the Verres needle. If the needle punctures the pregnant uterus, carbon dioxide may enter the venous circulation through the venous sinuses. Fatal carbon dioxide embolism can ensue. Although a safe technique for insertion, pregnancy must be excluded.

Most experienced surgeons agree that the lower edge of the umbilical depression is the area of choice. At this point the peritoneum joins the umbilical plate, thus considerably reducing the distance the Verres needle needs to traverse through the peritoneal fat. The incision should only be large enough to allow the insertion of the Verres needle in the first instance in case a pneumoperitoneum is not established and the alternative sites of insertion need to be considered.

Verres needle insertion

The insertion of the Verres needle should be made through the deepest part of the umbilicus, because at this point the abdominal wall is thin and the peritoneum is at the closest point to the skin. The area of the lower abdomen just above the symphysis pubis is grasped by the surgeon's left hand and elevated upward and cephalad at a 45° angle to the horizontal. This slightly elevates the umbilicus, placing its underlying peritoneum on a stretch in a plane roughly perpendicular to the axis of the true pelvis. The Verres needle is then grasped in the surgeon's right hand with the upper barrel between the thumb and index finger, and the fourth finger of the right hand resting down the shaft of the needle to prevent it being inserted too far into the peritoneal cavity.

The Verres needle can then be inserted at right angles to the skin (45° caudad off the vertical) straight into the axis of the true pelvis (see Figure 3.2).

Throughout the insertion of the Verres needle the patient should be kept horizontal, for only the horizontal plane provides reference to the underlying anatomy. In our opinion, the practice of tilting the patient in a Trendelenberg position before the establishment of a pneumoperitoneum is unsafe.

Confirmation of peritoneal entry

After the insertion of the Verres needle, there are various tests to ensure that the tip of the Verres needle is indeed within the peritoneal cavity.

Double click test

There are several disposable Verres needles now available. Some feature hollow chambers containing a small ball above the spring mechanism. These devices make an audible click on piercing the rectus sheath and then again on entering the peritoneum. This double click, though not an absolute test of peritoneal entry, is a useful addition to the tests outlined below.

Saline test

A 10 cc syringe is filled with saline and attached to the Verres needle. 5 cc is then injected and the plunger is then withdrawn. There should be no aspirate obtained if the needle is in the peritoneal cavity, as the fluid will have dispersed between loops of bowel. If the needle lies in the abdominal wall,

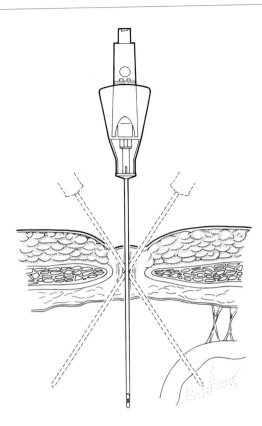

Figure 3.2: The Verres needle is inserted at right angles to the skin (45° caudad off the vertical) straight into the axis of the true pelvis. (Illustration courtesy of the Department of Medical Illustration, St. Bartholemew's Hospital, London)

clear fluid will be withdrawn. If the aspirate is stained red or brown, however, then perforation of bowel or blood vessel has occurred and the surgeon must decide how best to proceed with the operation.

As a continuation, the plunger is removed from the syringe and the residual saline is allowed to flow into the peritoneal cavity. If the needle is supraperitoneal the fluid may dissipate itself into the peritoneal fat but its flow will be much slower.

Direct Verres needle insertion with optical catheter

This is the last blind entry in laparoscopy. Recently optical catheters have been designed to fit inside a Verres needle and allow the surgeon to directly visualize entry into the abdominal cavity.

Problems encountered with insufflation

High pressure

The opening at the tip of the Verres needle is always on the same side as the valve lever, which should be directed downwards to avoid the peritoneum pressing against the opening (Figure 3.3). High insufflation pressures may also be caused by tissue blocking the needle tip. Flushing with 5 cc of saline should clear this problem. Erratic pressure readings can be caused by residual water in the insufflation tubing after rinsing, and will clear in due course. If irregular high pressures persist, a supraperitoneal insertion should be suspected. In these situations the insufflation should be discontinued, the pocket of gas evacuated, and a second effort made at reaching the peritoneum.

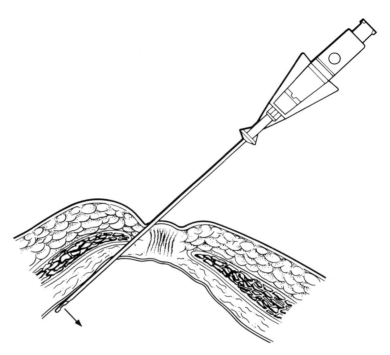

Figure 3.3: The opening at the tip of the Verres needle is always on the same side as the valve lever, which should be directed downwards to avoid the peritoneum pressing against the opening. (Illustration courtesy of the Department of Medical Illustration, St. Bartholemew's Hospital, London)

Repeated insertion attempt

Repeated unsuccessful attempts to enter the peritoneal cavity can result in the preperitoneal tissue being dissected away from the peritoneum. In such circumstances an alternative site of entry needs to be considered, eg via an incision in the left hypochondrium (1 cm lateral to the costo–chondral junction to avoid the superior epigastric vessels). This site is preferred as there are unlikely to be adhesions from previous intra-abdominal inflammation or surgery (ie cholecystitis or diverticular disease) and this point of entry avoids the dissected peritoneum in the lower abdomen. Alternative insertions can be made through the posterior fornix of the vagina or through the upper left margin of the umbilicus (to avoid the ligamentum teres). However, be careful to avoid the abdominal aorta lying directly underneath.

When the peritoneum is positively reached after such a scenario, it is advisable to inflate the abdomen beyond the normal 15 mmHg. This elevated intra-abdominal pressure will hold the dissected peritoneum against the preperitoneal fat and allow the first trocar to be inserted more easily. During this time the anaesthetist should be kept fully informed so that any respiratory difficulties caused by diaphragmatic pressure can be anticipated and compensated.

Failed entry

Inevitably we all have the occasional bad day when nothing seems to work! Since laparoscopy is usually an elective procedure, we should allow ourselves three attempts before considering abandoning it. At this point the patient's abdominal wall has been traversed repeatedly, and the surgeon has become increasingly disillusioned with each additional thrust of the Verres needle. At this juncture it is better to adjourn rather than compromise the patient's physical well-being and the surgeon's blood pressure. If a colleague is at hand, it may be prudent to let him make one more attempt. Open laparoscopy or mini-laparotomy may be an alternative, although most elective procedures can be postponed to another day.

Trocar insertion

Trocar insertion is the most hazardous part of the procedure. The principles involved are similar to those outlined previously relating to the insertion of the Verres needle. Trocars need to be extremely sharp to facilitate easy and unforced entry to the abdominal cavity. However, because of this property and the fact that the initial trocar is generally inserted blind, there is a risk of visceral trauma.

If there are suspected adhesions at the proposed site of entry of the trocar, the peritoneal space below the umbilicus can be explored with a needle or under direct visualization with an optical catheter. If gas cannot be aspirated freely after probing in several different directions, adhesions of bowel or omentum should be suspected. In these circumstances the surgeon should either consider an alternative site of trocar entry or perform an open laparoscopy.

The primary objective is to keep the trocar point as far away from the pelvic vessels as possible. This is achieved either by elevating the lower abdominal wall with the left hand or by pressing the left forearm against the patient's upper abdomen, forcing most of the intra-abdominal gas into the lower abdomen. Both of these techniques ensure that the distance between the trocar point and the major vessels is at its maximum.

The use of trocars which automatically guard their point when they meet no resistance should be encouraged.

A vertical incision is made from the deepest point of the umbilicus in an upward direction, the size of which depends on the laparoscope being used. The trocar should be aimed at the uterus and kept vertically in the mid-line as deviation to the left or right can result in damage to the pelvic vessels. When teaching laparoscopic techniques it is useful to observe the trainee from the foot of the operating table to ensure that the midline is being adhered to. Again it is worth emphasizing that the patient should be kept horizontal during this procedure as this is the operating surgeon's reference to the underlying anatomy (Figures 3.4, 3.5).

The trocar should be inserted in a zigzag path to avoid the risk of subsequent hernia formation (Figure 3.6).

As the trocar passes through the abdominal wall and enters the peritoneal cavity the surgeon should feel two distinct 'gives', the latter being the peritoneum. At this point the trocar should be held under a slight forward pressure and the trocar sleeve advanced on its own for about 5 cm, or, in obese women, when the trumpet valve touches the skin. This ensures that the sleeve is well within the peritoneal cavity and will not be inadvertently withdrawn above the peritoneum when the trocar is removed (Figure 3.7).

When the trocar is withdrawn, the trumpet valve is briefly kept open and the gush of gas confirms entry into the pneumoperitoneum. A laparoscope is then inserted past the trumpet valve but kept within the sleeve.

Laparoscopic inspection should first be directed downwards to observe any dripping of blood along the side of the sleeve which will suggest vessel damage at the insertion point. The laparoscope is then extended beyond the end of the sleeve enabling observation of the viscera directly below the trocar site. If adhesions are identified then the laparoscope should be advanced carefully into the abdominal cavity. Having passed through adhesions it is prudent to view your first portal of entry from another site to ensure that there is no bowel involved in the adhesions. If after these manoeuvres you are not in the abdominal cavity, the procedure should be abandoned. A laparotomy should be contemplated if there is any suspicion of damage to intra-abdominal organs.

Additional trocar sites

After careful inspection of the upper abdomen the patient is placed in a modified Trendelenberg position (25°) to facilitate the moving of bowel away from the pelvis. At this stage any additional trocar insertion points need to be considered and the plan of surgery established. The most usual points for insertion are shown in Figure 3.1.

One should bear in mind the location of the inferior epigastric vessels when inserting laterally placed trocars in the lower abdomen. These vessels are difficult to transilluminate except in exceptionally thin patients and may need to be visualized from within the peritoneal cavity. Their origin can be traced from the emergence of the round ligament from the deep inguinal ring, and the trocar can be inserted to either side of them under direct vision using the same technique as described previously to avoid subsequent hernia formation. If an abdominal wall vessel is injured, then a useful manoeuvre to arrest

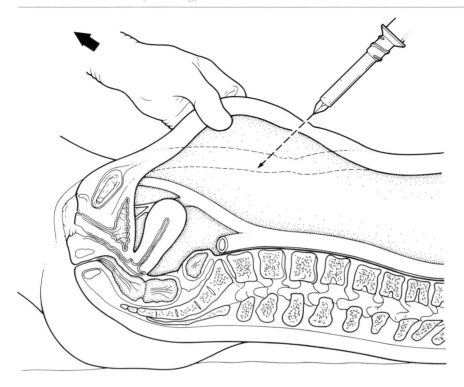

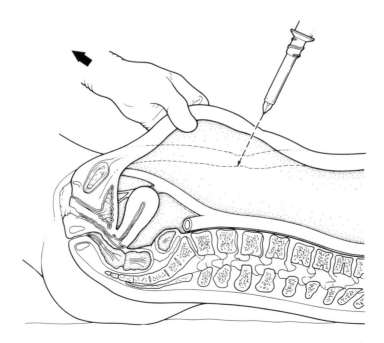

Figures 3.4 and 3.5: During trocar insertion the patient should be kept horizontal. (Illustrations courtesy of the Department of Medical Illustration, St. Bartholemew's Hospital, London)

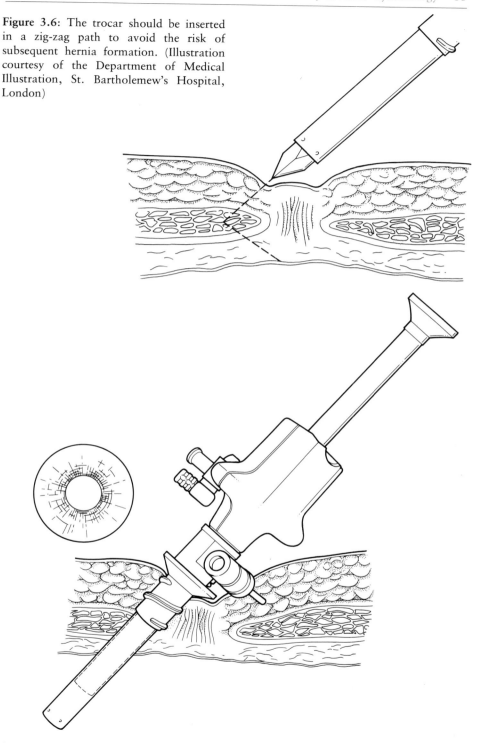

Figure 3.6: The trocar should be inserted in a zig-zag path to avoid the risk of subsequent hernia formation. (Illustration courtesy of the Department of Medical Illustration, St. Bartholemew's Hospital, London)

Figure 3.7: Insertion of the laparoscope. (Illustration courtesy of the Department of Medical Illustration, St. Bartholemew's Hospital, London)

bleeding is to pass a Foley catheter through the offending trocar and into the peritoneal cavity; its balloon can then be inflated and the trocar withdrawn until the catheter balloon tamponades the bleeding skin vessel. If this fails, a suture needs to be placed around the bleeding vessel, which is located laparoscopically.

The size of the skin incision should be checked using the trocar sleeve to ensure that undue force is not used to push the trocar past an incision which is too small. Again, keeping the forefinger extended on the sleeve prevents the trocar being inserted too deeply.

If a trocar is inadvertently inserted into adhesions or bowel, it should be removed, but the sleeve should remain in place so that if bowel has been perforated the site of perforation can be identified. It has been well described that when the trocar and sleeve have both been withdrawn after a suspected perforation, there has been great difficulty in locating the site of the perforation.

Wound closure

The additional trocar ports should be withdrawn under direct laparoscopic observation in case they have perforated a vessel in the anterior abdominal wall.

If a patient has a history of previous abdominal surgery, one should always be alert to bowel adhering to the anterior abdominal wall and in particular under the site of the scars. If the possibility of bowel perforation has not been excluded by viewing the primary site of entry from another trocar, the sleeve should be withdrawn slowly. It is important to maintain laparoscopic vision during this process so that one can make certain that the trocar has not perforated both walls of the bowel. It has been reported by several investigators that after a laparoscopic operation, at the point of removing the trocar it was discovered that the surgeon had perforated a loop of bowel that was adhering to the anterior abdominal wall under the umbilicus! Once you are confident that there is no evidence of bowel injury the trocar sleeve should be pushed back into the peritoneal cavity and the gas released.

Peritoneum and incisions smaller than 10 cm in the rectus sheath will heal spontaneously, as will many skin incisions along Langer's lines. At the site of larger trocar incisions, which are used for morcellating instruments, a deep absorbable suture should be inserted to close the deep fascia and thereby prevent hernia formation, which appears to be more common at the site of the laterally placed incisions. Approximation of the skin can be achieved using Steristrips, absorbable or nonabsorbable sutures. We have noted that several patients demonstrate significant development of ecchymosis as a result of the counter flexion required to insert large trocars > 15 mm in diameter (Figure 3.8). Despite their disconcerting appearance, they resolve spontaneously!

Practical manoeuvres and alternative methods

The techniques outlined above are our preferred methods of laparoscopic

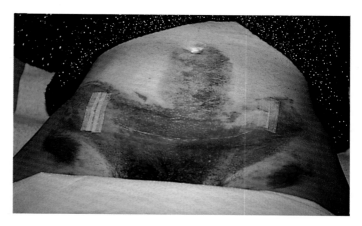

Figure 3.8: Extensive ecchymosis 48 hours postoperatively. Note the pattern of distribution caused by countertraction forces required to introduce large diameter trocars (> 15 mm). (Photo courtesy of Dr Grochmal)

surgery. These have been developed from personal experience and observation of the methods employed by several of the leading exponents of operative laparoscopy. There are many alternatives to the described techniques, and in experienced hands give excellent results; however they can be hazardous if performed by inexperienced operators. The methods which we have outlined will in our opinion result in safe practice and are easy to teach to the trainees. When necessary, the use of the open laparoscopic or Hasson technique should be considered.

Summary

Laparoscopic management of ectopic pregnancy, ovarian cysts, endometriosis and uterine fibroids should now be the norm, and will soon be demanded by our patients. Those who choose not to learn these simple techniques will not be able to meet the wishes of our consumers. As DeCherney wrote in 1985:

'The obituary for laparotomy for pelvic reconstructive surgery has been written; it is only its publication that remains... In the 80s, a burgeoning of reconstructive surgery with the use of the endoscope will revolutionize gynaecologic surgery.'

The majority of abdominal hysterectomies will be relegated to the history books, because the uterus which is not amenable to a vaginal hysterectomy by a properly trained surgeon will probably be removed by a laparoscopically assisted vaginal hysterectomy.

It should be borne in mind, however, that some of the new endoscopic surgical procedures require specialized training. The performance of these surgeons can be compared to that of a trapeze artiste in a circus, requiring dedication, intense training and excellent coordination, abilities given to few people, with the result that most will fall off the 'high wire'.

Endoscopic operative procedures that replace the standard laparotomy for common conditions must be simple and capable of being used effectively, repeatedly and safely by the majority of practising gynaecologists. If not, then the promised reduction in postoperative pain, reduced hospital stay and improved cosmetic results will not stand the test of time.

Bibliography

Bruhat MA, Mahnes H, Mage G and Pouly JL (1980) Treatment of ectopic pregnancy by means of laparoscopy. *Fertility and Sterility*. **33**:411.

Copeland C, Wing RR and Hulka JF (1983) Direct trocar insertion at laparoscopy. *Obstetrics and Gynecology*. **62**:655–9.

DeCherney AH (1985) The leader of the band is tired... *Fertility and Sterility*. **44**:299.

Hasson HM (1974) Open laparoscopy: a report of 150 cases. *Journal of Reproductive Medicine*. **12**:234–8.

Howard FM (1992) Breaking new ground or just digging a hole? An evaluation of gynecologic operative laparoscopy. *Journal of Gynecological Surgery*. **8**:143.

Kelman GR, Benzie RJ, Gordon NLM, Smith I and Swapp GH (1971) Cardiovascular effects of peritoneal carbon dioxide insufflation for laparoscopy. *British Journal of Anaesthesia*. **43**:719.

McMillan DL and Pesce A (1994) 'Foreveroscopies' and complications of gynaecological endoscopic surgery.

Nezhat C, Nezhat F and Nezhat C (1992) Operative laparoscopy (minimally invasive surgery): state of the art. *Journal of Gynecological Surgery*. **8**:111.

Ott DE (1991) Correction of laparoscopic insufflation hypothermia. *Journal of Laparoendoscopic Surgery*. **1**:183–6.

Puri GD and Singh H (1992) Ventilatory effects of laparoscopy under general anaesthesia. *British Journal of Anaesthesia*. **68**:211–13.

Shulman B and Aronson HB (1984) Caponography in the early diagnosis of carbon dioxide embolism during laparoscopy. *Canadian Anesthetists' Society Journal*. **31**:455–9.

4

Laser vs Electrosurgery: An Overview

GREGORY T. ABSTEN

High-energy surgery

Surgical instruments today span a wide variety of devices — from the simple sharp knife, at the 'low-tech' end, to the nanosecond pulsed surgical laser systems at the other extreme.

With the advent of high-energy surgical devices — electrosurgical tools, cavitational ultrasonic aspirators, harmonic (ultrasonic) knives, cryosurgery, various laser systems and endocoagulators — it is useful to view these various devices simply as different means of delivering energy to tissue. Even a simple scalpel may be viewed as delivering mechanical energy to tissue at a concentrated pressure point (the blade edge).

No single system is inherently better than the others for all surgical purposes. Each may have advantages in certain situations, and user preference is frequently only a personal bias, influenced by past familiarity with a system.

Both lasers and electrosurgical units use waves of high energy within the electromagnetic spectrum to produce surgical effects of cutting and coagulation by producing heat*. Light and laser beams simply use higher-frequency electromagnetic waves than the radio frequencies of electrosurgical units. Either way, energy is transferred into tissue to create heat.

Heat and heat transfer

The advantages of the high-energy modalities of electrosurgical electrodes or laser devices lie not only in their ability to create and localize enough heat to

---

* Some laser modalities work in other ways than by the effects of heat generation, but these are specialized applications that are not included in general surgical techniques of cutting, ablation or photocoagulation.

produce the desired surgical effects of cutting, ablation and photocoagulation, but also in the associated haemostasis. Laser effects may be more highly localized than electrosurgical ones. Laparoscopic dissection of a ureter, for instance, may be performed with more control with a laser than with electrosurgery. On the other hand, electrosurgery is usually very convenient when such precision is not required, such as for taking down thin filmy adhesions.

Heat was once thought to be a substance. It was believed that when a hot object was placed in contact with a cooler object, an invisible entity called phlogiston entered the cooler object to make it hotter. Now we know that heat is the result of continuous motion and vibration of the atoms and molecules that constitute all matter. The transfer of heat between objects of different temperatures involves a reduction in the average motion of the particles of the hotter object and an increase in the average motion of the particles of the cooler object. Therefore heat is not really an energy in itself, but the transfer of energy between objects.

Heat may be measured quantitatively as either calories or British thermal units (BTUs). Temperature is not heat. Temperature is a measurement of the intensity of heat, although an object at high temperature does not necessarily have more heat than an object at lower temperature. Larger or heavier objects can contain more heat, at the same temperature, than smaller objects. This is why larger-diameter laser fibres which are used in contact with tissue can contain more heat and accomplish more work than smaller-diameter devices at the same temperature. A 200 L drum of water at body temperature contains significantly more heat than a thimbleful of boiling water. The temperature of boiling water is higher (intensity), but the total heat content of the large drum is higher because of its size.

The transfer of heat from one object to another occurs through one or more of three basic mechanisms: conduction, convection and radiation. Lasers are used in one of two ways to generate heat: either 'non-contact' methods which rely on radiation transfer, or contact methods which rely on conduction transfer. Electrosurgery, when used correctly, relies only on radiation transfer.

Conduction

Conduction heat transfer is the flow of heat energy in matter as a result of molecular collisions. If a hot object touches tissue, therefore, it can burn it through direct conduction of heat. This is the mechanism of the classic 'cautery' of tissue by hot objects — not to be confused with electrosurgery.

'Contact' laser fibres and sapphire probes typically used on Nd:YAG lasers are another type of 'cautery' which work by direct conduction of heat from an object into tissue by direct contact. This might be called 'photocautery', since the laser supplies the energy required to heat the tip of the fibre or sapphire. This is much more effective than electrical methods of heating and means that devices can be significantly smaller (less than 1.0 mm). Laser light does transmit through these fibre and sapphire devices and, even though there may be some focusing of the energy right at the tip, the major mechanism of action is conduction heating from the crystal material to tissue directly through contact. The crystal, or contact laser fibre tip, gets very hot.

Conduction heating can become a problem when a laser is left in contact with tissue for long periods of time because of low power applications. Unwanted heat conducts from the target tissue into adjacent tissues and may cause thermal injury by heat conduction. Another problem with conduction is that irrigating fluid makes an excellent thermal conductor. This means that contact-type laser devices, although useful under fluid, are subject to significant diminuition of heat intensity at the tip because of the conductive cooling qualities of the fluid. During laparoscopy, in fact, irrigating an already hot laser fibre contact tip can make it crack.

Non-contact lasers, such as the carbon dioxide, excimer and Ho:YAG, do not operate in the 'cautery' mode since the beams of light themselves are not hot.

The green-light KTP and argon lasers can be contact or non-contact, depending on which fibre is selected and how it is used. The Nd:YAG laser is most commonly used with contact tips and fibres for laparoscopy. It could technically be used in a non-contact fashion, but this is fraught with hazards for laparoscopy.

Convection

Convection involves larger quantities of matter than conduction, such as when a saucepan of water is boiled. This has important implications in electrosurgery and laser technology because convection is what carries away the excess heat from the incision site through generation of steam (laser or electrosurgical plume). Although there does not have to be much plume, if either device is used to dissect in a manner which is too slow to allow any generation of steam, heat will build up in the tissue and conduct into lateral tissues. This usually occurs when the laser or electrode is used at such painfully low powers that vaporization cannot proceed immediately and the device just 'wallows' and burns in tissue. Adequate power levels for clean vaporization will generate the required 'steam envelope' around the device and carry away excess heat.

Radiation

Radiation is the primary mechanism of heat transfer for electrosurgical and non-contact laser modalities. This involves the transfer of thermal energy by electromagnetic waves. Materials do not have to touch to transfer heat in this way. Heat may even be transmitted across a vacuum by radiation since it does not depend on the presence of matter. This is the essential mechanism of the non-contact lasers mentioned above. If a laser fibre is used 'away' from the tissue, so that a high-power density spot creates the vaporization, then it is said to be non-contact. If a laser fibre or contact tip is actually stroked through the tissue, in contact with it, then the heat of the fibre tip itself does the work, and this is said to be a contact technique.

Radiation transfer means that laser beams contain no inherent heat in the light itself. They transmit only radiation energy. Heat is created only when the tissue absorbs the transmitted radiation and converts it to motion in its atoms and molecules. This is exactly the way a microwave oven works, but at different frequencies. Those lasers which rely on the cautery effect of a hot tip create the heat there when the laser radiation (semantics for light) is inefficiently transmitted from the tip; this inefficiency generates heat in the quartz or ceramic material of the tip. It can be a very effective and haemostatic cutting instrument.

The last pertinent concept of heat and heat transfer is that of the heat capacity of an object. Heat capacity and specific heats of objects are closely related, and have to do with how much heat is required to produce a certain temperature change. In other words, biological objects of high heat capacity require much more heat to effect any given surgical effect. Highly vascular tissues have a higher heat capacity than other tissues, and consequently require higher laser powers, or larger contact tips, to effect the same surgical effects.

Laser

Laser is an acronym which stands for light amplification by the stimulated emission of radiation*.

Light (made up of photons of energy) is contained within the forces that hold together atoms and molecules. By tapping into these atomic and molecular bonds we can release the light that is stored there. Regular light sources such as light-bulbs release this light energy in a random and chaotic process, spontaneously emitting photons of all energies (wavelengths or colours) in all directions and with no coordination between them. This results in incoherent white light.

Laser light consists of the same photons of light as from ordinary light sources, but released in an organized fashion called stimulated emission. The laser tube, with a mirror at each end, serves to propagate this process and build an intense beam of light. The light emitted is of one energy (wavelength and colour) and travels in one direction through space as a tight beam. The result is a coherent, bright beam of one colour, or at least pure colours.

Various materials emit characteristic colours of light, and the laser is named after the material used. The primary lasers used in gynaecology are the carbon dioxide (CO_2) laser, which emits far-infrared light at 10 600 nm; the Nd:YAG laser, which emits near-infrared light at 1064 nm; the KTP laser (sometimes combined with an Nd:YAG), which emits green light at 532 nm; and the argon laser, similar to the KTP but emitting blue/green light at 488 and 515 nm. The holmium:YAG, which emits mid-infrared light at 2100 nm, is used primarily in orthopaedic arthroscopies but may also be used in laparoscopic procedures.

---

* Radiation here does not refer to ionizing-type radiation such as X-ray. It refers to a 'radiant' body, or one which shines light. Conventional medical laser units do not produce any hazardous ionizing radiation.

Table 4.1 lists the common medical lasers and their associated wavelengths. Ones of particular importance in gynaecological surgery are marked with an asterisk.

*Carbon dioxide (CO$_2$)	Far-infrared	10 600 nm
— the best laser for cervical/vulvar/vaginal use; also has general laparoscopic use		
Erbium:YAG (Er:YAG)	Mid-infrared	2940 nm
— investigational: bone-cutting and drilling		
Hydrogen:fluoride	Mid-infrared	2940 nm
— investigational: bone-cutting and drilling		
*Holmium:YAG (Ho:YAG)	Mid-infrared	2100 nm
— general laparoscopic use; primary use in orthopaedic surgery		
Neodymium:YAG(harmonic) (Nd:YAG)	Mid-infrared	1318 nm
— investigational tissue welding (fusion)		
*Neodymium:YAG (Nd:YAG)	Near-infrared	1064 nm
— general laparoscopic use with contact fibres and devices, and for hysteroscopy		
Diode lasers	Variable with system	
Ruby	Deep red	694 nm
Krypton	Red	647 nm
	Yellow	568 nm
	Green	531 nm
Helium neon (HeNe)	Red	632 nm
Gold vapour	Red	632 nm
Tunable dye laser	Variable with dyes:	
	Red	632 nm
	Yellow	577 nm
	Green	504 nm
Copper vapour	Yellow	577 nm
	Green	510 nm
*Potassium titanyl phosphate (KTP)	Green	532 nm
— a frequency doubled YAG (which may include an Nd:YAG in the same machine); general laparoscopic use, either contact or non-contact		
*Argon	Blue	488 nm
	Green	515 nm
— general laparoscopic use, either contact or non-contact		
— excimers	Ultraviolet	
Investigational in ophthalmology, cardiovascular and orthopaedics		
ArF		193 nm
KrCl		222 nm
KrF		248 nm
XeCl		308 nm
XeF		351 nm

Table 4.1: Surgical lasers.

The infrared lasers are, by definition, invisible to our eyes. For this reason the very low-power red helium neon laser is usually coupled with these invisible lasers so that we can see where the beam is pointing. This is the same laser used in grocery checkout scanners. However, with most of the laser fibre and contact systems, the tip is so close to tissue that there is no real need for a guide light.

The process of stimulated emission gives rise to three properties of laser light that are distinct from ordinary light. Laser light is unique in that it is:

- coherent
- collimated
- monochromatic.

Not all of these parameters are used to create surgical effects. For the most part, surgical laser systems are used on quite a crude level for their heat-producing effects, even though those resulting surgical effects may be exceptionally precise. Tapping these unique characteristics of laser will give rise to a myriad of diagnostic and therapeutic applications in gynaecological surgery in the future.

Coherence

Coherence refers to the phasing of the wave patterns of light. Coherent waves are analogous to surf as it comes towards a beach in orderly rows. Ordinary light is incoherent and very disorganized. When all the waves are in phase (coherent), the effect is amplification and orderliness. This is the beginning of the light amplification process.

Another interesting phenomenon produced by the combination of the light's coherence and identical wavelengths is holography. Three-dimensional images may be produced by taking a picture of an object with a laser. Holograms contain information as small as the wavelength of light used to make the picture. In other words, you can look at a hologram through a microscope and see the actual microscopic structure. If a hologram is broken into a thousand pieces, each individual piece will contain the whole picture, although it will become less distinct the more pieces it is broken into.

Endoscopic holographic pathology is a technique which is in its early stages of development. A very small catheter with a capsule at the end is inserted into the patient. A fibre inside the catheter allows a holographic 'snapshot' on a small piece of microfilm within the capsule. When it is retrieved and developed, the pathologist may read the hologram microscopically in three dimensions.

Laser interferometry uses holographic principles to make precise measurements of target geometry. This is commercially useful now and will eventually have many medical applications.

Collimation

Collimation means that the laser creates a light beam that stays together tightly over long distances. This is partly due to the coherence of the waves, and partly due to the fact that the resonator is configured as a long slender tube.

For surgical purposes, collimation is important both for power delivery and for generating small spot sizes. Collimation allows the power to be retained wholly within the beam and does not fade with distance as with conventional light sources. The lamp in a laparoscopic light source, for instance, has a higher wattage than most surgical lasers, but loses the intensity rapidly with distance from the bulb. Collimation also allows the beam to be focused to very small spots, increasing the intensity and producing cutting, vaporizing and coagulating effects. This small spot also allows all of the energy to be focused into the ends of the typical 0.6 mm fibres. Regular light sources cannot be focused to such a degree. It is really collimation that creates the surgical effectiveness of the laser.

Monochromaticity

Monochromacity means that the laser produces pure colours of light. Contrary to popular conception this does not necessarily mean that only one colour is produced. Lasers can produce multiple colours in a narrow band, each being a pure colour by itself. Ordinary light sources produce white light that consists of all colours, with no definite separation and with broad bandwidths.

Lasers may be tuned to emit only one of the pure colours. Surgical lasers are used primarily for their thermal effects, and colour is only grossly important because it determines how well the energy of the light is coupled as heat into the tissue. This determines the gross tissue effects such as vaporization and coagulation. The range of colour is important — blue–green is very different from infrared — but absolute spectral purity is usually superfluous when using the laser to cut or vaporize tissue.

Another area in medicine where the spectral purity of the light is critical is in photodynamic therapy. This is currently an investigational technique that holds great promise for cancer patients. For this therapy a type of dihematoporphyrin ether (DHE) is administered systemically. About 72 hours later one can observe significant differences in residual drug levels between normal and malignant cells. By itself the drug is latent until activated by specific colours of light that the laser provides. This type of laser light produces no thermal effects and is used solely to initiate phototoxic processes in the cell via a photochemical reaction with the drug. The red wavelength is used because it penetrates farthest in tissue, rather than because it has the best absorption peak in DHE.

Dihematoporphyrin ether is the primary drug now used for this work, but other drugs are coming. Other photosensitizing drugs and light sources are being examined for possible applications in the diagnosis and treatment of cancer, atherosclerosis, viral infections such as human papilloma virus (HPV) and some dermatological conditions. This is an area of clinical photo-chemistry which utilizes the monochromaticity of the laser and has tremendous potential.

Energy concepts

Routine daily use of a laser does not usually require tedious calculation and quantification of the factors of power density, total energy or fluence. Control of the laser is generally based on visual cues, noting the geometries of the defects created and deciding to proceed faster or slower. These things can only be learnt by practice, not calculation; however, a knowledge of energy concepts is important to understand why a laser works as it does.

Power

This is simply the rate at which the energy is delivered. The faster a given amount of energy may be delivered, the more confined the resulting heat damage will be. As a general rule, therefore, the highest power with which one is comfortable should be used if precision is desired. This becomes very important when discussing pulsing modalities on CO_2 lasers such as superpulse and ultrapulse. Pulsing allows for controlled delivery of very high peak laser powers, which is desirable to eliminate burning or charring. Unlike laser, electrosurgery should not be used at powers much in excess of what is required to cut cleanly. This is because of incumbent higher voltages or current which could cause unseen damage elsewhere.

Power density

This is the single most important factor in the application of any laser or electrosurgical electrode. It is sometimes referred to as irradiance or spot brightness. With electrosurgery it is sometimes called current density. Power density is the relationship between the power and the spot size (surface area of an electrode) in which it is concentrated. It is a balance between these two parameters and is expressed in W cm^2 (power per surface area).

When the laser is operated as a continuously emitted beam, power density is the factor controlling eye/hand coordination, rather than the power itself as is commonly believed. This is the speed at which the laser beam can penetrate through tissue. The higher the power density, the faster the tissue removal within that size spot and hence the faster the penetration. High laser power densities are desirable in that they vaporize cleanly without char, but they can make surgical control difficult if they are too high. Too low a power density is very controllable surgically, but can create unwanted burning and charring of tissues.

As children discover when they try to burn a piece of paper, using a magnifying glass and sunlight, the smaller the area in which the light is concentrated the more intense it becomes. The relationship is described by the formula:

$$\text{power density} = \frac{\text{watts} \times 100}{\pi \times r^2} = \text{watts cm}^2$$

where r is the spot size in millimetres. Power density increases with either an increase in power or a decrease in spot size. Since the spot size equation contains a square function, this will more rapidly change the tissue effect than the power.

Since power density is a balance between spot size and power, it means that eye/hand coordination and control of penetration may be maintained at any power if it is balanced by the appropriate spot size. Spot size may be changed by the surgeon.

Power density is crucial for the correct use of electrodes with electrosurgical units. If the electricity is concentrated within a very small surface-contact area (like the fine tip of a needle electrode), then the intensity of the effect will increase, and the cut will be very clean at relatively low powers on the unit. If the electricity is spread out over a broader contact area (like the broad back of a spoon electrode), then the intensity of effect will be diminished at any given power and the electrode will probably coagulate and/or burn tissue. Controlling the haemostasis one achieves while using electrosurgical instrumentation is, in fact, best achieved by manipulating the contact area of the electrode in this way, rather than resorting to changing the 'cut' and 'coag' modes on the unit.

Energy

The total amount of light or electrical energy delivered to tissue is described in joules. This is simply the rate of delivery times the length of time of delivery, or:

$$joules = watts \times time = watts\ s^1$$

The argon, KTP and CO_2 lasers do not provide a readout of the number of joules delivered. The concept is important but the numbers are not. Most surgical Nd:YAG lasers do provide a readout of joules, and of the watts of power (as set by the operator). Lasers that are truly pulsed, such as the Ho:YAG, have readouts of the joules delivered, which is the parameter set by the operator. The average power then becomes a secondary readout determined by the joules per pulse and the pulse repetition rate.

Although the concept is important, complete surgical procedures are not based on a light 'dose' limit in joules. The procedure is terminated whenever the incision is finished or the correct amount of tissue vaporized, regardless of the number of joules required. Endometrial ablations are based on the visual observation of how well coagulated the endometrium is — not how many joules were required to achieve the effect.

When discussing the theoretical aspects of superpulsing and ultrapulsing of CO_2 lasers, the energy contained within each pulse becomes important. To optimize the superpulse or ultrapulse, the individual pulse must contain sufficient energy to vaporize tissue cleanly with each individual pulse.

Fluence

The concept of energy delivery is important because it allows us to trade off power for time, keeping total energy and extent of the impact constant, to limit heat damage.

Fluence actually combines the concepts of power density and total energy, and is expressed as joules cm^{-2}, or energy per unit area. This is sometimes referred to as the radiant energy of the beam. A high fluence is like a 'bolus' of light. A low fluence is like a 'drip' of light. We will see that high fluence creates surgical precision and thermal control. It is the critical concept in the use of superpulse and ultrapulse. Recently, a surgical Nd:YAG laser has been introduced for laparoscopic use which also employs the high fluences of fast pulsing. This creates better surgical control and cleaner dissection of tissue compared with using the laser in a lower fluence continuous wave setting.

Energy delivery and laser pulsing concepts

The way that laser energy is delivered to tissue may sometimes be more important to the tissue effect than the wavelength selected. The rate at which the light is delivered determines the lateral extent of a burn, ie its precision. If delivered quickly enough (very high fluence), one can bypass direct heating effects altogether and achieve minute 'sparking' and acoustical snapping effects with no thermal damage. These acoustical effects are not really used in gynaecological surgery. They are used to fragment kidney and biliary stones by laser lithotripsy and, at higher levels, used to 'snap' apart membranes within the eye with a cold-cutting effect.

It is useful for the practitioner to have a basic knowledge of the different modes of operation because of the variety of systems which are commercially promoted, and whose tissue effects depend a great deal upon the pulse configuration. In particular it is useful to understand the basic differences between continuous wave, gated pulses and true laser pulses, particularly with CO_2 lasers.

Continuous wave

Most of the CO_2 and surgical Nd:YAG (non-ophthalmic) lasers, and all argon lasers, operate in a continuous wave (CW) mode. This means that the power output (rate of energy delivery) is steady and constant over the time in which it is delivered. It is like filling a bathtub and allowing it to overflow. As it begins to overflow it does so at a steady rate as long as the tap is not turned off.

The identifying characteristic of this mode is that the maximum peak power delivered by the laser is never greater than the averaged power, which is what one reads on the power meter of the laser. In other words, a 40 W maximum power Nd:YAG laser, will never produce higher powers that the rated 40 Watts. The bathtub can never give you a greater 'gush' of water over the sides than the rate at which it comes through the tap. This is in contrast with true laser pulsing, where the peak powers may go much higher.

CW operation is also the most 'thermal' way to use a laser in that the relatively long times involved allow for more heat conduction to surrounding tissues. One gains haemostasis, but at the expense of tissue precision. When using contact-type laser fibres and tips, the CW mode is generally used.

A point of confusion on many lasers is that manufacturers sometimes label an operating button on the machine as 'continuous'. This does not necessarily mean a CW mode: instead it means that the beam will be emitted continuously as long as the foot pedal is depressed. In this way it is possible to operate some pulsed modes, like superpulse, in a continuous fashion with foot pedal control.

Gated (timed) pulse

When a laser such as CO_2, argon or CW Nd:YAG are set on a 'pulse' of fractions of a second to several seconds, it is generally a gated pulse and not a true laser pulse. Manufacturers of these lasers frequently label the button 'pulse' (either single or repeat). A gated pulse is simply a timer or shutter on a CW beam. The semantics are unimportant in most situations, but it is important to understand the difference between the two.

The characteristic of a gated (or timed) pulse is that the maximum peak power of the pulse is not any higher than the CW setting. In other words, if a CW CO_2 laser is set at 40 W for a 0.1 s pulse, the maximum power of that pulse will not exceed the 40 W. It is simply a timer on an otherwise CW mode beam. Using the bathtub analogy, if the tub was filled to the brim, and then the tap was turned on and off, the water would still overflow at the same rate, but in timed 'gushes' according to how the tap was controlled.

The advantage of using this type of timed pulse is primarily one of surgical control. Pulsing, either in single bursts or in a series of repeated pulses, gives the operator more time to react to change, so things may be slowed down.

This type of pulsing may be achieved either by 'pumping' the foot-pedal while the laser is operating in a CW mode, or by selecting a timer on the control panel. Using the foot-pedal control is a faster way to work, but does not provide the consistency of the control panel pulse timer. Pulsing a laser like this seems to be most useful in gynaecology with a CO_2 laser.

It should also be pointed out the 'pulse' buttons on most CO_2 laser control panels may serve equally as a timer for either a CW mode beam or a true pulse such as a superpulse. The latter would technically be gated pulsing of a superpulse. Gated pulsing is a time limit. Typical pulses are from 0.05 s to several seconds in length.

'True' pulse

True laser pulses are found on many of the pulsed dye lasers, excimers and superpulse CO_2, KTP, copper vapour and ophthalmic Nd:YAG lasers. They are frequently used to limit the zone of thermal damage, or to produce the 'sparking' and acoustical effects with little or no thermal damage. Much of the cold-cutting effects of excimer lasers have as much to do with their pulsing characteristics as with the wavelength of light (from 308 nm up). The Ho:YAG laser, or a superpulse or ultrapulse on CO_2 lasers, are gynaecological lasers which employ true pulsing.

The identifying characteristic of a true laser pulse is that the maximum power output of the pulse far exceeds the maximum obtainable in a CW mode. The power delivery is compressed to a short time frame. The Ho:YAG laser, for instance, will produce pulses of several thousand watts for only a few microseconds, which may be repeated up to 15 or 25 times per second to provide maximum average powers of around 20–30 W.

A recently introduced surgical Nd:YAG laser is also a truly pulsed system. This allows its use with contact-type fibres to provide very precise incisions, and possibly some bone cutting or drilling. This pulsed Nd:YAG laser should not be confused with other CW Nd:YAG lasers which are used with the contact tips.

A pulsed Nd:YAG used in ophthalmology may produce power spikes of tens of millions of watts, but for only billionths of a second! This extreme pulsing leads to photo-acoustic sparking effects.

True pulses may be emitted singularly, such as with the pulsed dye laser for stones, or as a rapid series of pulses, such as with the excimers in orthopaedics. The KTP laser also produces a series of pulses, but of less individual energy than a Ho:YAG laser. These rapid-series pulses are referred to as high-frequency pulsed lasers.

The principle may again be illustrated with the bathtub analogy. If one were to build a 'dam' around the walls of the tub, with a small door at the bottom, and let the tap run at a constant rate, the water level would continue to rise as the water was stored in the dam. When the dam is full and the door at the bottom is opened, the water gushes out at a much higher rate than which the tap filled the tub. The problem is that it gushes out very quickly, and then there is a delay while the dam is refilled; this is a refractory time or time between pulses. This is exactly how a true laser pulse works. Pulses may only last for millionths or billionths of a second, and may rapid-fire up to several thousand times per second, but the principle is the same.

It is possible to squeeze so much energy into such a short pulse that the damage threshold for a fibre is exceeded. This is why the ophthalmic Nd:YAG lasers, which produce a 'spark' and 'snap', cannot be delivered down a fibre as can an ordinary CW Nd:YAG laser used in gynaecology. The input energy would blow up the input end of the fibre.

Beam profiles, spot sizes and fibre use

A laser beam is unlike a physical instrument such as a scalpel blade, in that it does not have definite sides. The beam is a concentration of energy in a spot that tends to fade at the edges. This affects the sizes of spots created at different settings, and the precision of incisions.

Furthermore, beams are emitted differently from fibres (argon, KTP and

Ho:YAG lasers), and from articulated arms (CO_2 lasers, which preserve the true shape of the beam). Contact-type fibres or sapphire tips rely only on the physical size and shape of those materials themselves.

A CO_2 laser beam has a focusing/defocusing effect. When used through a laparoscope, the laser lens is contained within the coupler attachment on the top of the scope. This focuses the beam down through the hollow channel of the scope itself and converges to a focal spot. The biggest difference between this and a fibre system is that this focused CO_2 beam stays tightly focused for a greater distance than the beam from a fibre system.

Carbon dioxide laser waveguides are fibre-like devices which are actually slender, hollow tubing. The laser beam is focused into one end of the tube, through hundreds of internal glancing reflections down the inside walls of the waveguide, and delivered from the distal end. This destroys the focus/defocus aspects of the CO_2 laser and makes it behave more like a fibreoptically delivered system.

Laser fibres tend to scramble the input beam, resulting in a blended, homogeneous output, diverging immediately in a 10–15° cone. There is no focal point to a fibre. This means that power density, and hence tissue effect, is highest right at the tip of the fibre and falls off rapidly with short distances from the fibre tip. Cutting is achieved with the fibre just off tissue (less than 1.0 mm); another millimetre or two back creates sculpting and vaporization, another millimetre or two forward causes simple photocoagulation with no vaporization. No damage is possible much past 5–10 mm.

Handpieces designed to hold the laser fibres for laparoscopic use provide some mechanical stability to these slender fibres. It is possible simply to insert a fibre down another laparoscopic instrument, but the 'wobble' and lack of support usually make this awkward unless used in conjunction with some fibre-deflecting instrument.

Shooting the laser fibre while it is positioned perpendicularly at right angles to the tissue (shooting directly at it at 90°) is the usual method of handling the fibre. Occasionally firing tangentially to the tissue (shooting across the tissue mostly parallel to the surface) is necessary because of trocar placement. Slender fibres, 600 µm and smaller, may actually be inserted through a needle puncture in the abdomen to gain better positioning.

Non-contact fibres provide the option of cutting when placing the fibre onto tissue, sculpting or simply coagulating when pulling away. Contact-type fibres and probes can only be used by directly touching the tissue, though one company does make a combination-type fibre to achieve either effect.

Tissue effects of laser and use of fibres

The focus of our discussion of laser tissue effects in gynaecology is primarily on the photothermal effects of the light but there are other types of effects possible. At very low levels of light, lasers can actually stimulate cellular physiology — an area known as biostimulation. Very low-power laser beams are also used through research microscopes as tractor beams — surgical tweezers — to hold and move microscopic organisms such as bacteria or even sperm cells. Light may be used to initiate or mediate chemical reactions in the area known as photodynamic therapy discussed earlier. Once the light intensity is high enough to begin warming effects, it still may be used in a non-destructive manner. Tissue fusion, or welding, involves heating tissues to approximately 55–58°C to cause physiological bonding of proteins — which may be important in future reconstructive surgery.

At sufficient light intensities the tissue is heated to destructive levels by the photothermal effects of the laser. These effects include almost all of the current surgical applications of CO_2, argon, KTP, Ho:YAG and Nd:YAG lasers to cut, vaporize and photocoagulate tissue.

Once a certain higher intensity is achieved, other effects begin to take over. These are termed 'nonlinear laser effects', since they are more than simply a linear rise in tissue temperature with light intensity. At some point a plasma is generated by the high-intensity light. The small plasma 'sparks' create an acoustical snap or shock-wave which physically cuts or fragments an object.

When used as a surgical instrument to cut, vaporize or photocoagulate and destroy tissue, the laser depends primarily on the ability of the light to be absorbed by tissue, converting it into heat, much like the black asphalt on a hot day.

Effects of heat on tissue

To understand how tissues are heated by light, it is useful to know how light may interact with tissue, and what the tissue does to retain or dissipate this heat.

As heat energy builds within tissue, it is removed either through the energy of vaporization or conducted laterally into adjacent tissue or blood. Blood flow acts as a heat sink to dissipate heat to some degree, as we all have experienced when we touch a hot object momentarily: we are not burnt because the blood flow dissipates the heat and it is not applied for long enough to conduct into tissue. Irrigation fluid also serves to conduct away some of this excess heat.

We have already seen how heat can conduct between materials. Tissues have a characteristic thermal conductivity time. This is the rate at which heat may be conducted away. If laser energy can be applied quickly, the heat does not have enough time to conduct into adjacent tissue. If the laser is applied slowly, a significant lateral heat conduction can occur, potentially resulting in pain and scarring.

We can tie together the concept of pulsing, which we have already discussed, to that of thermal conductivity in tissue.

Tissue temperatures exceed 100°C before vaporization begins, regardless of whether the power applied is 1 or 3000 W. The lower powers mean that extra time must be spent to deliver the same amount of energy (low fluence) and therefore allow a significant lateral heat conduction and burn. Use of higher powers and shorter times (higher fluence) means that the heat will be dissipated in the energy of vaporization and not have time to conduct laterally: therefore pulsed laser energy will always be more precise than CW type systems.

Another approach to this problem is to move a high power density laser spot very quickly over tissue in a controlled, uniform fashion. The speed this requires dictates the use of an electro-optical scanning device. Since the high power density CW beam is not over any given spot except for a very brief time (a few microseconds), the clean tissue effects closely mimic a pulsed laser effect. The disadvantage with the scanner is that only vaporization of surfaces is possible, not tissue dissection.

In order for any heating to occur, the light must first be absorbed by tissue; but other interactions besides absorption are possible, such as reflection, transmission or scattering. It is in manipulating these characteristics that one can achieve very selective tissue effects with various lasers used in the non-contact mode.

Colour specificity

If the light is reflected from tissue, or transmitted through it, no heating effects will occur. Some of the lasers are colour-specific in their absorption. Argon and KTP absorb best into red or dark tissue (like haemoglobin), and the non-contact Nd:YAG into dark tissue. These lasers may reflect off or transmit through lightly coloured or non-pigmented tissue such as various types of cartilage. One must use hot tips, or attain exceptionally high intensity, to see satisfactory tissue effects on non-pigmented tissue. The CO_2 and Ho:YAG lasers are absorbed by the fluid in any soft tissue and produce highly localized absorption.

The material that serves as the absorbing target for the light is referred to as the target chromophore. This is what makes the light absorb and generate heat. For CO_2 and Ho:YAG lasers this is primarily water in tissue. For argon and KTP lasers it is primarily melanin, haemoglobin and proteins in tissue. For the Nd:YAG laser it is melanin and protein in general, especially if darkly pigmented.

Effects in fluid

The argon, KTP and Nd:YAG lasers transmit easily through water, so they may be used under fluid. CO_2 lasers are absorbed by even thin layers of fluid, including blood, and cannot be used under irrigation fluid. They work well for laparoscopy, but one should be aware that a thin sheet of irrigation solution over the target site will nullify the laser effect while the fluid is flowing.

Scattering of the light in tissue causes it to be absorbed over a more diffuse area. The Nd:YAG laser is the most highly scattered laser, and argon and KTP rather less so.

Tissue effects from one type of laser to another may overlap significantly due to varying powers, pulse widths and delivery systems. This creates part of the confusion generated when claims are made that one particular type of laser is the 'best' for overall surgical use. Though there is overlap between cutting, vaporizing and coagulation, no single laser is the best at everything and each has its particular strengths.

The CO_2 laser is so highly absorbed by water that it concentrates a lot of energy in a small volume of water. 30–90 µm of water will absorb about 90% of the incident beam. This creates immediate heating of the tissue to temperatures exceeding 100°C. It is an excellent cutting and vaporizing instrument, working from the surface down. It is possible to perforate tissues with the CO_2 laser beam if kept in one place long enough, but it is easy to avoid this hazard by pulsing the laser or moving the beam around. When used at lower power densities it will cause a thin film of coagulation. The lateral zone of damage may be confined to 0.5 mm or less, depending on how the energy is applied.

The argon and KTP lasers are, for all clinical purposes, equivalent in their tissue effects for laparoscopy. The differences have more to do with the features and benefits of the equipment than of the light, though there are some subtle differences between the two. They are of much lower power than the CO_2 or Nd:YAG lasers, delivering about 15–20 W maximum on medically available units, although a newer KTP unit produces up to 30 W. They may be used to cut or vaporize by placing the fibre tip in or very close to tissue, generating very high power densities.

The Ho:YAG laser is a truly pulsed, fibreoptically delivered laser which may be used under irrigation fluid. It produces average powers of up to about 22–30 W, though the surgeon actually selects the energy per pulse and repetition rate as the primary parameters. Its precise tissue effect closely approximates the CO_2 laser. If used at excessive pulse energies for laparoscopy it will produce a disconcerting 'popping' effect, and may 'splatter' tissue. The solution is to simply turn down the pulse energy.

The bare fibre Nd:YAG laser is absorbed over a depth of 4–6 mm in tissue. The effect is generally one of a delayed blanching or cooking of tissue. It may be used to vaporize at much higher powers, though the zone of coagulation necrosis will still be deep beyond the crater bottom. This bare fibre, non-contact approach is usually used for hysteroscopy. For laparoscopy it is ordinarily used with hot-tip devices such as sapphires or shaped fibres to prevent this deep coagulation effect and produce more intense cutting effects.

Sapphire tips

Sapphire probes (actually synthetic ceramics) have, within the last few years, significantly expanded the applications of Nd:YAG lasers in medicine by providing a high degree of control in cutting and vaporization of tissue. Sapphire probes do not transmit the laser energy like fibres. They must be held in contact with tissue and will quickly burn up if fired when not in tissue contact. Probes and tips come in a variety of physical geometries and sizes to produce various effects.

There has been much debate over whether the tissue effects created by a sapphire contact probe are from high power densities at the tip of the crystal, or simply from direct heat of the crystal itself. It is rather a moot point in that it is the observable tissue effect that matters — and these probes do cut and vaporize nicely — but there are many characteristics which indicate that the tissue effects are from the heating of the crystal itself and not the laser energy (cutting like a hot knife through butter). The laser light is used as the energy source physically to heat the crystal. Various terms are used to describe these sapphire probes such as crystals, tips, probes, contact probes and sapphires.

Sapphire tips have evolved for endoscopic use. Many tip shapes are possible (such as wedges, cone points and ballpoints), each dissecting or vaporizing tissue a little differently. Surgeons generally develop personal preferences for two or three shapes. One of the advantages of these tips over the sculpted fibres is that the sapphire tips have more thermal mass behind them. They are bulkier at their bases (not necessarily at their actual tips), and this acts as a kind of thermal 'flywheel' to store heat energy for sustained vaporization. This is not necessary in all situations, but the bloodier and thicker the tissue being dissected, the more sustained heat is required to cut, and the better these types of tips perform. Bulkier tips are used in thicker and bloodier tissues.

Special types of sculpted fibres reproduce the hot-tip cutting effects of the sapphire probes. These fibres are physically sharp and pointed at their tips or have rounded ball tips, unlike the flat cleaved end of a regular fibre. This altered tip destroys the optical transmission of the fibre and allows heat to build up at the tip. They function much like the sapphire probes and produce fine cutting effects with very little lateral damage, even though using the Nd:YAG wavelength. These fibres also seem to work very well to cut under fluid. When used in combination with the new pulsed Nd:YAG laser they produce very fine and quick cutting effects under fluid.

Practical electrosurgery

In electrosurgery, an understanding of basic electrical conduction, heating and vaporization of tissue allows these units to be used more safely in a wide variety of circumstances. The relative advantages of electrosurgery versus lasers have most recently come into question, particularly for laparoscopic use. Though it is true that electrosurgery is less expensive, easier to use and provides better haemostasis than lasers, it is not true that electrosurgery is an inherently 'safer' modality than lasers. The quintessential advantage of lasers lies in the very precise, predictable and controllable tissue effects. The question of whether this high degree of control is worth the added cost and encumbered use will vary from procedure to procedure and user to user.

Clarification of electrosurgical terminology

Learning the 'language' is the first step in developing a good understanding of a 'foreign' technology. The semantics involved with electrosurgery can become quite confusing, so it is useful to clarify several terms.

'Bovie' is not a generic term for electrosurgical units. It is frequently used this way but is actually the name of the originator of the electrosurgical unit. W.T. Bovie worked with a neurosurgeon by the name of Harvey Cushing to pioneer electrosurgery in the 1920s. Modern electrosurgical units (ESUs) are not the old, green 'Bovie' units and work in a technically different fashion.

'Electrocautery' or 'cautery' are not the correct terms for electrosurgical units, although they are commonly used. Cautery refers to a direct heating process, like a soldering iron, whereby the electricity does not flow through the tissue. Semm's endocoagulator is a type of cautery unit. The use of electrically created 'hot wire' cautery was first described in the 1890s. In the 1940s this 'hot wire' technique had a resurgence in cervical conizations. This should not be mistaken for current leep cervical excisions that use an ESU loop, which is not a hot wire.

Electrosurgical unit is the correct term for modern units that utilize either monopolar or bipolar electrosurgical elements. This involves an electrical current flow through tissue to generate the heating effects on tissue.

Monopolar or *unipolar* signify that the surgical instrument has only one contact surface or electrode. Instruments like graspers may still have two jaws but they are electrically the same surface or pole. Since electricity requires two electrodes in order to flow, the other electrode will be some type of ground pad (dispersive electrode) on the patient. Electricity will flow between the active electrode and the dispersive electrode. Heating and tissue damage can theoretically occur anywhere between the two electrodes. Monopolar is used for needle and hook electrode dissection in laparoscopy, loops and roller balls for hysteroscopy, fine wire loops for cervical excisions, and handheld scalpels (pens).

Bipolar signifies that both electrodes are contained within the surgical instrument itself, and the dispersive electrode is inactive or not used. This means that the flow of electricity is confined to the space between the two surfaces of the instrument. Tissue damage is theoretically confined to this direct space, but the current can 'mushroom' out peripherally around the instrument. Bipolar techniques have been used in the form of coagulating graspers which were unable to cut and dissect, though new bipolar cutting instruments used with their own specialized power supplies, are changing this.

Cutting current on an ESU does not refer to a setting designed to make a surgical incision or cut, but to one that accentuates the amperage, or current, aspects of the power setting with the lowest attendant voltages. Though the setting is most effective for cutting, deep desiccation of tissue is also best performed in this mode. The size of the electrodes and the way tissue is touched produce the difference in effects.

Coag current on an ESU does not refer to a setting which is required to obtain good haemostasis, but to one that accentuates the high voltage aspects of the power setting with the lowest attendant amperages or current. This creates the most fulgurative and 'burning' effect on the surface, but is not deep unless the electrode is firmly planted in tissue to eliminate the sparking. It is useful to obtain a haemostasis from a diffuse and oozing bed, such as a raw peritoneal surface. The attendant high voltages can create problems with unseen tissue damage, burns from trocar cannula, and 'zaps' through surgical gloves.

Desiccation of tissue refers to its being destroyed by drying and protein coagulation. Either the 'cut' or 'coag' modes will achieve good desiccation of tissue provided the electrode contact area is reasonably large and held in good firm contact with tissue, and that the probe is clean. Bipolar is safest for this, followed by the cutting mode on monopolar. The coag mode is the least safe and effective for gaining deep desiccation.

Fine point cautery or *microcautery* describe the use of very fine wire needle-like monopolar electrodes, frequently used in laparoscopy for haemostatic dissection. Microcautery for microsurgery uses different ESU power supplies.

Effects of electricity on biological tissue

The effect of electrosurgical instruments on tissue is due to heating in some form or another. Electrical principles are important to an understanding of how and where this heat may be created by the way it is delivered to an intended site, intensified and localized.

Electricity can have different effects on tissue, dependent primarily on the frequency of the current. Our direct experiences with electricity are generally in the 60 Hz range of household current. These 'shocks' produce muscle contraction and pain, and potentially can stop a heart. These are all termed faradic effects and are associated with the frequencies from about 60 Hz up to 200–300 KHz. Frequencies higher than this do not produce these types of effects: in fact at high frequencies — as long as the power density is not high — the electricity passes through the body with no effects at all. Faradic effects are caused by the depolarization of nerve and muscle tissue.

Sometimes faradic effects can be observed when using conventional ESUs, even though their frequencies are above this range. This is because the current can sometimes be 'rectified' by biological tissue to lower faradic frequencies. Rectification of AC electricity is a situation where the current is allowed to flow in one direction, but not the other. This lowers the frequency of the unit. Sparking from an electrode can also set up its own frequency lower than that of the ESU, again resulting in faradic effects. When faradic effects are observed the procedure should be stopped.

Electricity can also cause electrolysis in biological tissue, causing ions in solution to become polarized, or positive and negative ions to become separated. This polarization of ions within tissue can cause a chemical cauterization. These effects are minimal with electrosurgery because of the very high AC frequencies. Electrolysis would be more apparent with a direct current applied to tissue, and this does not apply to electrosurgery.

Heat generation

The actual surgical effects of electrosurgical cutting or coagulation are created by tissue heating, though an ESU electrode is not 'hot' in the way that a soldering iron is. The ESU causes a flow of electrons through the instruments and tissue, concentrated to small contact areas. This induces heat generation by creating molecular motion of the water molecules, rather like heating water in a microwave. Some of the cutting effects are caused by the intense heating which concentrated 'sparks' create within a thin steam envelope around the electrode. To use an ESU safely and effectively, it is best to localize the heat just where you want it and prevent it from forming or spreading elsewhere.

Lasers accomplish the same end but by a different mechanism. Lasers produce light as packets of energy, or photons. When photons shine on tissue they are absorbed by the tissue. This creates vibrational energy, which is heat. The localization of heat created in this fashion may be controlled to a much higher degree than the use of electricity, but at greater expense and complexity of instrumentation.

Heat is heat, whether induced by electricity, light or high-frequency vibration. Heating effects of electrosurgery are indicated by the following relationship:

$$Q = I^2 \times R \times T$$

where Q = quantity of heat, I = current intensity, R = resistance and T = time. A typical scenario might then be: 6 calories = $0.5A^2 \times 100$ohms $\times 1$ s.

One calorie is the amount of heat required to heat one cubic centimetre of water 1°C. If the current above is distributed over 1 cm^3 of tissue, there is a resulting rise in temperature of 6°C. If the same current is concentrated to 0.1 cm^3 of tissue, there is a 60°C rise in temperature (tissue temperature of over 100°C). The concentration of energy, as power density, is therefore very important and is exactly analogous to the spot size/power relationship with lasers. Power density with electrosurgery is controlled primarily by electrode size and how it is manipulated on tissue.

When used to incise tissue, the ESU is generating heat in the tissues which actually vaporizes cells, much the same way as the laser does. This is a sublimation process where the cells 'flash boil'.

The smoke-like steam rising from the incision is seen as the electrosurgical plume which has similar properties to a laser plume. Good smoke evacuation equipment should be used to remove the plume regardless of which instrument generates it. At the very least it is a respiratory irritant for the staff. At worst, there is some question about the viability of viruses carried away in this smoke plume. Good smoke evacuators have the ability to filter down to sub-viral sizes of around 0.1 μm.

Basic electrophysics

Electricity must have two poles in order to flow. In electrosurgical units, when these two poles are localized in one instrument or probe, it is referred to as a bipolar unit, since both poles are contained within the one instrument. When one of the poles is an instrument, and the other a remotely located ground pad (dispersive electrode), it is referred to as a monopolar, or unipolar instrument, since the instrument is only one of the two poles.

Direct and alternating current

Direct current is the most simple of circuits, such as contained in a flashlight using batteries. In an electrosurgical power supply where the switch is the foot or handswitch, the patient becomes the resistor (R) in the circuit, and the flow of electricity is the current (I, for induced current). Electricity must have the two poles to flow.

Alternating current takes the concept of positive and negative just one step further by quickly reversing the polarity, or order of positive and negative, back and forth. AC is the type of electricity we find in household electrical outlets. At home the AC circuit reverses about 60 times a second, or 60 Hz. This frequency of AC electricity can directly interfere with our own biological electrical frequencies and result in shocks or stopping of the heart. The ability of electricity to create this type of interference with our own bodies — muscle tetany and contraction, interference with normal heart rhythms, etc — is termed the faradic effect of electricity.

An actual monopolar ESU circuit shows the electrosurgical probe introducing the circuit which finds its way to the dispersive electrode and back to the power supply.

Electrosurgical units also utilize AC electricity but at significantly faster rates of reversal for the polarity. ESUs utilize frequencies of around 500 000 times per second; some go up to 3 or 4 MHz. This extremely high frequency does not interfere with our own biological processes to any significant degree, so faradic effects do not apply. These high frequencies are up in the range of AM radio station transmissions and beyond, and are referred to as RF, or radio frequency, current.

Choice of frequencies

The choice of frequencies for an ESU is more important in laparoscopy than office use. The patient is asleep in laparoscopy, and one is using electrodes in a more electrically complex area than involved with office leep procedures. Lower frequency units (350 000 to about 1 MHz) are inherently safer and more controllable for endoscopic surgery than are the higher frequency units that go to 3 and 4 MHz. Some of these higher-frequency units are relatively inexpensive and are fine for use in an office setting.

When one chooses parameters to operate an ESU, a choice of 'cut' or 'coag' is made, and the power setting selected. The first basic electrical relationship we have is that of power, or rate of energy delivery, expressed in watts:

$$\text{Power (watts)} = \text{voltage} \times \text{current (amps)}$$

From a practical standpoint you can apply this to your home electrical panel. For instance, a 1500 W hairdryer consumes about 14 A of electricity (1500 W divided by 110 V). A 1000 W microwave oven consumes about 9 A. If both are connected to a line with a 20 A circuit breaker, this means that your teenager cannot use a hairdryer while you are using the microwave oven; if they are on the same line the circuit breaker will 'pop' because it cannot cope with the 23 A.

One can see that voltage and current may be oppositely varied (balanced) and still deliver the same power output in watts. This is exactly the choice we make when choosing the 'cut' vs 'coag' modes on the ESU. 'Cut' accentuates the current aspects of the equation, and 'coag' that of the voltage. However, a mental association between these technical terms and the physiological terminology of cutting and coagulating creates the wrong impression of how each modality is best used.

Resistance

Before we examine more of the implications of 'cut' and 'coag' modes on an ESU, we need to look at one more fundamental electrical relationship which describes the three electrical parameters of voltage, current and resistance:

$$V = I \times R$$

This is a fundamental law of electricity called Ohm's law. The electrical units for measure of resistance are called ohms (Ω).

Remember that voltage and current are factors of the power you have selected on the ESU (watts = $V \times I$). Resistance is not controlled by the operator but is a function of the tissue. We will see that voltage 'drives' or pushes the current through tissue against the tendency for tissue to 'resist' this flow. As the flow is resisted, heat is generated in tissue.

Resistance varies in different tissues. It may vary from $100\,000\ \Omega$ for dry calloused palmar skin, to $2000\ \Omega$ for fat, and to $400\ \Omega$ for muscle. High-electrolyte tissues such as blood and muscle offer low resistance and easily transmit the electrical current. Skin and fat have higher resistance. More importantly, as electricity is applied to tissue and it begins to desiccate or char, the tissue resistance will begin to change immediately. A 40 W setting may remain constant, but the voltage and current are in constant flux as a function of this varying tissue resistance, and distance from electrode to tissue. Changing voltages will cause fluctuating levels of lateral damage from cut to cut, or even during the same excision. Some newer ESUs sense this changing resistance in tissue, and allow the power to adjust accordingly to allow for constant voltage application — providing more consistent margins of lateral damage.

Our understanding of the relevance of these electrical parameters of voltage, current and resistance is enhanced by the frequently used analogy of flowing water to the flow of electricity. Voltage is the driving pressure, or head, of the water and current refers to the actual flow of water in the pipe.

Voltage can be compared with the height of water in a water tower. The higher the tower, the better the pressure 'head' at the tap. Voltage drives the current though tissue in the same way that pressure drives water flow through the pipe. We have already mentioned that voltage is the parameter enhanced when choosing the 'coag' mode on an ESU.

The use of 'coag' with a monopolar instrument will allow for a higher driving force through all the tissues between the instrument and the dispersive electrode, and increases the probability of stray energy causing unintended damage to tissues somewhere outside the immediate target area. The higher driving force also allows sparks to jump farther in air. This is seen with the long sparking when fulgurating tissue in 'coag'. This high-voltage 'coag' is also the primary reason the current can 'jump' through a surgical glove and 'zap' the recipient. The hole you see in the glove was not there when the current first jumped — it was created by the heat of the spark. Electricity can jump right through insulators if given enough driving force of voltage*. This also applies to the insulation surrounding a monopolar instrument — particularly the disposable ones which have less insulation than reusables.

Resistance results from the diameter of the pipes in our analogy, and the outlet size of the tap. The greater the diameter, the less the resistance and the more the water will flow. One can increase water flow through the pipe by either increasing its diameter (lowering resistance) or increasing the height of the water tower (ie voltage or driving force).

Current is then the amount of water that flows in the pipes. With electricity, this is the actual number of electrons which are moved per unit time (amperes or amps). The 'cut' mode on an ESU accentuates the amperage aspects of the power setting. Its lower attendant voltages provide for better control over any stray energy, and cause less marginal damage on an incision.

Current density and electrode geometry

The intensity of power from a laser beam is described as power density. This applies equally to electricity and is sometimes referred to as current density, though the former is still more correct. The concept is the same: the amount of energy distributed over a certain contact area.

This remains the most important parameter controlling the quality of an electrosurgical cut and the level of haemostasis achieved. For instance, though the use of pure 'cut' with a fine wire electrode would probably provide inadequate haemostasis, using the same 'cut' setting with a broader spoon (spatula) electrode can provide good dissection and haemostasis together. This size of the electrode contact surface makes the difference.

Have you ever wondered why the electricity from an ESU will cause a cut at the active electrode, but does nothing at the dispersive electrode? It is not because of the direction of current flow — you could change the connections to the machine and still get the same effect. The difference is created because of the relative surface contact areas of the electrodes. The cutting electrode has a relatively small contact area. The electricity 'crowds' together at this point of contact, resulting in a high power density and intense thermal effect.

---

* The misconception of insulators totally blocking electricity is seen in the popular belief that rubber-soled shoes offer some protection from lightning, because you are insulated from the ground by the rubber soles. In truth, one would have to be wearing rubber soles more than one mile thick to gain any protection from the voltage levels in a bolt of lightning.

The dispersive electrode (ground pad) does just what the name implies: it collects the electricity over a wide surface contact area, allowing a 'dispersion' of the energy. This creates a very low power density and totally eliminates any induced heating of tissue. The current is harmlessly dispersed over this electrode. If this pad were to pull away from the patient, however, the surface contact area would get smaller and smaller, causing a bottleneck in the flow of electricity, increasing the power density, and resulting in a burn. Some units incorporate fail-safe devices — eg return electrode monitors (REMs) — to sense this.

Choice of electrode size

The choice of electrode size, and how one applies it to tissue, affects the cutting and haemostatic effect as much or more so than the choice of 'cut' and 'coag' modes.

The correct technique is to activate the electrode just before touching tissue. The small contact area of the initial point of contact allows clean cutting with a high power density. This activation just before touching actually applies to most situations where clean cutting is desired.

When using the ESU laparoscopically, power densities are varied by using different sizes and configurations of electrodes. A hook electrode, besides having a convenient geometry to handle tissue, has a moderate electrode size to allow haemostatic dissection. A finer needle point electrode will allow finer and cleaner incisions, but at some expense to haemostasis. Ball electrodes will be good for electrodesiccation and fulguration of oozing tissue beds. A spoon electrode, when brushed against tissue with its narrow side, will allow clean dissection. By angling the spoon slightly so that more and more surface area is used, various degrees of haemostasis may be achieved while leaving the ESU in a 'cut' setting.

The reason for this discussion of power density, electrode configuration and haemostasis, is that selecting and manipulating use of the electrode is the first step, and a far better way of obtaining desired haemostasis than using the ESU in the 'coag' or high blend modes.

High power densities can be a very real cause of pedicle type injuries which are unintentional and frequently unobserved. When tissue is grasped then put on a 'stretch', a small trunked pedicle may be created. Current applied to tissue at its end, sufficient to cause coagulation, may see an increase in power density where the electricity tries to 'dive' through the small pedicle trunk, resulting in an inadvertent burn.

Protecting intra-abdominal organs

Lowering power density may also be exploited as a technique to protect intra-abdominal organs from accidental injuries. The use of monopolar ESU is ineffective if you try to activate the electrode under a conductive solution such as saline. It is not particularly harmful: the conductive solution simply dissipates the energy so that it is ineffective. The same characteristic, however, may be used to provide electrical protection to all organs under the fluid — as long as the electrode is working out of the fluid. In laparoscopic surgery, if the target tissue may be lifted high anteriorly, then the cul-de-sac and posterior abdomen may be flooded under warmed saline. Organs which are entirely immersed in this pool of fluid would be totally protected from inadvertent electrical injury. The extremely large contact surface of all organs tied electrically together by the conductive saline will harmlessly disperse any current. (Non-conductive solutions such as sterile water or glycine will offer no protection.) This technique may also be applied during hysteroscopy when using monopolar ESU (roller ball or resectoscope) if there is any reason for concern about electrical injury to abdominal contents such as bowel in contact with the serosal surface of the uterus. Flooding the abdomen with the conductive solution, then ensuring that the patient is positioned so that the base of the pool envelopes the uterus, offers protection from stray current. The non-conductive solution is then used within the uterine cavity itself so that the electrode is effective here. Be advised, however, that physically penetrating the uterine wall too deeply with the electrode can still create bowel injury by bringing the electrode into close direct contact with the structure.

Cutting, fulguration and desiccation

So far we have learned the basics of an electrical circuit, examined parameters of voltage, current and resistance and seen how these are affected by choice of cut or coag modes, and discussed the relationship of electrode configurations to power density. Having examined the technical parameters of the ESU and the electricity itself, we should now look at electrosurgery from the point of view of the surgical effects.

The terms 'cut' and 'coag' have meaning only in terms in of voltage and current parameters. They should not be selected simply because one wants to cause an incision or achieve haemostasis. The surgical effect is achieved through a combination of the mode and power selected, the size and geometry of the electrode, and the technique by which the electrode is applied. A more detailed look at these surgical effects will allow us to use an ESU more effectively and safely.

Appendix A describes in more detail the AC waveforms of 'cut' and 'coag' modes. We previously oversimplified in order to describe the 'cut' mode as the one which accentuated the current aspects of the AC, and the 'coag' mode as accentuating the higher voltages. Appendix A explains in more detail how this is really related to a comparison of average and peak voltages called the 'crest factor' — even though actual peak voltages may vary between 'cut', 'coag' and bipolar modes. For our purposes, we simply want to look at the 'cut' mode as an uninterrupted emission of the AC sinusoidal waveform. It is emitted in an undampened fashion and is frequently called an undampened waveform. 'Coag', on the other hand, provides for interrupted bursts of the same AC waveform, and is frequently called a dampened waveform.

Bipolar vs monopolar

Cutting has traditionally been possible only with monopolar ESU. This is changing and several companies have developed cutting bipolar instruments. The physical mechanism of the cut is the same whether using bi- or monopolar, but techniques of use will vary. Theoretically a cut with bipolar instruments should be no different than a cut with monopolar ones, but in practice there is some difference in the feel and efficacy of the different instruments. Bipolar is most definitely a safer modality to use during laparoscopy, but that is not to say informed application of the monopolar mode is unsafe. The rest of the discussion on cutting and fulguration is applied primarily to monopolar ESU.

'Cut'

With an undampened waveform ('cut' mode), it makes sense that the water molecules will be most highly vibrated and generate more intense heat. The pure cutting mode, coupled with high power density from a small electrode, always gives the most controlled and precise tissue effects, but at the price of limited or non-existent haemostasis if the electrode geometry is not manipulated.

'Cut' works best when the electrode is lightly floating just above the tissue, but not making firm contact with it. A very narrow steam envelope is created in the small gap between tissue and electrode which allows intense, short sparking to tissue. If the envelope is lost by forcing the electrode into tissue, the cutting has changed to desiccation.

Combined with the undampened delivery of current, the small pinpoint tips of the sparks concentrate the current to even higher power densities and intensify the explosive vaporization effect. It is intense and unrelenting enough that the tissue is not given any chance to desiccate or char before more current continues driving through it. The steam plume further dissipates heat which would otherwise accumulate at the incision. The result is a very clean and narrow margin vaporization of tissue with very little lateral heat damage — translating into poor haemostasis.

Electrode size

The power should be set at a level just sufficient to obtain a smooth, clean cut. Unlike vaporization by laser, which is made more precise by short applications of very high power, use of excessive powers in electrosurgery is unnecessary and can bring the risk of injury from stray energy. If the electrode stalls and 'waddles' through tissue without being forced, try turning the power up until a clean incision results. With a fine wire, like a needle electrode, 20–30 W is frequently sufficient to obtain a good cut. With slightly larger electrodes, power settings of 45–75 W may be needed. Loop electrode excision varies considerably with the size and thickness of the electrode, and the site where it is used.

The very clean but bloody incision of 'cut' works only when the steam envelope is maintained, and a high power density electrode is utilized. The finer the edge or point on the electrode, the cleaner the incision and lower the power required to obtain it.

If the electrode is rushed through tissue rather than 'floating' it at its own rate, then the tissue will bunch up as it makes contact with the electrode and a 'stall' occurs. At this point the electrode should be removed from tissue and deactivated, and the incision restarted, preferably beginning just off tissue and using light stroking motions.

Altering the size of electrode and way it touches tissue is the first step in enhancing haemostasis when using the pure cut mode. Pure cut can often be used successfully throughout a laparoscopic procedure by using a spoon or similar electrode, and manipulating the edges which are allowed to stroke tissue. This approach of manipulating electrode use should be tried before resorting to blends or 'coag' settings on the ESU.

Traction

A key point in proper technique of electrosurgical cutting is the maintenance of good traction on tissue being incised. Tissue on stretch presents a smaller contact point to an electrode which increases power density. Tissue on stretch will be immediately removed from contact with the electrode when cut, allowing power density to be concentrated in the next segment of tissue. Good traction is an essential requirement of proper cutting with either laser or electrosurgery.

A large contact area electrode may be used in firm contact with tissue using the 'cut' mode, and the surgical effect will change entirely to that of deep desiccation discussed in a following section.

'Coag'

Voltage determines how far a spark can jump a gap. The 'coag' mode allows for longer sparking than the 'cut' mode. The damage is very superficial unless the electrode is held in contact with tissue so that no sparking occurs. This creates deeper damage.

Voltage determines the margins of damage surrounding an incision. Wider margins of thermal damage produce less precise incisions, but allow for better haemostasis. Use of cutting loop electrodes are frequently used in a blend setting to obtain this haemostasis.

The dampened aspect of the 'coag' waveform means that the RF current is applied for only about 6–10% of the actual time that the unit is on (though this varies among companies). This 'rest' time of motion of the tissue's water molecules, and the fact that heating can occur with no explosive vaporization of tissue to carry away this heat in the steam, allow a progressive thermal insult to build in tissue. Tissue desiccates and gradually builds up char on the surface. Tissue resistance continues to build until the current eventually stops entirely. Charring of the electrode surface will also stop the electrical flow.

Appropriate and inappropriate applications of 'coag'

In the author's experience, the 'coag' modality on ESUs is highly overused, and frequently for the wrong reasons. The best and most apparent use of 'coag' is to dry a diffuse, oozing bed (such as a raw peritoneal side wall) by fulguration. This involves holding the electrode just off tissue, allowing it to 'sparkle' over the surface. It is also sometimes used to 'spray' a surface lightly for a shallow burning effect. Some companies refer to this as 'spray' coagulation. This technique is also used with a ball electrode to 'spray' the raw surface left in the base of a cervical loop excision.

Inappropriate or unnecessary uses include stopping a bleeder by touching an electrode to the clamp, or achieving deep protein coagulation in structures such as fallopian tubes or infundibular pelvic ligaments. These are desiccation techniques where the pure 'cut' or undamped waveform should be used, as explained below.

Argon beam coagulator (ABC)

Though conventional spray coagulation will not result in very deep damage, it is rather destructive to the surface of the target. When fulgurating like this, the sparks carry quite a punch and the spray pattern can be rather erratic within the sparking area. Air, or in the case of laparoscopy the pneumoperitoneum, offers a fair amount of resistance which must be overcome before the spark can jump. This also limits the distances which the spark can jump and the uniformity of effect.

The argon beam coagulator is a conventional monopolar ESU used in the 'coag' mode for fulguration. The difference is that the probe delivers a purging flow of the inert argon gas while the unit is activated. Argon gas offers very low electrical resistance to the sparking and this alters the nature of the fulgurative sparking. Lower 'coag' powers may be used to generate the sparks. The sparking is more homogeneous and uniform, and produces a gentler effect on tissue. The gas flow has the added effect of blowing blood away from the surface as the fulguration coagulates the surface. Since the gas will penetrate irregular surfaces, the fulguration is more uniform even on an irregular surface. Some advocate its use even in bone for this reason. The sparks can seek out nooks and crannies.

The argon beam coagulator is not associated in any way with an argon laser, even though the word 'beam' is used. The laser uses argon gas internally in the tube to generate the blue/green laser beam, usually delivered laparoscopically by a fibre. The ABC actually blows the argon gas into the pathway of the fulguration inside the patient's abdomen.

Since the constant flow of the argon gas is an additional gas source during pneumoperitoneum, the abdominal pressure must be closely monitored to prevent overpressure.

Desiccation

Unlike techniques of cutting or fulguration, desiccation involves no sparking to tissue of any sort. The electrode, which must be clean, is held in firm contact with tissue and water is driven from tissue as it progressively heats from resistance to the electrical current.

Desiccation may be applied to a vessel to stop bleeding, or to a larger structure like a fallopian tube to cause deeper protein coagulation and tissue destruction. The 'cut' modality on an ESU is the safest and most effective way of obtaining desiccation. Bipolar is safest when this is possible.

Tubal sterilizations are now most frequently performed with bipolar rather than monopolar ESU. These principles of using 'cut' vs 'coag' apply equally to bipolar, but are more pronounced with monopolar because of the higher attendant voltages.

Either 'cut' or 'coag' could achieve deep tissue necrosis, but cut is definitely safer and frequently more effective.

Using the 'coag' mode involves higher voltages and interrupted current delivery (dampened current). When using monopolar these higher voltages are present throughout the entire circuit, therefore there is an increased risk of getting 'zapped' through your gloves. The chance of stray current causing unintended injury through downstream sparking or high current density burns increases. The chance of insulation breakdown and inadvertent burns increases in laparoscopic instruments; nor are these small theoretical increases in risk. They are clear and substantial safety problems.

Capacitance

Capacitance involves transferring electrical energy through intact insulating materials to nearby conductive instruments, such as laparoscopic suction irrigator probes, some trocar sleeves, or operating laparoscopes. This induced energy can then burn tissues which touch it, even though the instrument is not touching any live electrodes.

The flow of electricity down a conductor (your active electrode) produces a magnetic field around the device. The high voltages of 'coag' produce the strongest fields. Insulators like plastic are of course transparent to magnetic fields, so the magnetism will go through the insulator and set up the reverse process in closely situated metal instruments: ie the magnetic field will induce an electrical current in the nearby instrument even though it is not touching the conductor. Higher frequencies present more potential for capacitance. Some of the inexpensive 3 + MHz ESUs used for office work, although fine for those purposes, would present a significantly higher chance of capacitance than surgical ESUs operating in the 350–550 KHz range.

This happens all the time, but presents no problem when all-metal instruments are used. If an all-metal trocar sleeve is in contact with the abdominal wall, any induced current created in the sleeve (or any metal instrument in it such as the suction irrigator) will be harmlessly bled into the abdominal wall and back to the dispersive electrode. The surface contact area of the sleeve with the abdominal wall keeps the power density low enough for the electricity to be harmless here and cause no burns.

Problems with capacitance begin when using all-plastic or plastic/metal trocar sleeves. In a plastic/metal sleeve, the plastic is in contact with the abdominal wall and provides no means for conduction of electricity back to the dispersive electrode. The metal tip of this plastic sleeve is in electrical isolation. Any current that is induced here has no way to be harmlessly bled off. Instead a charge builds on the metal tip and when it lightly touches some internal organ (small contact area and high power density) it will discharge at this point, potentially causing a burn.

All-plastic sleeves are not a problem — until you put a metal instrument down them, and then put the electrode down a channel of this now isolated metal instrument. This would apply to a suction/irrigator, or even an operating laparoscope. The electrical current is induced by capacitance in the instrument the same way, and the all-plastic sleeve prevents it from being harmlessly bled off. A touch to internal tissues by the isolated instrument (suction/irrigator — operative laparoscope) allows the discharge to occur.

This is enough of a problem that one company has developed a 'shield', which slips over the electrode to protect from capacitance or insulation breakdown. The shield requires its own control unit and wiring to tie into the ESU, but eliminates many of the hazards with monopolar electrosurgery.

Deep protein coagulation

These are all some of the problems potentially created by using the 'coag' mode to achieve desiccation. The effectiveness of using straight 'coag' in order to achieve deep protein coagulation is also compromised. Two problems can occur.

The best way to use 'coag' to achieve deep coagulation would be to hold the tissue firmly with graspers as the current is applied. Stop the current when thoroughly desiccated and move the graspers to the next site before applying the current again. This should maintain good contact with tissue and eliminate sparking. Sparking (fulguration) will create a shallow zone of charred and desiccated tissue on the surface which would actually electrically insulate deeper structures from further damage. It is similar to cooking a steak on a very hot grill: the surface would be seared and sealed, but the inside would be raw.

The first problem occurs because the graspers are usually not applied in this manner if using 'coag' for deep coagulation. They are usually lightly run up and down the structure, causing significant sparking, or tissue is repeatedly regrasped without deactivating the electrode — again causing much sparking. This builds up the insulating barrier of desiccated surface tissue and decreases the chances of deep coagulation.

The second problem occurs even if good contact with tissue is maintained. Remember that the higher voltages will cause more tissue damage at the interface. Desiccation begins and deep coagulation proceeds as the electrode is held in firm contact. At some point the damage at the tissue/electrode interface will be enough to either stop electrical flow by char formation, or by steam vaporization at the interface. This terminal point in desiccation will occur more quickly with 'coag' settings than with 'cut', and prematurely limit the coagulation.

The best and safest way to obtain protein haemostasis, whether for clamping and 'buzzing' a bleeder, or performing tubal sterilization, is to grasp the tissue firmly with a large contact area electrode and use a straight 'cut' mode.

Bipolar ESU and electrodes

When using bipolar electrodes, the two poles are both in contact with the target tissue right at the active site. No remote dispersive electrode is needed. Less electrical energy is therefore needed to achieve the same effects since the current does not need to pass through the entire body to get back to the other electrode. Attendant voltages and currents are lower with bipolar than monopolar instrumentation. This, and the fact that the current stays roughly between the two active electrodes, makes it a much safer modality to use.

Capacitance is not a problem with bipolar instrumentation. Since both electrodes are contained in the same instrument their magnetic fields will cancel each other out. Electrical current will not be induced in other instruments, even if they are isolated.

The use of bipolar instruments in laparoscopy has traditionally been very limited and specific. It was used with flat-bladed graspers to achieve localized coagulation. It has been excellent for control of bleeders and for tubal sterilizations, but could not cut or dissect tissue. New instruments, however, are changing this.

New instrumentation allows for bipolar cutting and dissection with bipolar scissors, hook electrodes and the standby coagulation graspers. The power supplies on these cutting instruments are somewhat different from their old counterparts which were designed only for coagulation. This instrumentation should substantially increase the safety of laparoscopic ESU procedures.

When using bipolar for coagulation, hold the conductive portion of the forceps exactly where the coagulation should occur. If tissue is held too high up in the forceps, insulation will prevent any electrical contact from occurring. The forceps must be clean to achieve good electrical contact.

Remember that the tissue to be coagulated must be in between the two jaws of the forceps in order to make the tissue an integral part of the electrical circuit. Often the jaws of the forceps will be squeezed shut so tightly that the tips of the forceps actually meet. This causes a short-circuit to occur and allows electricity to flow directly from one jaw to another, entirely bypassing the tissue. This reduces or eliminates the desired effect, and may make the forceps look as though they are not working. The solution is to grasp the tissue lightly but firmly and avoid complete closure of the jaws.

Another characteristic of bipolar to be considered is its potential to create a 'mushrooming' coagulation effect around and outside the actual space between the jaws of the instrument. This is created because of the magnetic field-like nature of electrical conduction. It travels in curving lines between electrodes when not confined by a wire or other conductor. This means that a delicate structure, such as a ureter, is not immune from injury simply because it is not directly in the jaws of the instrument. The spread is not large, but it can go several millimetres around the tip of the device. This is usually seen as the tissue blanches white with coagulation.

In spite of this mushrooming, bipolar instruments offer much more control over the electrical current than does monopolar. For the most precise control, predictability and uniformity of thermal effect, one would make the transition to various laser modalities. Like anything else however, it is not just the selection of the instrument which increases the control and precision, but the knowledgeable use of the device.

Good surgeons perform good surgery with whatever tools they choose to use. The best surgeons make the effort to become very knowledgeable about the attributes of every technical tool from which they can choose.

5

Enhanced Precision and Tissue Selectivity in Laparoscopic Microsurgical Procedures

MICHAEL SLATKINE

Introduction

Surgical instruments which enable extremely precise incisions, with minimal thermal damage to surrounding tissue and good haemostasis, are a prerequisite for the longterm success of most laparoscopic surgical procedures. Typical examples of such procedures are linear salpingostomy, fimbrioplasty and adhesiolysis. Some other frequently encountered procedures require highly controlled charfree ablation of tissue, layer-by-layer. Char-free ablation provides visualization of the treated lesion, minimal thermal damage and postoperative adhesion-free healing. Major procedures which benefit from char-free ablation capability are the treatments of endometriosis and various ovarian cysts of endometrial origin. Finally, selective fragmentation and aspiration of tissue may be extremely useful for the inherent safety of many common laparoscopic procedures. For example, a surgical tool which selectively fragments water or fatty-rich tissue and spares elastic collagen and fibrin-rich tissue is useful in disection to expose clearly and later excise selected nerves as in presacral neurectomy or lymphodenectomy.

In this chapter we present an overview of three major laparoscopic surgical instruments which provide respectively: (1) precise and highly controlled haemostatic incisions; (2) layer-by-layer char-free ablation of tissue, and (3) selective fragmentation and skeletizing of tissue. Operating principles and clinical results will be discussed.

Sculptured fibres for high-precision contact surgery

A highly flexible surgical tool that performs comparable to a precise monopolar electrosurgical unit without its potential risks has long been the desire of gynaecologists and other surgeons. The recent flourishing of laparoscopic minimal access procedures has made the development of such a tool almost mandatory due to possible risks of fatal bowel perforation with electrosurgery. Shaped conical fibres provide an excellent cutting tool for minimal access surgery (MAS) without the above-mentioned possible risks of electrosurgery (Figure 5.1). Incisions are achieved with good haemostasis. The thermally affected zone is as small as 0.5 mm. Moreover, the fibres act only upon actual contact, thereby eliminating the possibility of damage to adjacent or forward tissue. Ease of use is comparable to or better than in the monopolar mode. Simultaneous cutting and irrigation are possible. Here we briefly present the operating principles of the conical shapers fibres and elucidate the origin of their inherent safety. We also describe a hemispherical contact fibre for incisions and surface ablation and a dual-effect fibre for contact incisions and non-contact coagulation.

Operating principles of contact conical Nd:YAG laser fibres

The operating principles of conical sculptured fibres are presented in Figures 5.2 and 5.3. Nd:YAG laser energy is focused on a 3 m long silica optical fibre of numerical aperture 0.4. The angle of incidence of internally reflected rays gradually increases along the 10° tapered end of the fibre until it exceeds the total internal reflection critical angle. An optical leakage emitting zone is thus created. Further scattering is obtained by frosting the conical tip. Contact of the leaking zone with tissue causes this zone to become hot and therefore active. At 15–40 W, Nd:YAG laser power levels, the sharp conical leaking zone reaches tissue ablation temperature, thus enabling dissection with a tissue-affected zone of less than 0.5 mm (Figure 5.4). Cutting speed can be increased by increasing the laser power level. Fast incisions in a liquid environment can be achieved at power levels up to 60 W. For lysis of adhesions in minimally invasive laparoscopic surgical procedures, power levels as low as 15 W may be used.

A remarkable feature of conical fibres (as well as hemispherical) is the very large angular divergence (80°) of the optical radiation emitted from the distal sharp end of the fibres. This provides clinical safety, since adjacent tissue will essentially not be affected immediately after lysis of adhesions although laser emission may be continued for a short time[1]. Figure 5.5 elucidates the origin of this fibre safety. A simple calculation shows that the temperature of subjacent tissue located at a distance greater than 3 mm from the fibre will not reach more than 30 °C rise at 40 W of power and 1 s irradiation time on a single tissue location. Practical incision conditions are far below these, thus ensuring no thermally irreversible denaturation of tissue. As shown in Figure 5.6, the conical fibre is suitable for coagulation by contact with bleeding tissue along the tapered end of the fibre.

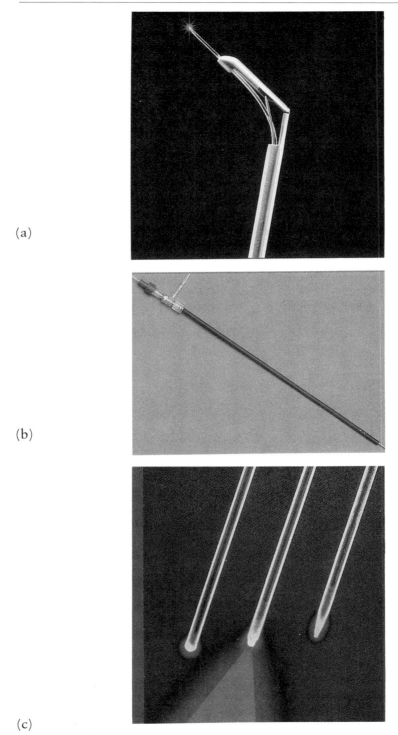

(a)

(b)

(c)

Figure 5.1: A sculpted fibre (a) can be used through a variety of laparoscopic channels (b). The fibre can be sculpted in three different shapes: hemispherical, flat and conical (c).

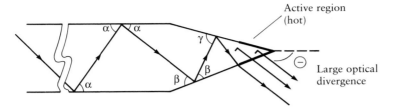

Figure 5.2: Optics of a conical sculpted fibre. (The fibre is frosted for additional scattering.)

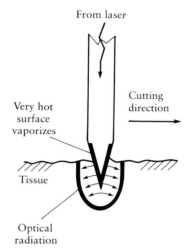

Figure 5.3: Origin of high incision efficiency of a conical sculpted fibre.

Additional sculptured fibres

Two additional contact fibres are frequently used in surgical procedures. The first is a hemispherical fibre (800 and 1000 μm), for coagulation and ablation (Figure 5.7). The second is a 'dual-effect' flat fibre which cuts and coagulates. This fibre (400 μm, 600 μm) is suitable for incisions of thin adhesions. Its forward radiation pattern enables coagulation of excessive bleeding in case of emergency. This fibre is very effective in myomectomy as well as laparoscopic cholecystectomy. For other laparoscopic procedures where subjacent tissues are critical, the hemispherical and conical fibres are recommended.

Instrumentation and applications

The contact fibres may be inserted in a variety of surgical probes. The most frequently used probes are the irrigator/aspirator for all laparoscopic procedures and a fibre deflector.

The contact fibre has been used in thousands of laparoscopic procedures with excellent results and without any complications. Recently, it has found interesting use in mini-laparoscopy where instrumentation with very small diameters are being used without the need of total anaesthesia[2]. Finally, non-contact fibres are extensively used in hysteroscopy for endometrial ablation. Deep uniform (6 mm) coagulation is achieved with no evident regeneration.

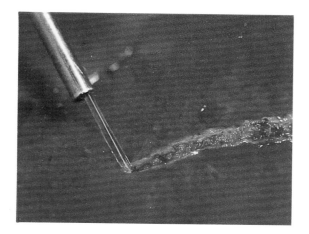

(a)

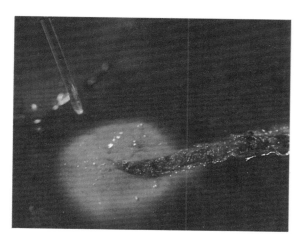

(b)

Figure 5.4: (a) Tissue incision with a sculpted fibre (power level 15 W). (b) Tissue coagulation with a dual-effect fibre in the non-contact mode (power level 40 W).

Long term follow-up show definitely better results than achieved with electrosurgical units, whether resectoscope or the roller ball[3].

Table 5.1 compares sculpted fibres and electrosurgical units used in laparoscopic MAS procedures. The comparison clearly indicates advantages of Nd:YAG fibres over electrosurgery. Shaped fibres will eventually play a key role in the success of the MAS revolution.

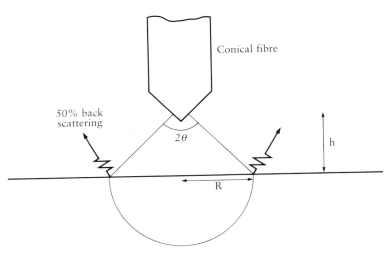

Figure 5.5: Temperature rise of tissue for non-contact irradiation is a source of safety. Assume an irreversible thermal effect for $\Delta T > 65°C - 37°C$, extinction coefficient ≈ 0.6 cm^{-1}, power input of 40 W (two times higher than in normal procedure), and 1 s irradiation (longer than normal). Calculations show lack of thermal effect for $2\theta \geqslant 50°$ at h $\geqslant 4$ mm. Since conical fibres are produced with $2\theta \geqslant 80°$, thermal effect on tissue is achieved at a distance less than ≈ 3 mm from tissue.

	Laser Surgery	Electrosurgery
Tissue effect	Assessable	Often unassessable
Safety	Typical problems	Typical problems
Miniaturization	No problem	Limited
Flexibility	High	Low
Education	Necessary	Necessary
Handling	Fair	Easy
Price	Currently high	Low

Table 5.1: Comparison between major benefits of laser surgery and electrosurgery.

Layer-by-layer char-free ablation of tissue

Layer by layer char-free ablation of tissue can be achieved with 10.6 micron CO_2 lasers operated in a high energy, short time duration pulsed, mode commercially known as the Sharpulse or the Ultrapulse, depending on the manufacturer. The Sharpulse is an ideal char-free ablator with good haemostasis both at low and high (70 Watts) power levels. In this paragraph, however, we shall describe an alternative technique to achieve

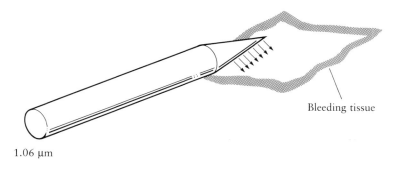

1.06 μm

Figure 5.6: Tissue coagulation with a conical fibre.

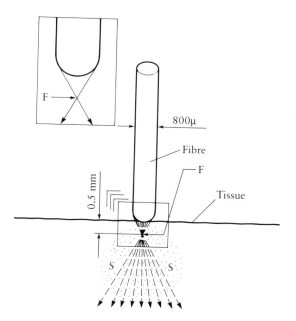

Figure 5.7: Operating principles of a hemispherical fibre. F is the point where the power density is maximal, and around which there is divergence of the radiation. S shows where radiation is scattered into the tissue.

char-free ablation even with a continuous wave CO_2 laser. The technique is based on a novel miniature fast scanner, the SwiftLase.

The SwiftLase flashscan is a unique new CO_2 laser modality which enables surgeons to obtain precise, char-free ablation of tissue, layer-by-layer, easily and safely. The concept behind it is simple: a focused laser beam of high-power density is scanned and delivered to the treatment site so rapidly that the tissue is vaporized before any thermal damage or carbonization can occur. As this process depends upon power density rather than actual power, any CO_2 laser, even at low power levels, can use it (Figure 5.8). It can also be used with

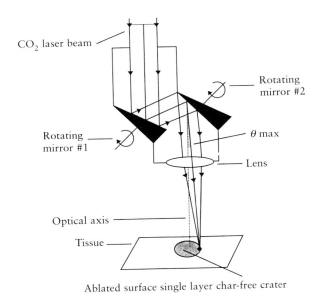

CO$_2$ laser beam

Rotating
mirror #2

Rotating
mirror #1

θ max

Lens

Optical axis

Tissue

Ablated surface single layer char-free crater

Figure 5.8: Operating principle of the SwiftLase for obtaining single-layer char-free ablation with any CO$_2$ laser.

any conventional operating laparoscope. Diseased tissue can be ablated very carefully, layer-by-layer, without any char or thermal damage to adjacent tissue. Histologies have indicated that thermal necrosis depth is smaller than 0.2 mm[4]. This is especially advantageous when working in delicate areas. Furthermore, as the SwiftLase technique creates no obstructive char, visualization of the treatment area is clear throughout the entire lasing process (Figure 5.9).

Applications in laparoscopy

The major application in laparoscopy is for the atraumatic vaporization of endometrial implants and endometriotic cysts[5]. Using SwiftLase, the surgeon can precisely vaporize endometrial implants and endometriotic cysts with a bloodless and char-free operating field. It also allows surgeons to work safely in very delicate areas such as the tubo-ovarian functional unit, the urethra and the bowel serosa.

The recommended laser power level for the effective use of the SwiftLase in

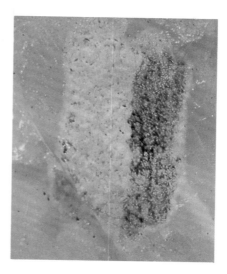

Figure 5.9: Single-layer char-free ablation with the SwiftLase scanner at 10 W power level. Left: With the SwiftLase. Right: Without the SwiftLase.

laparoscopy is 30–40 W. This is the same power level used in colposcopy for the treatment of vulvar lesions, where single layer char-free ablation is extremely significant[6].

Quantitative analysis of char-free ablation in laparoscopy

As already mentioned, the SwiftLase is a miniature opto-mechanical scanner compatible with any CO_2 laser. It consists of two almost parallel folding mirrors. Optical reflections of the CO_2 laser optical beam from the mirrors cause the beam to deviate from its original direction by an angle θ (Figure 5.8). The mirrors constantly rotate at a slightly different angular velocity, thereby rapidly varying with time between zero and a maximal value θ_{max}. By attaching the laparoscope focusing coupler of focal length F to the SwiftLase, the CO_2 laser generates a focal spot which rapidly and homogeneously scans and covers a round area of diameter $2F \tan\theta_{max}$ at the distal end of the laparoscope. For a single puncture laparoscope F = 300 mm, θ_{max} was selected to provide a round treatment area of 2.5 mm diameter. The rapid movement of the beam over the tissue ensures a short duration of exposure on individual sites within the area and very shallow ablation.

Since therapeutic CO_2 medical lasers typically generate a focused beam smaller than 0.9 mm diameter at the laparoscope working distance, using the SwiftLase with a laser power level of 30 W will generate an optical power density of about 50 W mm^2 on tissue. This is considerably higher than the threshold for vaporization of tissue without residual carbon char (the threshold for char-free tissue ablation is about 30 W mm^2)[8]. The time required for the SwiftLase homogeneously to cover a 2.5 mm round area is about 100 ms. During this time, the 30 W operating laser will deliver 3000 mjoules to the tissue. Since the typical energy required to completely ablate tissue is about 3000 mjoules mm^{-2}, keeping the laparoscope precisely on a single site for 0.1 s will generate a clean char-free crater of 0.2 mm depth.

However, the laparoscope can be smoothly and evenly moved across an extended lesion intended for treatment, consequently ablating a tissue layer as thin as 0.05–0.1 mm. Histologies of tissues irradiated with a SwiftLase show a thermal necrosis depth of 0.15 mm (Figure 5.10)[4].

Selective fragmentation of tissue with an ultrasonic aspirator

The selective mechanical fragmentation of tissue with ultrasonic aspirators has been used extensively in the debulking of brain tumours in the proximity of blood vessels and nerves since its introduction in the early 1980s.

Ultrasonic aspiration has been used successfully in open laparotomy since the late 1980s[9,10]. The recent availability of ultrasonic aspirator laparoscopic handpieces has paved the way for a wide range of new possibilities in MAS, where proximity to critical structures such as bowels, blood vessels, nerves and ureters have so far limited safety. Although relatively limited clinical experience has been accumulated so far with ultrasonic aspirators in laparoscopy, we believe that this new modality will help the surgeon to expose delicate organs by aspirating adipose tissue and adventitia and consequently increasing safety[7].

Operating principles

An ultrasonic aspirator consists of a hollow metal (titanium) vibrating tip, an irrigation channel around the tip and aspiration through the tip (Figure 5.11). Modern ultrasonic aspirators use piezoelectric crystals to vibrate the tip. An alternating frequency exciting voltage is applied to the crystal; consequently the crystal vibrates at the same frequency. A tapered titanium hollow tube amplifies the piezoelectric transducer vibrations to a typically 200–300 µm amplitude. The length of the operating tip is selected to mechanically respond at the excitation operating frequency (Figure 5.12).

The selectivity of the tissue response to the ultrasonic aspirator tip vibrations is based on the cavitation effect in water: positive excursion of the tip in non-compressible water which is part of most nonelastic tissues, followed by a sudden negative pressure formation during the negative excursion of the tip, causes micro-bubbles in the tissue to explode intensively and collapse at ultrasonic speed. These abrupt explosions and collapses produce extremely high pressures which are responsible for the fragmentation of water-rich tissue such as most tumours, liver and kidneys.

On the other hand, collagen and other elastic protein fibres yield to the ultrasonic aspirator vibrations and start to vibrate. Consequently tissues rich with collagen, such as blood vessels, nerves and bowels, are not fragmented and remain intact.

Figures 5.13 and 5.14 show an ultrasonic aspirator unit and a laparoscopic

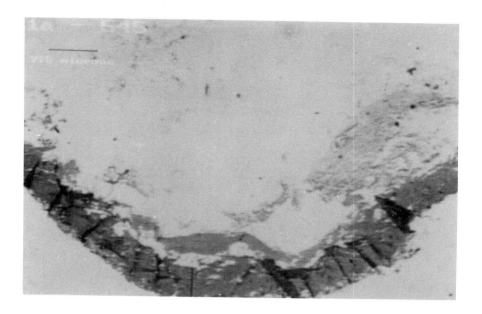

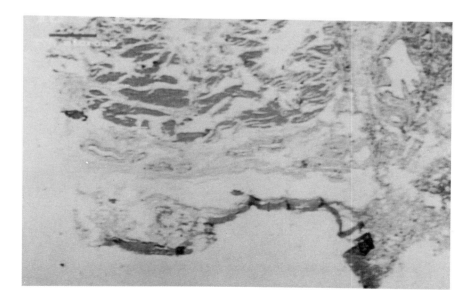

Figure 5.10: (a) (Top) Histology of a laser-irradiated skin of a New Zealand white rabbit. Necrosis as the result from irradiation by a 3 mm defocused C.W. CO_2 laser beam at 15 W is 545 microns deep. (b) Tissue irradiate with the SwiftLase under same conditions. Thermal necrosis depth is 152 microns.

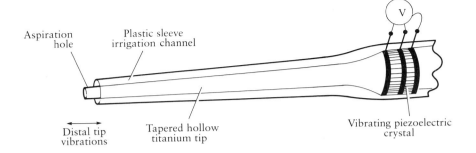

Figure 5.11: General schematics of an ultrasonic aspirator tip.

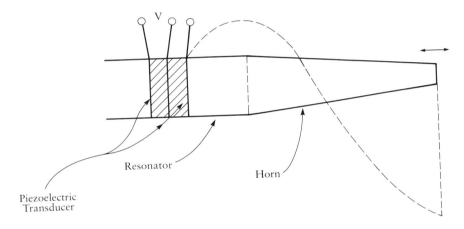

Figure 5.12: Acoustic excitation of an ultrasonic aspirator tip.

handpiece. Table 5.2 presents the specifications of a typical ultrasonic aspirator.

Tip material	Titanium
Tip length	275 mm
Tip diameter	3 mm
Operating frequency	23 KHz
Maximal vibration amplitude	250 μm
Compatibility with trocars	Any 10/11 mm trocar

Table 5.2: Typical specifications of an ultrasonic aspirator for laparoscopy.

Clinical results

As already mentioned, ultrasonic aspirators have frequently been used in open laparotomies. Applications included debulking of tumours around nerve

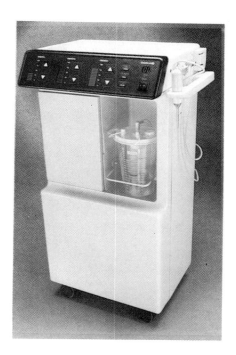

Figure 5.13: Ultrasonic aspirator unit (Sharplan 4300).

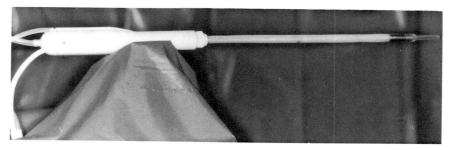

Figure 5.14: Laparoscopic ultrasonic aspirator handpiece.

fibres, urinary tracts, bowels, ovaries and other tissues. One of the most appealing applications of ultrasonic aspirators is lymphadenectomy. A direct extension of this technique to laparoscopy seems natural. As an example, initial use of the ultrasonic aspirator for selective presacral neurectomies enabled the aspiration of adipose tissue and adventitia surrounding blood vessels and the presacral nerve plexus[7]. Soft tissue was aspirated, enabling the accurate exposure of the presacral plexus. The time required for the procedure strongly depended on tissue type and amplitude parameters. In addition to assisting in neurectomies and lymphadenectomies, the ultrasonic aspirator seems to have a great potential in other laparoscopic specialties such as nephrectomies with minimal bleeding.

References

1   Tadir Y *et al.* (1994) Safety characteristics of the conically sculpted Nd:YAG fiber for operative laparoscopy. *Journal of Gynecologic Surgery.* In press.

2   Lomano J and Grochmal S (1991) New Microendoscopic Techniques Reduce Scars, Recuperation Time. *Clinical Laser Monthly.*

3   Donnez J and Nisolle M (1988) Laser hysteroscopy in uterine bleeding: endometrial ablation and polypectomy. In Donnez J ed. *Laser operative laparoscopy and hysteroscopy.* Louvain.

4   Raif J and Zair E (1993) SwiftLase – a new CO_2 laser scanner for reduced tissue carbonization. *Lasers in Surgery and Medicine.* Suppl. **5**:28.

5   Donnez J *et al.* (1993) The SwiftLase – a new method for the treatment of endometriosis and ovarian cysts. In press.

6   Reid R (1991) Physical and surgical principles of laser surgery in the lower genital tract. *Obstetrics and Gynecology Clinics of North America.* **18**:429–74.

7   Grochmal SA, Weekes A, Garratt D, Slatkine M, Hanson E (1993) Applications of the laparoscopic ultrasound aspirator for advanced gynecologic operative endoscopic procedures. *The Journal of the American Association of Gynecologic Laparoscopists.* **1**:43–7.

8   Carruth JAS and McKenzie AL (1984) *Medical lasers — science and clinical practice.* Adam Hilgen, Bristol.

9   Deppe G *et al.* (1990) Debulking of pelvic and para aortic lymph node metastases in ovarian cancer with the Cavitron ultrasonic surgical aspirator. *Obstretics and Gynecology.* **76**:1140–2.

10 Adelson MD *et al.* (1988) Cytoreduction of ovarian cancer with the Cavitron ultrasonic surgical aspirator. *Obstetrics and Gynecology.* **72**:140–3.

6

Organization of the Minimally Invasive Surgery Unit and Trouble-Shooting for Operative Endoscopy

CHARLES E. CONNANT

Minimally invasive surgery

The recent progress in gynaecological endoscopy and other fields of endoscopic surgery to improve both diagnosis and treatment has been due primarily to the improved technology[1]. The instrumentation has become so specialized that the lack of even the simplest piece of ancillary equipment — a small rubber stopper or tiny screw — can mean that the procedure can no longer be carried out laparoscopically. As Benjamin Franklin wrote: 'A little neglect may breed mischief . . . For want of a nail, the shoe was lost; for want of a shoe the horse was lost; for want of a horse the rider was lost.'[2]

The development of advanced instrumentation has led to the creation of the minimally invasive surgery unit (MISU). As the decade ends, such units are likely to become the standard not only for modern gynaecology, but also for other surgical specialties as well. It is in these units that all the specialized equipment and back-up systems are kept, and where the surgical procedures are performed. This is also where members of the surgical team are trained and based: scrub technicians and scrub nurses, biomedical technicians, electronic engineers, anaesthetists, videographers and specialists in medical photography.

Currently most hospitals store all their endoscopic equipment in ordinary operating room suites, cluttering up the room where ease of movement is all-important. Figure 6.1 shows how an ideal minimally invasive surgical unit might be designed, and where the equipment, personnel and ancillary personnel would be located. One-third of the room is set aside for the anaesthetist, one-third is devoted to the main surgical team and their equipment — video, insufflators, light sources, etc, and the other third is set aside for the instrumentation nurse and ancillary personnel who operate lasers, electrocautery units and suction-irrigation and supply the required primary and secondary instrumentation for the surgical procedure. This basic plan can be adapted for almost any surgical requirement.

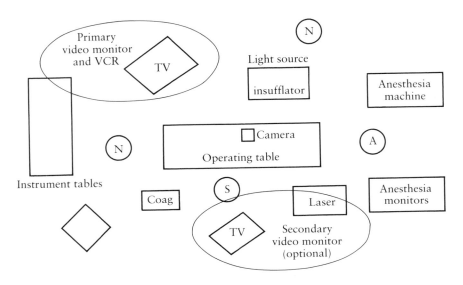

Figure 6.1: Basic floor plan for MISU suite, designed for maximum efficiency. (Illustration by courtesy of J. Leventhal, MD.)

The surgical team

The surgical team consists of surgeon and assistant, nurse or scrub nurse and assistant, biomedical technician, circulating room nurse (or nurses — ideally there should be two), anaesthetist and postoperative recovery nurse. Each person has assigned duties and responsibilities, such as preparing and providing the appropriate instrumentation and anticipating the manoeuvres of the surgeon, as well as his specific requirements and preferences. The biomedical technician establishes control of all the electronic equipment including light source, lasers, video, and instruments for insufflation, electrocautery and suction-irrigation. His role may also include that of a still-photographer as well as video editor and titler for each surgical procedure as required. The circulating room nurses are the backbone of the team; they must be aware of possible last-minute changes, sorting out additional small items of equipment that may be needed, checking irrigation fluids, input and output in the case of hysteroscopic procedures for fluid balance, monitoring the patient's condition for crepitus, pressure points on the extremities, and overall well-being. The postoperative recovery nurses should also be prepared for all eventualities. They should be told if fluid has been left in the abdomen for the prevention of adhesions, or if an intrauterine catheter has been left in the uterus to prevent postoperative adhesions. They should also understand why the procedure is being performed and be aware of any signs of complications or sequelae which the surgeon needs to be notified of immediately.

A laparotomy set-up should be available at all times for minimally invasive procedures. This is not only excellent planning, but also improves the outcome of patients who may not be able to be successfully treated totally endoscopically[3].

Fire prevention should always be a concern of the two circulating nurses within the MISU. There should be a plan of action for each operating room suite, developed and governed by its own special committee. The plan should include specific responsibilities for each designated team member of the MISU and there should also be excellent communication between the anaesthetist and the personnel of the MISU concerning the plan of evacuation should a flash-fire occur during the surgical procedure. There should be regular fire drills and reviews of patient safety.

Patient positioning is of paramount importance during surgery since different procedures require different positions. Injuries can result from hyperextension of the ligaments or from compression of nerves due to poor patient positioning on the operating room table[5]. Operating room personnel should be aware of the patient's past surgical history, including any previous problems with extremities and previous joint and abdominal surgery. During intraoperative and postoperative care, firm support of the patient's body should receive due consideration. Extreme overflexion of the legs, for example in 'candy canes', should be avoided because it tilts the pelvis in such a way that a pelvic mass often recoils and might not be found during examination under anaesthesia[6]. Liberal use of table-tilting and manipulation helps to emphasize a particular area of the abdominal cavity which is being explored[7].

Trouble-shooting for operative endoscopy

Although the emphasis is on a team approach, it is the ultimate responsibility of the endoscopic surgeon to have a basic understanding of all the applications, small quirks and problems that may develop during an endoscopic procedure from a technical point of view. An endoscopic surgeon must be prepared to break scrub in order to correct any problems with the equipment.

The video system

One of the most important components of the endoscopic approach is the visualization that the surgeon obtains via the video system. All too often, problems arise with image quality during the endoscopic procedure. The endoscopic surgeon must be sufficiently familiar with the electronics to solve some of these problems himself, and indeed to spend a few minutes before the operation to check the equipment. Whether using an electronic video laparoscope or hysteroscopic eyepiece, it is important to attach the camera before sterilization of the equipment in order to check the connections and the image on the video monitor. It is not unknown for a procedure to be under way before it is discovered that the camera does not work, just because the cables have been removed during cleaning.

It is always best to insert the hook-up of a video printer or recorder in the middle of the electronic system, and the primary or secondary video monitor should be the last item to be connected. No output video signal should come from the primary or secondary monitors, in order to allow proper video signal transmission within the system. By placing the VCR or printer in line between the cameras and the video monitors, there will be no degradation of the video image. If the camera system has both S-video and composite video terminals, these can run both the VCR and video printer directly from the back of the TV camera unit itself. S-video gives a much cleaner image and separates both luminance and chrominance in the video signal. Composite video may be used as a second recording source, should the need arise. They give exceptional quality to the picture but do not provide a higher separation for chrominance and luminance (Figure 6.2). Whenever possible, one should use the S-video connections for a brilliant on-line monitor display as well as to record exact colour interpretation from the operative site picture.

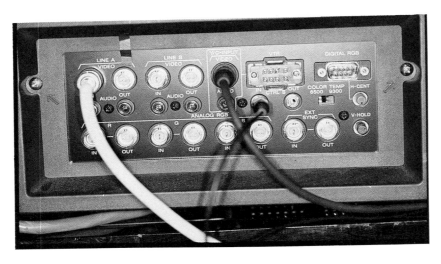

Figure 6.2: Composite or BNC terminals (white cable) and S-video terminal (black cable) are standard configuration for video signal transmission. With new digital videotape recorders, serial RS232 ports (*right*) will provide maximum image quality on high-definition television systems.

All power switches should be on, because situations do arise where no video image is obtained on the monitor because someone has forgotten to power up one of the printers or VCRs. When the entire TV tower or stand is plugged into the wall outlet and powered up, all components should register power immediately, thus avoiding any possible confusion later in the surgical procedure. Also of importance is the transmission of video signals from primary monitors to secondary and tertiary monitors, or monitors located remotely.

So far no manufacturer has successfully addressed the issue of remote (ie cableless) video transmission of images. There are some consumer products which can transmit video signals through walls and floors to a secondary TV monitor; however, this has not proved to be effective within the operating room setting, due to the significant amount of radio interference that is generated by the various other electrical components.

Proper cabling terminating in British Nut Connector (BNC) terminals should be utilized to avoid accidental pull-outs when equipment is moved, as well as to transmit signals satisfactorily from one monitor to another. In semi-permanent installations the commercial-grade cable may be channelled up the walls, across the ceiling and down across the other side of the room. On occasion, cables are taped and secured to the floor so that they will be more secure and less likely to become entangled in the feet of the people scurrying around the operating room during the procedure. (Figure 6.3)

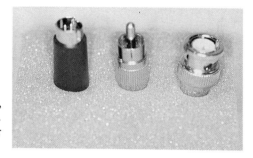

Figure 6.3: *From left to right:* S-video, RCA pin plug and BNC video terminals. RCA pin plugs are usually designated for audio signals.

Remember that the VCR or video printer can be utilized to disperse a single video image from the camera unit to various monitors or recording devices. Commercial-grade VCRs and printers have both S-video and composite BNC video terminals. These are marked 'video in' and 'video out' and also have video or S-video selections. By hooking up the main camera to one of the video inputs on the back of the VCR or printer, several different video outputs can be generated through one component, and with the flick of a switch can be sent anywhere in the room or outside it without any additional expensive video wiring system. On older recording equipment, which does not offer S-video/composite BNC inputs and outputs, a video switcher system may be utilized to disperse video images to several other receivers.

As new video systems become available, it is increasingly important to attach the specific type of camera terminal to a dedicated electronic output device. For example, the electronic video laparoscope (EVL) requires a dedicated cable output device. Should the cable termination be inserted into a camera unit of a similar but non-compatible terminal type, significant damage will result to the male and female receptacles in the electronics of the EVL. It should also be noted that newer digitally enhanced conventional camera heads are not interchangeable with analogue camera units. Connections should be clearly marked and labelled so that there will be no opportunity for error or camera damage. It may also be wise for the endoscopic surgeon to spend some time instructing his nursing staff and dedicated operating room personnel. He may inform them about his preferences for the set-up of the video equipment and the quality of the video image. The controls for colour, brightness, hue, contrast and sharpness are all independent of each other and must be properly adjusted for the best image on the monitor. The surgeon's preferences should be noted down in a record book for future reference.

Video images are best displayed in a dark environment so shades, blinds or window shutters should be installed in the operating room. Often an entire endoscopic procedure occurs with a very bright ambient light in the operating room and only at the end does the surgeon realize why he could not see clearly. Someone should be in charge of darkening the room to a degree which is satisfactory to everyone involved, and controlling this throughout the procedure.

Instrumentation

Perhaps the best way to organize instrumentation is to treat an endoscopic procedure as if it were a conventional open surgical approach. The instruments should be arranged according to the frequency of use on the primary table, which the scrub nurse must have immediate access to. Additional specialized instrumentation should be located on a secondary tray or table close to the scrub nurse (Figure 6.4). Instrumentation that may not be required on a regular basis for a standard endoscopic procedure should be sterile-wrapped, packed and available within the operating room itself. This avoids unnecessary resterilization of instrumentation that may not be used in every endoscopic procedure: eg myomectomy morcellators and tissue extractors.

The surgeon should be familiar with the fact that instrumentation is available in both the ratchet and the spring-loaded format, and the two formats should be easily interchangeable. Also of importance (but too often forgotten) are the small end-caps which are located near the finger grips of the instruments. These end-caps which are used during cleaning of the instrumentation and allow jets of water to travel down the internal mechanism of the instruments, can cause a loss of pneumoperitoneum during an endoscopic procedure. Therefore every instrument should have an end-cap attached to its Luer lock at the proximal end.

Some instruments need rubber stoppers, bulbs or gasket sleeves to allow them to function properly. An assortment of these should be readily available on the primary endoscopic instrument table in case of instrument malfunction (eg leaking of air, backflow of fluid or jammed trocar valves). Re-usable trocars, especially those required for tissue morcellation and extraction, should be thoroughly inspected and properly lubricated on a regular basis. High-temperature autoclaving tends to expand brass-lined jackets and sleeves, making trocar trumpet valves and trap doors difficult to operate and leading to undesirable rapid desufflation of pneumoperitoneum. For this reason, some of the larger trocars are now available in a disposable format with interchangeable reducing sleeves and extraction tubes.

(a)

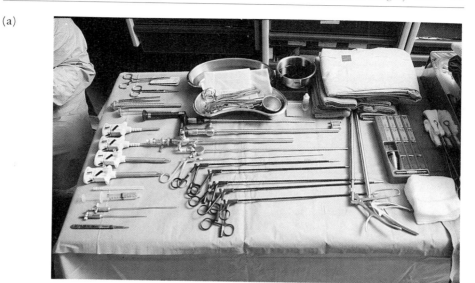

(b)

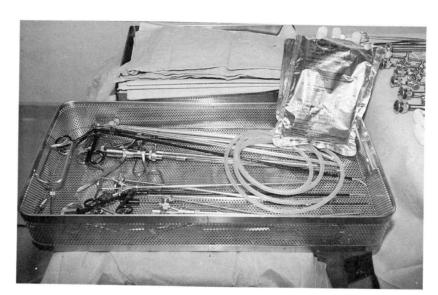

Figure 6.4: a The primary surgical table is arranged conventionally. All instrumentation is available based on frequency of use, specialized use or emergency needs. **b** Ancillary (large-diameter) instrumentation deserves a separate table in proximity to the main table.

Consideration should also be given to a situation where large trocars (20 mm or greater in diameter) are being used for the endoscopic procedure. Often it is not convenient to remove a large trocar at the end of its specific application and step down to a smaller size to complete the procedure. A wide variety of extraction tubes (also known as reducer tubes) of various lengths should be available. This will allow a step down (eg from 20 to 10 mm or from 5 to 3 mm as necessary) to avoid removal or reinsertion of instrumentation, or repair of the abdominal wall prematurely in order to close a large gaping defect from a large diameter trocar. All these small items should be on the table for every endoscopic procedure as they may be required at any time (Figure 6.5).

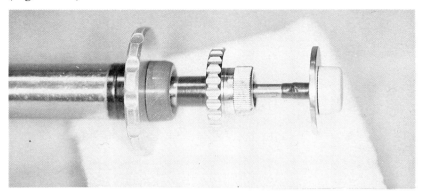

Figure 6.5: Reduction in size (here from 20 mm to 3 mm) is simple if these extraction tubes are readily available. This conversion prevents unnecessary removal of large trocars prematurely.

Insufflation equipment

The insufflator is essential to the endoscopic procedure. Although a gasless type of laparoscopic surgery is now being developed, using robotic arm and abdominal wall retraction devices, most endoscopic procedures are still done with gas. The gas cylinders should be checked before the start of the procedure, and a half-empty tank replaced with a full one. The inconvenience of changing tanks during a critical portion of an endoscopic procedure only leads to increased risk and anxiety. In-line filters should be utilized between the gas tank and insufflator, and again from the insufflator to the site of insufflation on the trocar. Disposable large-diameter insufflation tubes are now being manufactured with built-in filters. Recent evidence demonstrates that there is a significant amount of particulate matter which can be passed into the patient from the bottom of gas cylinders or bottles. This has also become increasingly important in the oxygen and nitrous oxide lines used for inhalation anaesthesia.

At our institute, we are utilizing a prototype in-line heater to warm the gas as it leaves the insufflator. The heater maintains the ambient CO_2 gas at a comfortable warmer temperature before it enters the abdominal cavity. This leads to a reduction in postoperative pain and diaphragmatic discomfort. However, until specifically designed apparatus is manufactured, makeshift devices will have to be utilized.

At least 10-15 feet of insufflation tubing should be available to provide greater distance between the operating surgeon and the insufflator itself. Often a surgeon has to work with the insufflator directly next to his back, making it uncomfortable to manoeuvre around the operating table. Longer insufflation tubing also allows the tubing to be channelled away from the surgeon (perhaps over his head), down into the middle of the operative site. This prevents insufflation tubing from getting tangled along the side of the patient, hanging down onto the floor or being stepped on, decreasing the CO_2 flow during the procedure. Large-diameter tubing also permits a less restricted air flow from the insufflator.

Every member of the surgical team should also be aware of the surgeon's specific requirements for intra-abdominal pressure (generally around 12–15 mmHg). This information should be passed to the anaesthetist who may need to make specific adjustments to his patient's anaesthesia, should there be a need to increase the abdominal pressure above 15 mmHg. One simple way of establishing continuity for the proper settings of insufflation can be to put a small label, marked with the specific amounts of intra-abdominal pressure required, on or near the control buttons. This is especially useful when more than one surgeon is using the same endoscopic equipment with different operating room teams.

The current state-of-the-art endoscopic insufflators provide a maximum of 15 l per minute of gas flow (Figure 6.6). Generally 1–2 l should be used for the initial approach to the endoscopic procedure, but once surgery is well under way, a slow increase in the flow rate may be needed to maintain adequate pneumoperitoneum. With a dedicated operating room staff, a team member may be responsible for adjusting the amount of insufflation flow according to the needs of the surgeon.

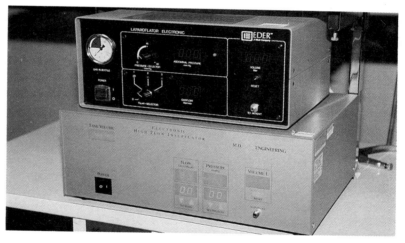

Figure 6.6: High-flow 15 l min^{-1} insufflation is controlled by a CPU, filtering the CO_2 gas for particulate matter and warming the gas via heater coils. Older equipment should be kept for back-up purposes.

In order to prevent excessive diaphragmatic irritation in patients post-operatively, all the pneumoperitoneum should be expelled at the end of the procedure by leaving the multiple trocar valves open during desufflation and taking the patient out of steep Trendelenburg, or even utilizing reverse Trendelenburg. Alternatively, wall suction may be utilized to desufflate rapidly the pneumoperitoneum, paying careful attention to surrounding structures near the suction cannula tip intraperitoneally. Especially during microlaparoscopic procedures, when patients are only under intravenous sedation, postoperative shoulder pain may be avoided by gently massaging the upper abdominal wall below the ribs, forcing the air under the diaphragm to come closer to the level of the umbilicus, where it can be expelled through negative pressure.

Particular attention should also be paid to the presence of subcutaneous emphysema. This is the responsibility of not only the operating surgeon, but of the circulating personnel and anaesthetist as well. It is embarrassing to have to tell the patient's family that the surgery went extremely well except that she now looks somewhat different. Subcutaneous emphysema is apparently occurring with decreasing frequency since coaxial cooled fibre delivery systems were replaced by sculptured laser fibres, especially in the case of Nd:YAG and KTP laser fibres; however, crepitus and its location should be documented and careful follow-up of this in the acute recovery phase should be emphasized.

Sources of illumination

The gold standard of illumination is the xenon light source. Available in 150 and 300 Watt configurations, recent prototypes tested in our institution have reached the maximum output of over 550 Watts of power. The advantage of xenon light is that it is almost like daylight, unlike halogen or metal halide illumination sources. This type of illumination is excellent both for still photography and video imaging. Third-generation auto-iris capability, either at the video-chip end of the camera or in the electronics of the light source itself, provides almost immediate automatic control of exact illumination required based upon the distance of the light source from its target. This effect is further enhanced by newer prototypes utilizing microprocessor circuitry to effect these minutely accurate auto-iris changes in a matter of milliseconds.

Often the source of illumination is adequate, but the switches and dials are not in their proper sequence. For most video applications, today's light sources have a switch marked 'video'. In most circumstances this switch must not be changed from this video setting, which allows complete automatic operation to occur while the light source is in use. These positions should be marked, just as on the insufflators, so that the correct illumination and auto-iris settings can be selected prior to the onset of the procedure.

The fibreoptic light cables must be properly inspected and maintained. Most manufacturers now produce fibreoptic large-diameter cables (10–12 mm) of various lengths, up to as much as 12 feet. The terminal ends of the cable should be checked to make sure that the proper cable has been selected for the particular laparoscope or hysteroscope. Light cables have similar couplings, but they are not interchangeable when it comes to getting them into the source of illumination. A large selection of interchangeable couplers and reducing sleeves should be readily available to adapt to different types of connecting sleeve on the laparoscope, hysteroscope or light source. Ideally, a dedicated light cable should be utilized for each particular scope and light source combination. This should all be planned, selected and checked in advance. A back-up fibre light cable should also be available for immediate use if required. Periodic inspection of the fibre cables themselves should be done by transilluminating the cables with a flashlight in order to evaluate proper fibre alignment and to discard any broken or cracked fibre cables. Along with the additional light cable, older (perhaps non-xenon) light sources should be maintained in good working order and used for back-up when a xenon bulb fails and changing the bulb is inappropriate during the surgical procedure.

At the end of the procedure, the first item away from the operating site is the light cable. On occasion, the light cable is removed from the end of the laparoscope or hysteroscope and placed on the drapes, which are only flame-retardant. It takes a matter of seconds to burn a hole through the drapes and onto the patient (and perhaps members of the team nearby) from the intense heat at the distal tip of the light cable. This is especially true when using liquid light cables. Our protocol calls for the immediate removal of the light cable and powering down of the light source upon completion of the endoscopic procedure. This will prevent accidents, which could result not only in burning the patient but also in expensive lawsuits.

Irrigation systems

Almost every endoscopic procedure today requires adequate irrigation and aspiration of fluids throughout. Despite the fact that numerous manufacturers have provided 'high-pressure' irrigation systems, they have all been disappointingly ineffective. Any irrigation system that the endoscopic surgeon is familiar with will be satisfactory for the purpose of irrigating and aspirating fluids. A 5 mm cannula, which allows for both aspiration and irrigation, usually with a thumb-switch or finger-activated control button, will suffice for most purposes. In more complex operative procedures (such as LAVH, myomectomy and the removal of dermoid cysts) a larger-bore 10 mm irrigation cannula is preferable, because their interchangeable distal tips allow for pool suction as well as manoeuvres which require an open cannula configuration.

There are various types of irrigation fluid, but our best results have been achieved with warmed lactated Ringer's solution. Generally, we use a 1 l bag or bottle of fluid, to which we add 1000 units of heparin. This appears to be the best way to keep blood clots soft enough to be evacuated under high-pressure suction. The high-pressure irrigation systems (1000–1500 mmHg) have been disappointingly ineffective in breaking up large clots and removing them quickly. More recent prototypes approaching 3500 mmHg, allowing for true aqua dissection, show promise but have not yet received FDA approval.

The irrigation system should be adequately tested and adjusted before the procedure commences. This is important where deep dissection will occur in a highly vascularized area, such as in the case of laparoscopic lymphadenect-omy or presacral neurectomy. The amount of tubing which is required for the suction irrigation system can be annoying on the operative site during the procedure. We have found it helpful to run both irrigation and suction tubing up and over the operative site, and then down along the side of the table in order to prevent it taking up too much space in the surgical area. This can easily be accomplished with the use of one or two intravenous stands. The proximal end of the cannula should also be checked for leaks in order to avoid flooding of the operative site and particularly where the surgeon is standing.

Hysteroscopic apparatus

There are some special considerations for diagnostic and operative hysteroscopic procedures. Although far less instrumentation is needed than for operative laparoscopy, appropriate measures should nevertheless be taken to maintain the equipment in good working order and to have all the specialized components available in order for the procedure to be carried out successfully. In no other area of operative endoscopy can a disaster occur more quickly than in operative hysteroscopic procedures[8].

Since the majority of operative hysteroscopy procedures are now performed under video surveillance, the same trouble-shooting concepts as discussed for laparoscopy apply to hysteroscopy. There are three areas of major consideration for trouble-shooting for hysteroscopic procedures:

- scopes, sheaths and specialized instrumentation
- uterine distension and fluid balance
- miscellaneous equipment.

Scopes, sheaths and specialized instrumentation

A general rule for operative hysteroscopy is that, for procedures performed with an electrical energy source, the hysteroscope usually has a 12° or 25° viewing angle. For basic diagnostic applications and other operative hysteroscopic procedures using lasers, a 30° telescope is the universal choice. With these combinations, the operative hysteroscopist can perform every procedure for treating intrauterine pathology.

The advantage of the 12° or 25° telescope for procedures performed with an electrical energy source is that it maintains the ball or loop electrode in a consistently close field of vision throughout the entire range that the electrode travels on the working element of the hysteroscopic sheath. This is important when one is trying to cope with decreased depth perception and field of vision within the uterine cavity. On the other hand, a wider angle of vision is required when utilizing laser energy, as the fibre is utilized relatively close to the distal end of the hysteroscope in a more stand-off approach. Care should be taken that the distal ends of the telescopes are not in too close proximity to the source of energy (either laser or electricity). Flashback and excessive heat from the energy source can damage the tip of the hysteroscope, perhaps clouding the optical lens or melting the distal portions of the light-transmitting fibres within the scope itself. The distal tips of telescopes have been seen to melt and crack when exposed to excessive heat from one of these energy sources or from a short-circuit from worn insulation on a ball or loop electrode.

For the majority of hysteroscopic procedures, a single operating channel sheath should suffice for both diagnostic and simple operative techniques. This operating sheath may be utilized to pass the biopsy sample, scissor instrumentation or laser fibre down into the uterine cavity. For electrical procedures, care should be taken to check the working element of the hysteroscope. This working sheath positions the electrode within the operative field in the uterine cavity. The connections to the working element should be checked periodically to ensure that connecting loops and wire connections are not loose, which might lead to short-circuits. The finger grip should rotate properly and the spring action of the working element should be checked for complete length of travel along its extended axis. The outer sheath, where the electrode is attached and which is placed over the entire hysteroscopic apparatus, has typical fenestrations at its distal tip. These fenestrations aid in the circulation of fluid throughout the uterine cavity and in mobilizing debris away from the operative site. If distension is not adequately achieved during the initiation of the procedure, these fenestrations may be blocked with tissue debris from insertion through the endocervical canal. The cannula should be withdrawn and the fenestrations cleared in order to allow optimal flow within the uterine cavity. A thorough working knowledge of how the entire hysteroscopic apparatus fits together is of paramount importance. Attempting to lock or unlock segments of the hysteroscope during the procedure wastes valuable anaesthesia time and can create a major flood of distension medium in the surrounding operative area.

Specialized instrumentation generally includes biopsy forceps, graspers and scissors. Recently, with the onset of video hysteroscopy, the instrumentation has been lengthened an additional 4-5 cm in order to clear an adequate working distance behind the camera head attached to the hysteroscopic eyepiece. Unfortunately, these are semi-rigid or flexible instrument shafts which can eventually bend or break. It is important to check these instruments frequently and take special care when using them. In the case of laser endometrial ablation, a laser fibre can be redirected down the operating channel of the hysteroscope with greater ease if a simple laser fibre guide is utilized. This is a flexible aluminium metal sheath which makes the laser fibre much more rigid, so that its manoeuvreability within the uterine cavity is easier.

Extra rubber stoppers should be available. Backflow and wash from the distension medium can occur through multiple operating channel ports, but this can be minimized by adding a rubber stopper on the end of the Luer lock.

Uterine distension and fluid balance

Although diagnostic hysteroscopy can be performed with a variety of distension mediums (eg CO_2, Hyscon and saline), most operative procedures are done in fluid. This may either be saline, as in the case of laser energy, or glycine, sorbitol or mannitol, in the case of electrical energy. With both solutions an adequate system is needed to instil, distend and extract the fluid on a continuous basis. Currently the various hysteroscopic distension pumps for operative procedures all require an adequate inflow and outflow channel, and a continuous-flow hysteroscope. These pumps utilize a strain gauge for measurement of the intrauterine pressure, and use this measurement for regulation of the total intrauterine pressure, which is designed not to exceed 90 mmHg. To accomplish this, certain accessory pieces of equipment may be necessary for proper monitoring and electronic feedback in the hysteroscopic pump. For older hysteroscopic equipment with only two channels, an additional overlying sheath may be required to provide an outflow channel for these specially designed pumps.

Other hysteroscopic designs provide three ports, but due to the location of the operating channel, one port may not be suitable for monitoring the intrauterine pressure. In these instances, a small T adaptor may be used to provide two access routes from one port (Figure 6.7).

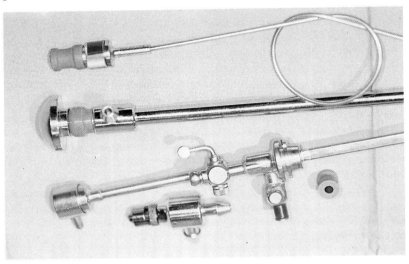

Figure 6.7: Accessory items for successful hysteroscopy. **a** T-adapter for intrauterine pressure monitor. **b** Single-channel operating sheath. **c** Outflow cannula for single-port hysteroscope. **d** Flexible laser fibre guide.

The operating team must be in command of the total amount of fluid used for distension of the cavity during operative procedures[9]. Electronic hysteroscopic pumps offer improved ability to monitor fluid inflow and outflow: proper management and special consideration for these particular situations are addressed elsewhere in this book. The disposable tubing utilized for the hysteroscopic pumps should be checked for proper attachment to the pumps, and the entire system must be primed with the distension medium prior to the onset of the procedure. As these tubing systems are disposable there are sometimes faults in the seals of the joints and insertions of the various tubes which may lead to leaks and decrease in intrauterine pressure. Checking the tubing system thoroughly before use will avoid any unnecessary delays once the procedure has commenced.

Miscellaneous equipment

We recommend the use of an in-dwelling Foley catheter during operative procedures. This keeps the bladder empty and so allows greater mobilization of the uterus. It also enables evaluation of fluid output during the operative procedure, especially if diuretics are given intraoperatively for a suspected early onset of fluid overload syndrome. The Foley may be removed in the acute recovery phase. A moistened sponge should be put into the rectum if the use of laser energy is contemplated, because laser energy (especially Nd:YAG energy) is extremely flammable in the presence of methane gas.

A fluid pouch may also be used to trap additional backflow and excessive fluid during distension of the uterine cavity, and then drain it so that it can be included in the measurement and estimation of total fluid output during the procedure. Care should be taken when utilizing these particular items during a laser endometrial ablation as the majority of the disposable products are not flame-retardant.

Most operative hysteroscopists prefer to stabilize the cervix with some type of tenaculum during the procedure. However, it can be difficult to hold the tenaculum while operating the hysteroscope with two hands, so a Martin arm retractor or other multi-articulated robotic device may be attached to the side of the table. This Martin arm can also be utilized for fixation and stabilization of instruments in other laparoscopic procedures.

Dilation of the endocervix at times may be perplexing, especially in patients who have never gone through childbirth or a hysteroscopic procedure. Their cervical stenosis may be difficult to manage, and many a hysteroscopic procedure has been aborted because of difficulty dilating the endocervical canal or because of inadvertent perforation in the lower uterine segment due to the creation of a false channel. Small graduated dilators (3–10 mm) are more satisfactory than the standard dilators utilized for dilatation and curettage. Where cervical openings are very small due to stenosis, 1 and 2 mm straight dilators are available for exploration of the stenotic canal. Also useful in instances of extreme cervical stenosis is the passage of a small 0.5 mm optical catheter (*see* Chapter 18). This the optical catheter may be utilized to visualize the stenotic endocervical canal while simultaneously dilating the canal with small dilators.

Inadvertent uterine perforation may happen to the best of operative hysteroscopists. It is always advisable to have a laparoscope and trocar ready for use. With these on the table, immediate entry into the abdominal cavity may be achieved, and any suspected perforation or bleeding confirmed and managed quickly. Inexperienced surgeons can perform the initial operative hysteroscopic procedure under laparoscopic surveillance while they gain confidence and skill. Picture-in-picture (PIP) circuitry built into the recording VCR projects both laparoscopic and hysteroscopic views simultaneously on the same video monitor.

Development of instrumentation and equipment

Verres needle

Verres needles are now available in both reusable and disposable form. Soon Verres needles will be complemented by the addition of a visual component which allows direct insertion of the Verres needle. As this is currently still a blind technique, this visual Verres needle will make a significant contribution to the safety of endoscopic surgery.

Video enhancement

Almost every manufacturer can now produce a single-chip video camera that either equals or surpasses the quality of the more cumbersome three-chip camera configurations. Beyond this, the camera chip has already been localized at the distal portion of the laparoscope, as seen in the electronic video laparoscope. The advantage of this configuration is that there are no optical solid glass lenses in the body of the scope, which add to weight and cost. Instead there are two small wires which transmit the video image from the distal chip to the remotely located camera unit. With this advanced design there can be an increased number of fibreoptic cables within the telescope, and thus more light at the target site. The ability to place the chips so close to the target also increases the resolution of the video image, approaching 800 lines in NTSC signal format.

Currently the electronic video laparoscope is offered in both a diagnostic (10 mm) and operative (12 and 14 mm) version. The operating laparoscope allows the extended visualization achieved with a diagnostic scope, plus the added convenience of an operating channel measuring either 3 mm (12 mm OD) or 5.5 (14 mm OD) telescopes. This EVL design will also become the prototype for 3D visualization as the next generation of video enhancement equipment becomes available.

Virtual reality systems are being developed to enhance and improve the skills of the operating endoscopic surgeon[10]. Recent technology of 3D imaging is actually quite simple, and since 1985 several major commercial corporations have made a significant investment in research to improve the technology. Two separate video images, right and left, gathered by two individual video cameras, are transmitted and compressed by a digital imaging processor. The image is then recorded or projected through a mirror box of polarization screens onto either videotape or a video monitor.

Several medical specialties are investigating the use of 3D enhancement for their various surgical procedures. Major investigation and research programmes including clinical trials and applications, have already been put into place in such medical centres as the University Hospital in St Louis, Missouri.

This three-dimensional technology will have applications in four areas[11]. First, it will help in the development of better teaching methods (see for instance the use of rapid access laser disc technology. This method has been used in jet flight simulators and in medicine, providing the surgeon with immediate feedback of information, including tactile stimulation). The second area of development will be in better imaging technology. Within the next 18 months, high-definition television will become commonplace. Unfortunately high-definition television components are still extremely expensive, but the cost will be driven downwards as the technology improves. This equipment will then provide an image close to perfect optical resolution. Thirdly, procedures which are now seen in two dimensions will be adapted to three dimensions. Finally, with the use of special computer arrays, 3D images will be able to be created and manoeuvred (though this is not a real-time visual 3D display). The system is similar to that developed for fighter pilots, the so-called 'head-up' system. All the important data would be displayed directly in front of the surgeon, including information from computerized tomography scans, ultrasound, etc. This image would then be superimposed over the visual image in front of the surgeon, so that he knows exactly what topography or pathology he will encounter next during the procedure. Additional information concerning the intra-abdominal pressure (in mmHg), flow rate of CO_2 gas (in L min^{-1}), magnification of the video images and angle of tilt in the Trendelenburg position may also be displayed in front of him. A further description of 3D technology can be found in Chapter 26.

Insufflation devices

With the rapid development of advanced endoscopic procedures to replace conventional surgical techniques, the need for absolute maintenance of pneumoperitoneum is critical. Current insufflators can produce a maximum output of 15 L min^{-1}. Recent developments in improved flow of computer-enhanced microprocessors have allowed this breakthrough to occur. Microprocessors also allow accurate maintenance of the intra-abdominal pressure and make minute adjustments to the flow rate in milliseconds. Recently, attention has been paid to modifying insufflators to address the issue of warming the CO_2 gas prior to its entry into the abdominal cavity. This tends to produce less abdominal discomfort in the postoperative phase due to the decrease in diaphragmatic irritation. Prototypes with line heaters and warmers for gas are under development.

Endoscopic light source

The prevalence of the xenon light source in endoscopic theatres has established it as the standard. The development of electronic video laparoscopes, image-sensitive individual pixel arrays and computer-enhanced relays now make these two advanced technologies excellent for providing a light source which not only adjusts the light intensity automatically, but does so in milliseconds. Improved construction of xenon bulbs has prolonged their lifespan and made their purchase a practical long-term investment. Compact and well ventilated xenon light-source units are being designed for in-office use and the coming of operative laparoscopy and hysteroscopy to the confines of the physician's office and consulting rooms.

Hand-held instrumentation

In no area has there been more rapid growth and development of prototype instrumentation for the endoscopic surgeon (Figure 6.8). Despite early

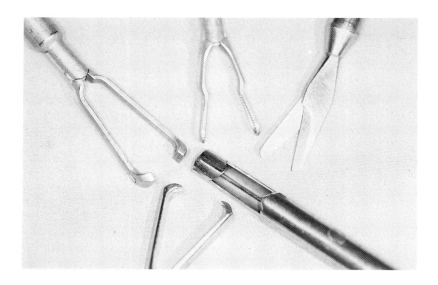

Figure 6.8: 10 mm instruments required for advanced surgical procedures. *Clockwise*: Allis forceps, claw forceps, morcellator, scissors and Babcock clamp.

attempts by corporations to encourage the use of disposable instrumentation, the realities of their cost have had an impact on health-care systems worldwide. More practically oriented instrument companies now provide reusable handles and/or shafts with disposable scissor tips, cautery tips, bipolar forceps tips and semi-reusable forceps. Dissecting scissors and atraumatic graspers are also available in semi-reusable design. Most endoscopic surgeons attempting advanced procedures have an array of 5 mm instrumentation, but a large selection of 10 mm instrumentation is just as crucial.

As these instruments are more intricate and costly to develop and produce, they are less likely to have disposability built into their design. As the need arises, the sizes will become even larger. 15, 20, 25 and 33 mm trocars are already being used for the extraction of tissue and the introduction of large instruments into the abdominal cavity. Some of these items are even offered in a disposable format (Figure 6.9). Instrument design is obviously based on surgical need. As the need arises, more and more specialized instrumentation will continue to appear in the endoscopic armamentarium.

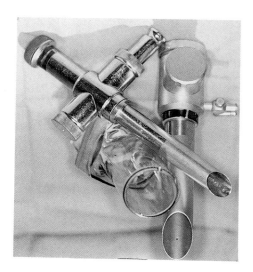

Figure 6.9: Large-diameter trocars (reusable or disposable) are necessary for myomectomy, total laparoscopic hysterectomy and oophorectomy.

References

1 Luciano A (1990) Getting started and becoming proficient in operative endoscopy. AAGL Abstracts, San Francisco.

2 Franklin B (1758) *Poor Richard's Almanack 1733–58*. Paddington Press, New York.

3 Corfman M (1990) Getting started and becoming proficient in operative endoscopy. AAGL Abstracts, San Francisco.

4 Hall F (ed). (1994) *Minimal Access Surgery for Nurses and Technicians*. Radcliffe Medical Press, Oxford. pp. 183–4.

5 Davis R *et al.* (1991) Deep venous thrombosis and pulmonary embolism. *Complications of General Surgery. Surgical Clinics of North America, Vol. 71, No.6.*

6 Gomes V *et al.* (1986) *Laparoscopy and Hysteroscopy in Gynecologic Practice.* Yearbook Publishers, Chicago. pp.7–31.

7 Corfman RS *et al.* (1993) *Complications of Laparoscopy and Hysteroscopy.* Blackwell Scientific Publications, Oxford.

8 Garry R *et al.* (1992) A uterine distension system to prevent fluid absorption during Nd-YAG laser endometrial ablation. *Gynaecol Endosc.* 1:23–7.

9 Hasham F *et al.* (1992) Fluid absorption during laser ablation of the endometrium in the treatment of menorrhagia. *Br J Anaesth.* 88:151–4.

10 Heinricks WL (1993) *Medical Surgical Training in Real and Virtual Environments*. Stanford Endoscopy Center for Training and Technology, Stanford, CA.

11 Bailey G (1993) Three-dimensional imaging in microsurgery. *Bull Am Coll Surg.*

Part II: Non Gynaecological Associated Procedures

Anaesthesia for Laparoscopy

Non-Gynaecological Complications of Laparoscopy

Appendectomy

Urological Considerations and Complications of Operative Endoscopy

7

Anaesthesia for Laparoscopy

ERVIN MOSS

Introduction

The history of gynaecological laparoscopy dates back to 1806 when Phillip Bozzini first described the use of candlelight through a urethral catheter[1,2]. In 1867 Segeles and Dormeaux described the use of a mirror to focus light through a genito-urinary speculum in a dog. It was at this time that the term endoscopy first appeared in the literature[2,3].

In 1902 a Dresden physician performed abdominal endoscopy on a dog using the light and mirror technique[1,2]. Jacobeus, from Stockholm, first described laparoscopy in a human in 1910[1,2]. Since then there have been numerous reports on the technique in the literature[3,4].

In England, Short used a cystoscope to visualize the abdominal organs through a small vertical incision[2,5]. In 1944 Decker and Cherry described culdoscopy as a technique to visualize the pelvis[2,6].

The development of the fibreoptic instruments, and the realization that an actual surgical procedure could be performed using multiple small entrance wounds has resulted in an explosion of technology and an increasing list of procedures that can be performed without long and painful incisions through the abdominal wall. Now the gynaecologist, with better visualization, fibreoptics, lasers, customized instruments and safer anaesthesia can do more extensive gynaecological procedures (including hysterectomies) requiring shorter hospital stays and less debilitating recovery periods.

In the late 1980s, the general surgeon began to use laparoscopy to remove gallbladders, and quickly extended his repertoire to include hernia repair, bowel resection, appendectomy and vagotomy[7,8]. Soon urologists were performing inguinal node dissections and nephrectomies through the scope. All specialists recognized the advantages of the technique for exploratory examination of the abdominal cavity through a scope, either by direct visualization or by the use of a camera attached or built into the eyepiece, which can magnify the image on television monitors for all within the operating room to observe, and then record it on VCR equipment for documentation. There is one camera that can be threaded through a Verres needle, thus enabling an exploration of the abdominal cavity without the use of a single suture to close a wound.

In routine surgical procedures, when an anaesthetic is administered, there are always inherent risks[9]. The procedure is also influenced by factors such as the skill of the anaesthetist, the equipment used to deliver the anaesthetic, and the availability and use of monitors to recognize untoward events such as hypoxia and hypercarbia. The patient also bears some responsibility, and a lifetime of bad habits such as smoking, drug ingestion and nutritional folly resulting in obesity contribute to the risk. The medical investigation may be performed by the internist without knowing the actual procedure to be performed, its risks or the anaesthetic agents to be used.

Although laparoscopic surgery results in a shorter hospital stay, less postoperative pain in most cases and a wound that can be covered with a sticking plaster, it increases the problems for the anaesthetist.

There was a time when the surgeon, as captain of the ship, assumed all responsibility for the patient's morbidity and mortality. It soon became evident that there was a co-captain, the anaesthetist, who was responsible for the administration of the anaesthetic and its complications. Juries soon learned to separate the responsibility of the surgeon from that of the anaesthetist and to judge accordingly.

However, in laparoscopy there has been a return to conditions, uncontrolled by the anaesthetist, that are the direct responsibility of the surgeon and which now add to the risks of anaesthesia and the procedure in general.

Credentialling of the endoscopic surgeon

High on the list of uncontrolled factors is the failure to set adequate credentialling standards for those performing endoscopic surgery. One contributing factor is the rush of various specialists to jump on the bandwagon and offer the highly publicized technique to their patients. Manufacturers of endoscopy equipment sponsor training programmes lasting a few days in which operations are performed on pigs and on training models. The surgeons then return to their communities where, in many cases, there has been a failure to set credentialling guidelines. The risks are compounded by the willingness of hospitals and ambulatory care centres to offer credentialling quickly in the hope of generating additional revenue and remain competitive in the hospital community.

On 4th May 1992, the American Medical Association published a feature article that was devoted to this ever-growing problem[10]. The most common non-gynaecological procedure performed today is laparoscopic cholecystectomy. While many centres are reporting no complications, others are reporting botched cholecystectomies and these have raised questions about the profession's system of disseminating new surgical techniques. Some surgeons in the USA fear that the profession has lost control of the process and that malpractice lawyers will move into the breach. This impacts on the anaesthetist because he will be named and implicated for not dealing properly with the complications created by the surgeon, eg an air or gas embolism or massive haemorrhage due to large vessel trauma.

In a very short time, laparoscopy has become the preferred method for the 500 000–600 000 cholecystectomies performed in the United States each year. At some centres 80% are done laparoscopically. By 1992, 10 000 surgeons had taken courses and laparoscopy is now becoming standard in surgical residencies.

Mortality and morbidity

In one 18-month period ending in May 1992, the New York State Department of Health found six deaths and 122 injuries related to laparoscopic cholecystectomy in at least 73 hospitals. It is estimated that half the injuries were to the common bile duct. An unusual number of injuries to the aorta, bladder, intestines, liver and other organs and vessels were found, according to Harry Bernard, MD, Senior Surgical Advisor to the New York Department of Health. 'I never heard of these injuries with open cholecystectomy,' he commented[10].

In New York State overall, 2% of all laparoscopic cholecystectomy patients were injured because of surgeons' errors, according to the New York Department of Health. The *New England Journal of Medicine* in 1991 reported on 1 518 cases; there was a 2.2% rate of bile duct injury, although the incidence dropped with the experience of the surgeon[11]. The data are incomplete because at least half of the complications go undetected at the time of the operation. According to Thomas Dent MD, of Temple University in Philadelphia, Pennsylvania: 'It is likely that the published complications for laparoscopic cholecystectomy are but the tip of the iceberg.'

Other reports from *Annals of Surgery* and from centres such as the University of Nashville, where the procedure was pioneered, report less mortality and morbidity based on their long experience[10].

Credentialling criteria

There is no question that training and experience play the major role in patient safety. The Society of American Gastrointestinal Endoscopic Surgeons recommend the following credentialling criteria:

- attendance at a general surgery residency
- attendance on a recognized laparoscopy course with animal practice, or training under laparoscopic surgeon
- written confirmation of competency from trainer
- proctoring under experienced laparoscopist (desirable, but not essential).

The Hospital Association of New York State recommends the following credentialling criteria:

- satisfactory performance of 10 procedures under direct supervision of experienced laparoscopist
- monitoring of operating record for first three months.

Within a month of the original warning in the *American Medical News*, a second article reported that there had been 158 injuries, 24 of them permanent or life-threatening, in 85 hospitals in the same 18-month period[12].

This report estimated that half the complications were injuries to the common bile duct. Many of the others were punctures to the aorta, inferior vena cava, hepatic artery, intestines, stomach and liver. These injuries occurred in New York State alone. The article further stated that there was a learning curve, as with all new procedures, but that (according to Thomas Hartman, Director of Health Care Standards and Analysis in New York State) the learning curve was not a valid justification for patient injury.

In addition, teaching centres are reporting a dramatic increase in referrals for difficult ductal reconstructive surgery after laparoscopic cholecystectomy complications. In the USA, this is likely to bring a huge increase in litigation[12].

New York State's credentialling recommendations are more specific than the guidelines issued by the Society of American Gastrointestinal Endoscopic Surgeons. They recommend a specific number of cases as an assistant and as the lead surgeon. Also recommended is a return to provisional status and preceptorship following any serious mishap.

Informed consent should be obtained, stating the risks of the procedure. The advisory document recommends the introduction of the trocar through an open technique using a mini incision, and insertion under direct vision of the scope. Because of the high incidence of ductal damage, an intraoperative cystic duct cholangiogram should be performed routinely in order to identify the anatomy.

Length of surgery as related to patient morbidity and mortality

In the days of open-drop ether administered by a variety of anaesthesia providers, surgeons learned to work fast out of necessity. Time was recognized as a factor contributing to mortality and morbidity. It was not unusual to see a 10-minute appendectomy, a 60-minute gastrectomy or a 20-minute gallbladder operation. With trained anaesthesia providers, new agents, monitors and machines, the younger generation of surgeons dropped the time factor out of the patient safety formula. However, the anaesthetist still relates time to morbidity and even mortality. Is it appropriate to take eight hours to remove a uterus using the laparoscopic technique? Does the advantage of a small incision outweigh the risks of an eight-hour procedure?

In the first 10 hysterectomies performed laparoscopically by one gynaecologist, one patient suffered a severe haemorrhage requiring exploratory laparotomy and transfusions, and two patients suffered cut ureters that required repair. Does the technique warrant the risk? Which patient shall be at the beginning of the learning curve?

Anaesthesia for laparoscopy

Numerous articles have been published describing various techniques and agents to be used by the anaesthesia provider during laparoscopy[13]. As the specialty of anaesthesiology developed after the Second World War, and as halothane replaced ether and chloroform (to be soon replaced by Penthrane, Ethrane, Forane and Desflurane), a philosophy was developed by anaesthetists that all agents were good when used in the hands of those experienced and trained in their use.

With a few exceptions, the same can apply today. The following factors should be considered when deciding on the technique or agents.

The planned procedure

A tubal ligation with an average duration of 10–15 minutes does not require the same anaesthesia plan as a nephrectomy or hysterectomy.

Where is the procedure being performed?

With 60% of surgical cases being performed in ambulatory care centres, from which patients are discharged the same day, an anaesthesia plan including use of short-acting, reversible drugs must be developed. The same-day setting does not preclude the use of a general endotracheal intubation.

Who is performing the surgery?

The anaesthetist must know his surgeon and his ability and experience. Thus a short procedure in the hands of an inexperienced surgeon may require general endotracheal anaesthesia to guarantee oxygenation, elimination of CO_2, protection of the airway from aspiration and monitoring to recognize the rare but dreaded gas embolism.

The condition of the patient

As time passes, the original contraindication list of those who were not candidates for endoscopy has shortened. No longer are obesity, the presence of hernia or previous surgery contraindications. The anaesthetist must tailor his technique to the patient, resorting to general endotracheal anaesthesia when there is any question about the ability to ventilate a patient in the Trendelenburg position. The physiological impact of the pneumoperitoneum upon the patient must always be a prime consideration. The mortality and morbidity statistics which appear in the literature were based on procedures performed on millions of healthy women undergoing tubal ligations. These statistics do not apply to the wide variation in physical status and age of patients now undergoing a variety of laparoscopic procedures.

Creation of a pneumoperitoneum

The creation of a pneumoperitoneum during laparoscopy brings an additional risk to the patient and increases the anaesthetist's chances of being accused of malpractice. The term 'pneumoperitoneum' is universally used to describe the insufflation of gases into the peritoneal cavity in order to separate the bowel and the abdominal wall from the bowel for better visualization. However, the term 'tension pneumoperitoneum' would be more descriptive and analogous to the term 'tension pneumothorax'. When air is described by the radiologist as being under the diaphragm after a perforated ulcer, it is accurate to refer to a pneumoperitoneum or air in the abdominal cavity. However, when air under pressure is pumped into the abdominal cavity, distending the abdominal wall and exerting pressure against vessels, upwards against the diaphragm, compressing the stomach wall, with the threat of regurgitation and aspiration, would not a more descriptive term be tension pneumoperitoneum?

Historically, five gases have been used to create the pneumoperitoneum. In 1903, Brainbridge used oxygen with its danger of support of combustion during cauterization[14]. Air was also used for insufflation[15]. However, air embolism may be fatal even in small volumes because of its low solubility in plasma. Nitrogen requires days for absorption from the peritoneal cavity and causes discomfort and shoulder pain[16]. As a result, the insufflation gas most commonly used today is CO_2 or N_2O.

Carbon dioxide

Carbon dioxide is the most common gas used for insufflation today. It is five times more soluble than air in plasma, and therefore the incidence and degree of gas emboli are decreased. The Royal College of Obstetricians and Gynaecologists (RCOG)[17] reported that 95% of 50 000 laparoscopies were performed using CO_2. Besides being soluble in plasma, it is rapidly excreted and does not support combustion. A volume of 200 cc slowly injected into a vein is not lethal, while 20 cc of air can cause death[18].

Rapid absorption of CO_2 may cause minimal shoulder pain. However, rapid absorption can also cause hypercarbia with increased respiratory acidosis. This was a concern in patients with heart and lung disease. It has been clearly demonstrated that this excess CO_2 can be blown off by increasing the rate and depth of respiration. This is most easily accomplished with the patient intubated, with controlled respiration and on a ventilator which allows the depth and rate of respiration to be adjusted.

A study by Diamant *et al.* found no significant hypercarbia in 21 women undergoing tubal ligation using CO_2 for insufflation under local anaesthetic[19]. The short duration of the procedure and the low pressures of CO_2 used could account for their findings.

Nitrous oxide

Nitrous oxide is purer than CO_2 and it absorbs at a slower rate from the peritoneal cavity[2]. It is non-irritating to the peritoneum and does not cause hypercarbia[20]. In 1975, a survey of laparoscopies was conducted by the American Association of Gynecological Laparoscopists. In 20 000 procedures, N_2O was used without any incidents related to gas[21].

The danger of explosion using N_2O has been reported, based on the theoretical possibility of methane gas from the bowel, hydrogen and N_2O (which can support combustion) causing a dangerous mixture[22]. Only one report appears in the literature during tubal ligation resulting in death[23].

The use of N_2O over CO_2 was recommended because of the possibility of the physiological effects of hypercarbia in patients with cardiac disease. However, the hypercarbia can be eliminated by controlled ventilation. The use of halothane was discouraged because of cardiac arrhythmias in the presence of elevated CO_2.

Another combination of gases used in harvesting eggs by laparoscopy is a mixture of CO_2 (5%), O_2 (5%) and nitrogen (90%)[24].

This gas mixture is used during fertilization and the growth of the embryo in vitro. However, at the end of laparoscopy the gas mixture is washed out using CO_2 in order to decrease pain.

Physiological effects of the pneumoperitoneum

The production of the pneumoperitoneum is an example of the potential negative physiologic changes produced by the surgeon, and impacting on the course of the anaesthesia. After the Verres needle has been inserted, and assuming that it has not perforated a viscus, torn a major vessel or caused a gas embolism by its being placed in a low lying liver, gas is pumped into the peritoneal cavity to a pressure of 15–20 mmHg[1]. Usually 2–4 l is needed and the rate of insufflation is 1 l min^{-1}. At a pressure of 25 mmHg there is an increase in airway pressure, intrathoracic pressure, central venous pressure, femoral venous pressure and decreased cardiac return to the heart with decreased cardiac output. Early on, the decreased cardiac return could cause a tachycardia with eventual fall in blood pressure if cardiac output is reduced[25,26].

When intra-abdominal pressure is increased above 30 mmHg, venous return from the legs can be reduced as a result of the pressure on the thin-walled iliac vessels and the vena cava[26]. As venous return is decreased, pressure builds up in the venous circulation resulting in increased peripheral resistance as much as twofold. As a result, there is an increase in cardiac afterload and decreased pre-load (venous return).

In addition, Scott and Julian[27] found that there were cardiac arrhythmias in 17% of patients when CO_2 was used to produce pneumoperitoneum, while only 0.5% of the patients had cardiac arrhythmias when N_2O was used.

Their results were based on the unphysiological technique of using a muscle relaxant plus halothane, with the patient in the Trendelenburg position and breathing spontaneously using a face mask.

Smith *et al.*[28] carried out laparoscopy with an endotracheal tube, and assisted respiration in a head-down position in which the PCO_2 never exceeded 40 mmHg, without evidence of cardiac arrhythmias.

The production of a pneumoperitoneum will also exert pressure upon the diaphragm, decreasing the compliance of the lung[29]. Pressure will be exerted upon the stomach and the oesophagus causing regurgitation of whatever is in the stomach. Thus a rule was established to pass a Levin tube after intubation in all patients undergoing laparoscopy (Figure 7.1). Under local anaesthesia, the passage of a Levin tube can be an unpleasant experience unless the patient is under i.v. conscious sedation, which then translates into not being a local anaesthesia.

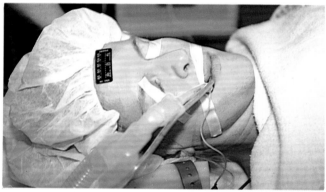

Figure 7.1: Levin tube in place and temperature monitoring on patient. If laser energy is utilized, the anaesthetist will cover the eyes with protection specific for the energy wavelength selected by the surgeon.

Contraindications

As surgeons, gynaecologists and urologists gain experience with the techniques, the list of historical contraindications has been shortened. However, this means again that the anaesthetist's reputation is at the mercy of the surgeon. For example, obesity is no longer a contraindication to laparoscopic cholecystectomy. Hernias were a contraindication to laparoscopic procedures and now are repaired through a scope. A history of peritonitis was once a contraindication. With the microcamera that fits through a Verres needle, a visual exploratory may be performed and the introduction of a laparoscopy through a site free of adhesions is now possible. However, the presence of advanced cardiac and pulmonary diseases is still a contraindication because of the physiological effects of a pneumoperitoneum and the need for a steep head-down position[30,31].

Complications

The purpose of this chapter is not to list all the anaesthetic combinations that may be used in laparoscopy. The anaesthetist and the endoscopic surgeon must be aware of the numerous complications that may arise during laparoscopy. Failure to diagnose and properly treat a gas embolism, for example, would lead a court of law to find the anaesthetist at fault for failing to treat a complication created by the operating physician. Theoretically, even if an anaesthetic were to be administered to a patient with no surgery being performed, other factors would influence the outcome despite the proper choice and administration of the anaesthetic. For example, did the internist evaluating the patient diagnose and treat the patient's medical diseases? Did the patient, through a lifetime of smoking, ingestion of alcohol or the use of drugs, decrease his chances of survival? Did the anaesthetist take a detailed history and examine the patient? Is his anaesthesia machine capable of administering hypoxia mixtures or more than one vapour? Was the machine serviced by authorized personnel? There can also be complications such as haemorrhage, perforation of an organ, subcutaneous emphysema, regurgitation of stomach contents, cardiovascular collapse, burn and gas embolism[17,32]. Of all the complications listed, haemorrhage and gas embolism top the list.

Haemorrhage

Today a large percentage of laparoscopy procedures are performed in the same-day setting. In the USA in 1992, for the first time, more procedures were performed with the patient being discharged on the same day of surgery than as a hospital in-patient. Whenever a Verres needle or a trocar is thrust through the abdominal wall, haemorrhage may result. Therefore instruments must be available for immediate conversion to laparotomy. Once serious bleeding is suspected, the abdomen must be explored and the bleeding controlled. In free-standing ambulatory care centres, blood and the ability to type and cross-match blood may not be available. Therefore it is crucial to control the bleeding early.

Bleeding can show itself as an abdominal wall haematoma and is not serious in most cases. A skilled laparoscopist can ligate a vessel in the abdominal wall using instruments already in place in the abdomen. More serious is direct trauma to major vessels including the aorta, iliac arteries, epigastric artery, splenic artery and vena cava[33].

Peterson et al.[34], reported on three deaths due to haemorrhage during sterilization. The introduction of laparoscopy for cholecystectomy and other surgical procedures in the last few years must certainly have resulted in other deaths by haemorrhage, but unfortunately the mechanisms for reporting and collecting data have failed to keep us updated.

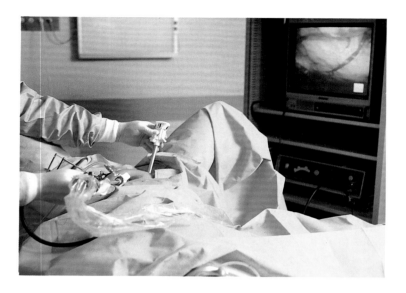

Figure 7.2: To avoid abdominal wall trauma or haematoma, insertion of·trocars should be accomplished under direct visual surveillance. As seen in the photo, ·large blood vessels can be avoided as they are viewed on the video monitor.

Gas embolism

Fortunately, gas embolism is an uncommon event, according to the literature. The RCOG study of 50 000 laparoscopies reported only one death following a proven gas embolism[17]. Since 1978, however, and the explosion of laparoscopy procedures, the danger of gas embolism must be constantly on the mind of the surgeon and the anaesthetist. The availability of more sophisticated monitoring has revealed that the incidence of gas embolism is higher than originally suspected. The reports of the incidence of gas embolism during caesarean section have called the gynaecologist's and the anaesthetist's attention to the presence of gas emboli and amniotic fluid emboli in the circulation during what has been accepted as a routine operation.

Fong *et al.*[35] reported a 26% overall incidence of venous embolism during caesarean section. Their lower incidence (compared to the 52% and 65% reported by Vartikar) was the result of defining Doppler detected emboli as a change lasting longer than 5 seconds.

Obviously gas and amniotic fluid embolism had occurred during the centuries that caesarean sections have been performed, and went unrecognized until the use of such monitors as the Doppler, the transoesophageal echocardiogram (TEE), the end-tidal PCO_2 monitor and the oximeter[34,36].

The simple use of a chest stethoscope for routine monitoring during a section would reveal the millwheel murmur associated with gas embolism, but unfortunately the diagnosis based on the millwheel murmur would be late as a result of the murmur being created by a large volume of gas mixing with blood in the right atrium. The earlier the diagnosis, the better the prognosis. Early diagnosis is the result of monitoring with instruments that detect minute gas bubbles[35]. Prevention of continuing embolism is the result of early detection and can prevent further embolism in volumes that may prove fatal or crippling. The low incidence reported by Peterson et al.[34] may not reflect the true statistics on mortality and morbidity between 1977 and 1981. The diagnosis of gas embolism is not always made. Reports of non-awakening after general anaesthesia may well have been attributed to hypoxia rather than neurological damage from an arterial embolism to the brain. Cardiac arrhythmia developing during anaesthesia and leading to fatality could have been caused by arterial emboli to the coronary arteries, instead of by the multitude of possibilities that are invariably discussed after an anaesthetic tragedy.

Fall in blood pressure, cardiac arrhythmia[38], hypoxia, hypercardia and cardiovascular collapse could all be the result of gas embolism and unless the diagnosis is made the true incidence cannot be a matter of record. A differential diagnosis must be made between a gas embolism and a vagal reflex, hypercarbia and haemorrhage[38–42].

Origin of venous gas embolism

Gas can enter the venous circulation in numerous ways[43]. The neurosurgeon was the first to recognize the danger, and the use of the Doppler became standard practice whenever a neurosurgical procedure was performed in a sitting position[44]. When an incision is above the level of the heart, negative pressure within the veins can result in air entering the venous circulation. In addition the large sinuses created during craniotomy provide access of air to the venous circulation. Air emboli have been reported in a multitude of procedures when air or gas is used such as in open heart surgery, renal dialysis, therapeutic pneumothorax, pneumoencephalography, arteriography, pressurized blood transfusions, epidural catheter placement, main line placement[45], and in the female, during sexual foreplay[46], equipment failure during vacuum abortion, caesarian section, hysteroscopy, thoracic trauma (as during a blast injury) and as a result of positive pressure airway. Thus any procedure that provides continuity between the atmosphere and low-pressure venous circulation can result in a venous embolism. The reverse position of sitting (ie steep Trendelenburg) can result in the pelvic veins being higher than the level of the heart, with the same possibility of venous emboli as when the head is higher than the heart in the sitting position[47–50].

An added source of gas embolism is the use of the gas cooled laser which is frequently used in laparoscopy today. Cases have been reported of gas embolism resulting from the gas-cooled tip of the laser being thrust into the liver bed during cholecystectomy[51–53]. Another reported case occurred as the result of a low-lying liver being entered by a Verres needle during insufflation of the abdomen. The liver was in this position as a result of the downward position of the diaphragm due to chronic obstructive lung disease and emphysema[54].

Gas can enter the venous circulation by inadvertent placement of the Verres needle in a vein and in the liver. More commonly a rent in a vein caused by the Verres needle or trocar can give the insufflation gas access to the low-pressure circulation. As the gas distends the abdomen, the increased pressure will exceed the pressure within the veins and the pressure gradient can result in gas entering the venous circulation. The Venturi Principle can also explain venous gas embolism[55]. As the pressure is increased within the peritoneal cavity, partial collapse of the thin walled abdominal venous circulation results. As the diameter of the veins narrows, the flow rate through the veins increases in order to maintain cardiac return. This faster flow through the vein (pipe) results in gas being sucked in from the peritoneal cavity through any rent in the vein wall.

Origin of arterial gas embolism

With regard to venous gas embolism, the lung has always been seen as a barrier between the venous and arterial circulation. Gas entering the venous circulation often remains trapped in the liver and is then released in a large volume to the vena cava and the right heart. In the right heart, if the volume is small, it may pass through the heart into the pulmonary bed without being recognized. When a large amount of air mixes with blood in the right heart, it forms a frothy mixture which can result in right sided heart failure as a result of the heart's failure to pump the frothy mixture out of the right atrium. When positive pressure is put on the airway, eg during resuscitation and when drugs are given to increase the contractile force of the heart, it is possible that the right atrium pressure will exceed the left atrium pressure, and in 30% of the population the foramen ovale will open and permit gas to enter the left heart[56]. The paradoxic flow will result in gas entering the brain, resulting in coma, delayed awakening or neurological deficit. If the gas embolism enters the coronary circulation, arrhythmia can occur (usually ventricular) and may even result in myocardial infarction and death. Arterial gas embolism can only be treated in a hyperbaric chamber. Under increased atmospheric pressure the emboli can be forced back into the plasma, followed by slow decompression as in the treatment of the bends. Unfortunately the availability of a hyperbaric chamber is rare. However, McGrath *et al.*[57] described a successful result in a 38-year-old female undergoing laparoscopy and hysterectomy who developed a gas embolism resulting in neurological damage. Although 140 minutes had elapsed since surgery, she was transported to a hyperbaric chamber and underwent compression to 3 atmospheres for 30 minutes and then 2.5 atmospheres for 60 minutes. The patient was eventually discharged with no neurological deficit.

Although arterial embolization most commonly occurs through the potentially foramen ovale patent in 30% of the population, it can also occur as a result of gas passing through the lungs as minute bubbles that then come together to form the larger and more dangerous bubbles[58].

In 1991, Black *et al.*[59] reported a fatal paradoxic air embolism in the absence of an intracardiac defect. This was attributed to pulmonary fibrosis concomitant with severe pulmonary arterial hypertension. Air may pass across the pulmonary capillary bed or through pulmonary arteriovenous shunts in the lung which are not grossly or microscopically appreciable using standard methods.

Choice of anaesthetic techniques for laparoscopy

There are three traditional types of anaesthesia: general, regional and local. However, frequently 'local' is used to describe a technique in which potent narcotics and other depressant and amnesiac drugs are used. Once such drugs have been given intravenously, for example, it is an error to classify the technique as local. Therefore a fourth technique should be described: conscious sedation. Although the most common use of such drugs is intravenously, it is possible to administer conscious sedation by the rectal or intramuscular routes.

When a general anaesthetic is administered using inhalation agents, the target organ of the Forane, Halothane or Ethrane is the central nervous system. In order to reach the central nervous system, the agents must cross through the pulmonary alveolar walls to the pulmonary circulation and hence to the brain. When potent intravenous drugs are given, the agents bypass the lungs and reach the central nervous system directly via the circulation. Although agents vary in their physiological action on the central nervous system, the target organ is the same. The difference is in the route of administration. The estimated 160 Versed deaths is grim testimony to the danger of the intravenous route when the method, dosage and action of these drugs are not fully understood by the person administering them. While all recognize that general or regional anaesthesia must be administered by trained and credentialled anaesthesia providers, the fact that lethal drugs can be given intravenously – thus bypassing the conventional lung route – is not universally appreciated.

Millions of tubal ligations have been performed throughout the world using local anaesthetics. The time required to perform these procedures is in the order of 10–15 minutes. Nevertheless, the fact that conditions in some areas of the world necessitate the use of only local anaesthesia does not mean that it is the best and safest method[60,61]. 3000 such procedures were reported in an article from Baylor University in Texas[62]. However, the article mentions the use of Versed and Fentanyl. Therefore it is not accurate to say that the procedure was performed under 'local' anaesthetic.

The choice of anaesthetic techniques should be based upon the operation proposed, the estimated time required by the surgeon to complete the operation, the patient's physical condition, and the required and available recovery times (outpatient surgery).

The technique of choice of most anaesthetists is general endotracheal anaesthesia even when performed on an outpatient basis. In expert hands, the often-described trauma of intubation is minimal or non-existent. The routine use of an oximeter is an indication of adequate oxygenation while the end-tidal PCO_2 monitor confirms the placement of the endotracheal tube in the trachea. The chest stethoscope verifies the placement of the endotracheal tube above the carina. The proper inflation of the balloon protects the airway from aspiration while making controlled ventilation with the resultant control of hypercarbia safe and efficient. The technique of using a mask combined with some muscle relaxation and spontaneous respiration is to be discouraged.

After intubation, a Levin tube should be passed to evacuate any gastric contents and decompress air that may have entered the stomach during preoxygenation and intubation. Without this simple exercise it is possible for a trocar to perforate a low-lying inflated stomach or for gastric juice to be silently regurgitated during the procedure, especially in the required head-down position. The general endotracheal intubation will provide a method to counterbalance physiologic effects of the diaphragm which is elevated by the pneumoperitoneum and by abdominal contents pressing on the diaphragm in the head-down position. Hypercarbia, as evidenced by an elevated end-tidal PCO_2, can be quickly corrected by a change in rate or tidal volume through adjustments of the ventilator[63,64].

The agents available today can consist of short-acting induction agents such as Diprivan[63]. Intubation can follow the use of extremely short-acting non-depolarizing muscle relaxants, thus eliminating the use of succinylcholine and the postoperative complaint of muscle aches. Maintenance can be by potent intravenous narcotics combined with other intravenous agents[65], such as Versed or Diprivan. Low concentration of Forane combined with intravenous agents can result in rapid awakening and recovery. Narcotics and muscle relaxants can be reversed and now Versed can also be reversed[66,67].

While N_2O has been recently implicated in postoperative nausea, it is suggested that, if used, it be turned off early in the case in an attempt to prevent bowel distension. It should also be discontinued if venous air embolism (VAE) is suspected.

However, if a procedure is expected to take many hours on an inpatient basis, the use of expensive shortacting drugs is not necessary. The use of pancuronium, for example, with an inhalation agent such as Ethrane supplemented by lesser quantities of intravenous narcotics, would be perfectly in order and much less expensive. In other words, the anaesthesia can be tailored to the requirements of the procedure, to the patient and the facility.

Regional anaesthesia, epidural and spinal

Regional anaesthesia (epidural and spinal) is not as commonly used in the 60% of all surgery which is now performed in the USA on an outpatient basis. In some procedures, such as knee arthroscopy or hernia repair, some anaesthetists use regional anaesthesia carefully titrating the dosage to assure early discharge. The set-up time for regional is longer than for general anaesthesia, and recovery is not as predictable.

Epidural or spinal anaesthesia would require a level in upper abdominal laparoscopy surgery that would result in a sympathetic blockade as well as the need for sedation. The patient may experience discomfort from the pneumoperitoneum and the need for a Levin tube is still present.

Local anaesthesia

Spielman *et al.*[68], discussing local anaesthesia for laparoscopy, stated that numerous drugs and drug combinations have served to supplement local anaesthesia and that the administration of drugs in appropriate doses with proper patient monitoring is most important[69]. As previously discussed, when local anaesthetics are combined with potent narcotics and sedatives, the anaesthesia is not local, but local plus i.v. conscious sedation. There is no question that local anaesthesia offers many advantages including:

- reduced anaesthesia time
- faster postoperative recovery
- less nausea and vomiting
- fewer postoperative complications
- lower costs.

Disadvantages to local anaesthesia include:

- patient discomfort
- anxiety
- delayed treatment of certain complications (eg haemorrhage or organ perforation)
- necessity to explain procedure during operation
- increased risk from electrical system if the patient moves or breathes deeply during cautery
- finally, inability to control respiration if hypercarbia develops[70].

The procedure proposed must be taken into consideration when local anaesthesia is used. It is possible to do a tubal ligation, D & C, hysteroscopy and even uterine ablation under local with careful sedation of the patient. When i.v. drugs are used, the procedures can be performed more easily. However, the use of these drugs classifies the procedure not as local but as intravenous conscious sedation, which means that the drug is titrated so that the patient retains control of the airway and cough reflex and responds to verbal commands. The danger is an overdose or relative overdose of the drug which places the patient into deep sedation when reflexes are lost. In the New Jersey regulations, monitoring for i.v. conscious sedation requires the use of an EKG, oximeter, chest stethoscope, and the monitoring of blood pressure and even temperature[71]. Whenever there is the possibility of drugs that can cause loss of reflex, anaesthesia and sedation often become indistinguishable.

Monitoring

During laparoscopy, as in the case of malignant hyperthermia, the earlier the diagnosis of a VAE the better the chance of survival. In the case of malignant hyperthermia, the American Society of Anesthesiologists recommends that temperature monitoring is available. In New Jersey, temperature monitoring is mandatory by state regulations whenever an anaesthetic is administered, and therefore a malignant hyperthermia (MH) would be recognized earlier[71].

The early recognition of a VAE is determined by the ability of the monitor to identify the smallest of gas bubbles that have entered the venous circulation. While small volumes are not lethal and do not even cause symptoms, early recognition alerts the anaesthetist and action can be taken to find the source of the gas or to decompress the pneumoperitoneum.

TEE

The most sophisticated monitor is the TEE, which is capable of identifying a gas bubble less than 0.2 cc in size. Currently anaesthetists use this instrument only during cardiac anaesthesia[72]. The number of anaesthetists knowledgeable in its use is minimal. However, there have recently been TEE workshops sponsored by the American Society of Anesthesiologists.

Doppler monitor

The Doppler monitor is based on a principle of physics first described by Doppler in the 1840s. It explains why the pitch of a train whistle changes as it approaches and then leaves an observer[73,74].

Neurosurgeons have long used the Doppler for monitoring patients during procedures performed in the sitting position. (Incidentally, a great amount of our present knowledge on the identification and treatment of venous air embolisms comes from anaesthetists who specialize in neurological anaesthesia.) The microphone of this relatively simple and inexpensive monitor is placed to the right of the sternum, usually between the third and fourth ribs. The best position can be found by injecting saline or even a few cubic centimetres of air into a vein and listening for the maximum 'whooshing' sound as the saline or air passes through the right atrium.

It has been predicted that, as TEE instrumentation is miniaturized and simplified in the next 10 years, TEE and the Doppler will become the standard of care during procedures in which VAE is a possibility. In the USA, at least, such monitoring is known to the trial lawyers. The use of a Doppler does not preclude the routine use of a chest stethoscope taped to the left chest. While an oesophageal stethoscope or a chest stethoscope placed on the right chest in place of a Doppler is used by many, its efficiency for early recognition is low.

End-tidal PCO$_2$ monitor

The end-tidal PCO$_2$ monitor ranks just below the TEE and the Doppler in its ability to identify early VAE. When a VAE reaches the lungs, having passed through the right heart, there is interference of gas exchange across the alveolar membranes. End-tidal PCO$_2$ suddenly drops because CO$_2$ is not crossing into the alvoli and being expired. A sudden drop of end-tidal PCO$_2$ during laparoscopy is a good indication of VAE. However, by this time the VAE has reached the pulmonary circulation, and the warning is later than the TEE or Doppler could have provided[75].

Other monitors

The oximeter is a late warning monitor when it comes to identifying VAE. While PCO$_2$ will drop early, the oxygen reserve in the body will result in a normal oximeter reading for two or three minutes. Although the oximeter has proved itself in the USA and is a standard of care, often regulated into use, it is a late warning monitor in the case of VAE.

Blood pressure monitors today are most commonly automatic and will document the blockage created by a gas embolism trapped in the right heart. With decreased cardiac return, there will be a decrease in cardiac output and blood pressure will fall.

The EKG monitor, again, is a standard of care in anaesthesia monitoring. In the case of paradoxic emboli, in which emboli reach the coronary circulation, ventricular arrhythmias are the ones seen most commonly. The EKG is also of value in monitoring how long it takes to create the pneumoperitoneum. Stretching of the peritoneum can lead to reflex brachycardia due to vagal stimulation.

Central venous pressure monitoring is not routine during most laparoscopic procedures. It is not used during tubal ligation or other abdominal procedures, including cholecystectomy; yet central venous pressure will rise when the VAE reaches the right atrium. The use of a main line has been discussed as a method of aspirating air from the right heart which may be life-saving. As longer and more complicated procedures are attempted through the laparoscope, it is possible that a main line will be routinely inserted. Early in the learning curve of a surgeon whose first hysterectomies may require eight hours of operating time, it may be wise to insert a main line.

Treatment of VAE

Prevention of VAE is the primary method of treatment of VAE. Early recognition by the use of high-tech monitors can avert a tragedy. Once VAE is recognized, immediate steps should be taken to identify the source[75].

The pneumoperitoneum should be reduced and exploration through the scope for a lacerated vessel should be undertaken. As the pressure within the peritoneum is reduced, the vessels will bleed and can be ligated or repaired. Since the Doppler or TEE will identify minute and non-life threatening VAE early, the customary methods of treating massive VAE need not necessarily be instituted at this time.

Once massive VAE is identified as a result of the use of less sensitive monitors such as the chest stethoscope, a fall in end-tidal PCO_2, or oxygen saturation, then immediate efforts to treat the condition must be instituted. Remember that the success of the treatment is directly related to the volume of the VAE and also the time factor. It has been shown that VAE in small volumes over a long period of time will result in minimal or no damage.

The same volume over a short period of time can be lethal. In many cases the treatments are theoretical in that, for example, aspiration of the VAE through a central venous line has been shown to be difficult and not always successful. In some cases the prescribed treatment such as positive pressure ventilation or drugs that will increase the contractile force of the myocardium will result in the frothing mass of gas and blood being forced out of the right atrium into the right ventricle and into the pulmonary circulation with resultant interference, not only of elimination of CO_2, but also of obstruction of the oxygen transfer across the alveoli, resulting in hypoxia.

Aspiration of gas

The placement of a main line into the right heart is a controversial treatment because of its questionable success rate[75]. During most gynaecological surgical procedures in which a pneumoperitoneum is created, the placement of a main line is not routine. When an anaesthetist makes the diagnosis of VAE, therefore, the main line must be placed under emergency conditions, with its risk of haemorrhage and pneumothorax, with the patient draped and theoretically turned on the left side in the Durand position.

A standard CVP line is inadequate with regard to the volume of gas that can be aspirated when placed at the junction of the superior vena cava and the right atrium. The single lumen catheter returns 16% of the VAE while the multiorifice catheter, placed at the same location, successfully aspirates 60% of the VAE. Using the central venous port of a pulmonary artery catheter, the return is 4%. The key to successful aspiration is the properly placed and properly selected catheter[76]. A multi-orifice catheter should be kept in the emergency crash cart. The downside of the story is that a VAE can reach the pulmonary arterial circulation in a few heartbeats assisted by the ionotropic drugs and positive end expiratory pressure (PEEP) given early in the treatment. This is the damaging location that cannot be reached by a catheter for aspiration; thus the timing is crucial. If the catheter is in place and in position, then aspiration is feasible. If the catheter is not in place, and the patient is given ionotropic drugs and PEEP while the insertion of the catheter is attempted, the VAE will probably reach the pulmonary arterial circulation.

Patient positioning

There is universal agreement, according to Lucas[75], that the gradient between the wound and the right heart in situations of VAE should be decreased. Therefore the patient should be placed with the heart elevated in the case of abdominal laparoscopic surgery[69]. As venous pressure rises due to the right atrial obstruction, there will be increased venous bleeding and a decrease in the further entrainment of air. Durand recommended the left lateral decubitus position to prevent an 'airlock' phenomenon and to keep the air in the right atrium, thus allowing a flow of blood into the right ventricle based on the flow of gravity when the patient is tilted head-up. However, this position may jeopardize and delay other treatment options[77].

Positive end expiratory pressure

The purpose of increased airway pressure is to reduce the gradient between the point of gas entrainment and the right atrium. If venous pressure can be increased, gas entrainment will be stopped or significantly reduced. PEEP produces increased airway pressure which is transmitted to the thoracic cavity, heart and intrathoracic vasculature, resulting in increased venous pressure. This in turn can decrease cardiac output which, in the case of hypotension due to massive gas embolism, further lowers the blood pressure. In addition, the increase in PEEP may result in producing paradoxic air embolism. As already mentioned, approximately 30% of the population have a probe patent foramen ovale. An increase in right over left atrial pressure can result in a paradoxic gas embolism with gas passing from the right to the left atrium. The use of PEEP has its advocates and its opponents. Perkins and Bedford have shown the incidence of Doppler detected air embolism without PEEP to be 36%[78] compared with the 51% of Doppler-detected VAE reported by Voorhees[79] who felt that, although the chances of paradoxic air embolism may be increased with PEEP, the overall decreased incidence of VAE more than offsets the theoretical disadvantage[80].

Nitrous oxide

When the diagnosis of VAE is made, N_2O (if in use) should be discontinued, to prevent the size of the gas emboli from increasing due to the solubility of N_2O. 100% oxygen should be used.

Other anaesthetic considerations

Neurological damage

The incidence of neurological damage in patients undergoing all types of surgery is surprisingly high. Many injuries are related to the upper extremities. In laparoscopic surgery, the arm extended on the armboard may be pushed upwards by assistants or the operating surgeon resulting in brachial plexus damage. The Trendelenburg position adds to this risk. The arm, kept at the side, must be cushioned against contact with the metal of the operating table with resultant ulnar nerve damage.

Subcutaneous emphysema[81]

When the Verres needle is inserted superficially, gas may dissect in all directions resulting in subcutaneous emphysema evidenced by crepitation on palpation[33]. Gas may dissect upwards to the neck and even to the face. This condition resolves itself through absorption of the gas. Pressure in the neck, however, if allowed to build up, could present an airway problem and should be watched carefully.

Postoperative recovery

The anaesthetist's responsibility does not end with the transfer of the patient to the PACU. The extent of the surgery will determine the patient's postoperative needs. Nausea and vomiting is the most common complaint seen after pneumoperitoneum[82]. The wide variety of drugs on the market is testimony to the lack of success of any of them to cure the problem. Patients who have undergone same-day procedures must be ready to go home that day. During the last hour of surgery, early treatment of pain by the administration of long-acting non-narcotic agents and anti-emetic agents will expedite early discharge. If patients are still in severe pain, it is a good policy to treat the patient early with 3 mg dosages of morphine intravenously. The patient will go back to sleep, then awake in less pain, and discharge will not be delayed.

In procedures that require overnight admission, the age and physical status of the patients will vary from young healthy women (upon whom the early statistics on mortality and morbidity were based) to the higher-risk elderly patients who are now undergoing laparoscopic surgery for a multitude of indications. This latter group will eventually provide the updated data on mortality and morbidity.

Monitoring in the PACU should consist of EKG, oximetry, automated blood pressure and temperature monitoring. In New Jersey, by regulation, end-tidal PCO_2 must be available for any patient who is brought to the operating room on a ventilator[70].

Conclusion

Laparoscopic surgery shortens the recovery period, makes procedures less invasive due to the small incisions required, possibly decreases the cost and is cosmetically more acceptable to the patients; however, it also adds to the inherent risks of the procedure and the anaesthesia involved. The anaesthetists must be alert for VAE and quick to treat it. Haemorrhage is the most common complication of the technique, caused by the insertion of the trocars needed to position the instruments. When lasers are used, burns have been reported, sometimes resulting from the igniting of drapes. The adequate credentialling of surgeons must be in place and the operating room team must be trained in the use and care of sophisticated and expensive instruments. When lasers are used, extra personnel are needed, one of whom should be assigned specifically to the laser equipment. There is no question that the technique is here to stay and that more and more procedures will be performed through the laparoscope. The anaesthetist must recognize the physiology involved in the creation of the pneumoperitoneum and the danger of gas emboli. As an increasing number of procedures are performed in the sameday surgery facility, the anaesthetic drugs used should be tailored to the requirement of discharge within hours of surgery.

References

1   Horwits ST (1972) Laparoscopy in gynecology. *Obstetrics and Gynecological Survey.* **27**:1.

2   Ohlegesser M *et al.* (1985) Gynecologic laproscopy, a review article. *Obstetrics and Gynecological Survey.* **40**:385–96.

3   Steiner OP (1924) Abdominoscopy. *Surgery in Gynecology and Obstetrics.* **28**:266.

4   Nadeau OE and Kampmeir OF (1925) Endoscopy of the abdomen. *Abdominoscopy.* **41**:624.

5   Short AR (1925) The use of celioscopy. *British Medical Journal.* **2**:254.

6   Decker A and Cherry T (1944) Culdoscopy: a new method in the diagnosis of pelvic disease. *American Journal of Surgery.* **64**:40.

7   Haiken BN (1991) Laser laparoscopic cholecystectomy in the ambulatory setting. *Journal of Post-Anesthesia Nursing.* **6**:33–9.

8   Salky BA *et al.* (1991) Laparoscopic cholecystectomy: an initial report. *Gastrointestinal Endoscopy.* **37**:

9   Smith BE (1985) Anesthetic emergencies, clinical obstetrics, and gynecology. **28**: No.2, June.

10   American Medical Association (1992) *American Medical News.* **4 May**:1.

11   (1991) *New England Journal of Medicine.*

12 Meyer H (1992) *American Medical News*. **1 June**.

13 de Grood PM *et al.* (1987) Anaesthesia for laparoscopy. A comparison of five techniques including propofol, etomidate, thiopentone, and isoflurane. *Anaesthesia*. **42**:815–23.

14 Brainbridge WS (1913) Techniques of the intraabdominal administration of oxygen. *American Journal of Surgery*. **27**:364.

15 Chaturachinda K (1973) Laparoscopic sterilization: an outpatient procedure. *American Journal of Obstetrics and Gynecology*. **115**:487.

16 Marlow J (1974) Creation of pneumoperitoneum and trocar insertion. In Phillips JM and Keith L (eds) *Gynecological laparoscopy*. Symposia Specialists, Miami. pp.101–15.

17 Carron Brown JA *et al.* (1978) Gynaecological laparoscopy. The report of the working part of the confidential enquiry into gynaecological laparoscopy. Conducted by The Royal College of Obstetricians and Gynaecologists, 1978.

18 Palmer R (1974) Security in laparoscopy. In Phillips JM and Keith L (eds) *Gynecological laparoscopy*. Symposia Specialists, Miami. pp.17–26.

19 Diamant M *et al.* (1977) Laparoscopic sterilization with local anaesthesia; complications and blood gases changes. *Anesthesia and Analgesia*. **56**:334.

20 Cohen MR (1982) Gynecologic laparoscopy. In Sciarra JJ (ed.) *Gynecology and Obstetrics*. Harper & Row, Hagerstown.

21 Soderstrom RM (1976) Danger of nitrous oxide pneumoperitoneum. *American Journal of Obstetrics and Gynecology*. **124**:668.

22 Robinson JS *et al.* (1975) Laparoscopy explosion hazards with nitrous oxide. *British Medical Journal*. **3**:764.

23 Robinson JS *et al.* (1979) Fire and explosion hazards in operating theatres: a replay and new evidence. *British Journal of Anaesthesia*. **51**:908.

24 Edwards RG *et al.* (1980) Establishing full term human pregnancies using cleaving embryos growing in vitro. *British Journal of Obstetrics and Gynaecology*. **87**:737.

25 Marshall RL *et al.* (1972) Circulatory effects of carbon dioxide insufflation of the peritoneal cavity for laparoscopy. *British Journal of Anaesthesia*. **44**:68.

26 Ivanovich AD *et al.* (1975) Cardiovascular effects of intraperitoneal insufflation with carbon dioxide and nitrous oxide in dogs. *Anaesthesiology*. **42**:281.

27 Scott B and Julian DG (1972) Observations on cardiac arrhythmias during laparoscopy. *British Medical Journal*. **1**:411.

28 Smith I *et al.* (1971) Cardiovascular effects of peritoneal insufflation of carbon dioxide for laparoscopy. *British Medical Journal*. **3**:410.

29 Alexander GD and Brown EM (1969) Physiological alterations during pelvic laparoscopy. *American Journal of Obstetrics and Gynecology.* **105**:1078.

30 Alexander TD *et al.* (1969) Anesthesia for pelvic laparoscopy. *Anesthesia and Analgesia.* **48**:14.

31 Fear RE (1968) Laparoscopy, a valuable aid in gynecologic diagnosis. *Obstetrics and Gynecology.* **31**:297.

32 Balin H *et al.* (1966) Recent advance in pelvic endoscopy. *Obstetrics and Gynecology.* **27**:30.

33 Vilardell F *et al.* (1968) Complications of peritoneoscopy. A survey of 1455 examinations. *Gastrointestinal Endoscopy.* **14**:178.

34 Peterson HB *et al.* (1983) Deaths attributable to tubal sterilization in the United States 1977 to 1981. *American Journal of Obstetrics and Gynecology.* **146**:131.

35 Fong J *et al.* (1990) Are Doppler-detected venous emboli during cesarean section air emboli? *Anesthesia and Analgesia.* **71**:254–7.

36 Matthews NC *et al.* (1990) Forum-embolism during cesarean section. *Anaesthesia.* **45**:964–5.

37 Symons NL, Leaver HK (1985) Air embolism during craniotomy in the seated position: a comparison of methods for detection. *Canadian Anaesthetists Society Journal.* **32**:174–7.

38 Harris MN *et al.* (1984) Cardiac arrhythmias during anaesthesia for laparoscopy. *British Journal of Anaesthesia.* **56**:1213–17.

39 Carmichael DE (1971) Laparoscopy — cardiac considerations. *Fertility and Sterility.* **22**:690.

40 Ostman PL *et al.* (1990) Circulatory collapse during laparoscopy. *Journal of Clinical Anesthesia.* **2**:129–32.

41 Williams EL *et al.* (1991) Sudden cardiac arrest during epidural anesthesia: venous air embolism? *Anesthesiology.* **71**:1171.

42 Myles PS (1991) Bradyarrhythmias and laparoscopy: a prospective study of heart rate changes with laparoscopy. *Australian and New Zealand Journal of Obstetrics and Gynaecology.* **31**:171–3.

43 Vacanti CA and Lodhia KL (1991) Fatal massive air embolism during transurethral resection of the prostate. *Anesthesiology.* **74**:186–7.

44 Matjasko J *et al.* (1985) Anesthesia and surgery in the seated position: analysis of 554 cases. *Journal of Neurosurgery.* **17**:695–702.

45 Dilkes MG *et al.* (1991) A case of intracerebral air embolism secondary to the insertion of a Hickman Line. *Journal of Parenteral and Enteral Nutrition.* **15**:488–90.

46 Eckert WG *et al.* (1991) The unusual accidental death of a pregnant woman by sexual foreplay. *American Journal of Forensic Medicine and Pathology.* **12**:24–9.

47 de Plater RM and Jones IS (1989) Non-fatal carbon dioxide embolism during laparoscopy. *Anaesthesia and Intensive Care.* **17**:359–61.

48 Sadan O *et al.* (1991) Air embolism due to pulmonary barotrauma in a patient undergoing cesarean section. *Acta Obstetricia et Gynecologica Scandinavica.* **70**:511–13.

49 Bradfield ST (1991) Gas embolism during laparoscopy (Letter.) *Anaesthesia and Intensive Care.* **19**:474.

50 Davies JM and Armstrong JN (1990) Fatal embolism (Letter.) *Canadian Journal of Anaesthesia.* **37**:709.

51 Greville AC *et al.* (1991) Pulmonary air embolism during laparoscopic laser cholecystectomy. *Anaesthesia.* **46**:113–14.

52 Baggish MS and Daniell JF (1989) Catastrophic injury secondary to the use of coaxial gas-cooled fibers and artificial sapphire tips for intrauterine surgery. *Lasers in Surgery and Medicine.* **9**:581–4.

53 FDA (1990) Warning gas embolism. *Journal of the American Medical Association.* **264**.

54 Bradfield ST (1991) Gas embolism during laparoscopy. *Anaesthesia and Intensive Care.* **19**:474.

55 Wadhwa RK and McKenzie R (1978) Gas embolism during laparoscopy. *Anesthesiology.* **48**:74.

56 Gottdiener J *et al.* (1968) Incidence and cardiac effects of systemic venous air embolism. *Archives of Internal Medicine.* **184**:795–800.

57 McGrath BJ *et al.* (1989) Carbon dioxide embolism treated with hyperbaric oxygen [see comments]. *Canadian Journal of Anaesthesia.* **36**:586–9.

58 Layon AJ (1991) Hyperbaric oxygen treatment for cerebral air embolism — where are the data? (Editorial.) *Mayo Clinic Proceedings.* **66**:641–6.

59 Black M *et al.* (1991) Paradox air embolism in the absence of an intracardiac defect.

60 Gordon AG (1984) Laparoscopy under local anaesthesia. (Editorial.) *Journal of the Royal Society of Medicine.* **77**:540–1.

61 Peterson HB *et al.* (1987) Local versus general anesthesia for laparoscopic sterilization: a randomized study. *Obstetrics and Gynecology.* **70**:903–8.

62 Poindexter AN *et al.* (1990) Laparoscopic tubal sterilization under local obstetrical gynecology. **75**.

63 Johannsen G *et al.* (1989) The effect of general anaesthesia on the haemodynamic events during laparoscopy with CO_2 insufflation. *Acta Anaesthesiologica Scandinavica.* **33**:132–6.

64 Versichelen L *et al.* (1984) Physiopathologic changes during anesthesia administration for gynecologic laparoscopy. *Journal of Reproductive Medicine.* **29**.

65 Cummings GC *et al.* (1984) Dose requirements of ICI 35868 (Propofol, 'Diprivan') in a new formulation for induction of anaesthesia. *Anaesthesia.* **39**:1168–71.

66 Marco AP *et al.* (1990) Anesthesia for a patient undergoing laparoscopic cholecystectomy. *Anesthesiology.* **73**:1268–70.

67 de Grood PM *et al.* (1987) Anaesthesia for laparoscopy. A comparison of five techniques including propofol, etomidate, thiopentone, and isoflurane. *Anaesthesia.* **42**:815–23.

68 Spielman *et al.* (1987) Local versus general anesthesia for laparoscopic tubal sterilization. A randomized study. *Obstetrics and Gynecology.*

69 Fong J *et al.* (1991) Venous emboli occurring during cesarean section: the effects of patient position. *Canadian Journal of Anaesthesia.* **38**:191–5.

70 Keith L *et al.* (1974) Anesthesia for laparoscopy. In Phillips JM and Keith L (eds) *Gynecological laparoscopy.* Symposia Specialists, Miami. pp.91–100.

71 New Jersey Register, *N.J.A.C.,* 8:43G–63(g) 10/15/91.

72 Marcus RH *et al.* (1991) Venous air embolism diagnosis by spontaneous right-sided contrast echocardiography chest. **99**:784–5.

73 Edmonds-Sea J and Maroon JC (1969) Air embolism diagnosed with ultrasound: a new monitoring technique. *Anaesthesia.* **24**:438–40.

74 Fong J *et al.* (1990) Are Doppler-detected venous emboli during cesaraean section air emboli? *Anesthesia and Analgesia.* **71**:254–7.

75 Lucas WD (1987) How to manage air embolism problems in anesthesia. **1**.

76 Hanna PG (1991) In vitro comparison of central venous catheters for aspiration of VAE. *Journal of Clinical Anesthesia.* **3**:290.

77 Gomar C *et al.* (1985) Carbon dioxide embolism during laparoscopy and hysteroscopy. *Annales Francaises d'Anesthesie Reanimation.* **4**:380–2.

78 Perkins-Pearson N *et al.* (1982) Atrial pressures in the seated position. *Anesthesiology.* **57**:493.

79 Perkins NAK *et al.* (1989) Hemodynamic consequences of PEEP in seated neurological patients. *Anesthesiology and Analgesia.* **63**:429.

80 Lucas WJ (1987) How to manage air embolism. *Problems in Anesthesia.* **1**.

81 Mumford ST *et al.* (1980) Laparoscopic and minilaparotomy female sterilization compared in 15,176 cases. *Lancet* **ii**:1066.

82 Hovorka J *et al.* (1983) Recovery after general anesthesia for laparoscopy. *Acta Anaesthesiologica Scandinavica.* **23**:396.

8

Non-Gynaecological Complications of Laparoscopy

CARLOS A. SUAREZ

Introduction

Laparoscopy can be considered to be a safe procedure. In large surveys, rates of major and minor complications are reported to be about 1%, while mortality rates are around 0.03–0.49% (Table 8.1)[1].

Reports	Total procedures	Complications		Mortality
		Minor	Major	
Dallas,1976–1983[2]	603	31 (5.1%)	14 (2.3%)	3 (0.49%)
Literature[27]	63 845	590 (1.0%)	174 (0.3%)	18 (0.03%)
p value		<0.01	<0.01	

Table 8.1: Frequency of complications of laparoscopy.

Every surgeon performing operative laparoscopy must strive to offer his or her patients the safest and most effective procedure possible, by becoming thoroughly familiar with the possible dangers and pitfalls and thereby minimizing them.

A wide array of complications associated with laparoscopy have been described, although most of these fortunately do not result in serious or life-threatening conditions[2]. However, for any patient who suffers a major complication, the effects can be devastating.

The following review will describe the complications that can occur during the course of a laparoscopic procedure and demonstrate methods of repair to damaged tissue or how to avoid pitfalls which may lead to potentially serious consequences (Tables 8.2–8.4).

Type of complication	No.
Minor	
Leakage of ascitic fluid	16
Abdominal wall haematoma	3
Wound dehiscence after suture removal	2
Transient bradycardia and hypotension	2
Severe abdominal pain	2
Transient oliguria	1
Mild decrease in haematocrit (no transfusions)	1
Inadvertent kidney biopsy	1
Cellulitis at trocar insertion site	1
Incisional hernia	1
Transient Ileus	1
Total	31
Major	
Haemorrhage from liver biopsy site	8
Perforation of colon	4
Peritonitis	1
Mistaken diagnosis of infection with gas forming organism	1
Total	14

Table 8.2: Complications of laparoscopy (from Kane and Krejs)[2].

	Rate/1000 cases
Pneumoperitoneum	7.4
Bleeding	6.4
Conversion to laparotomy	5.6
Perforation injuries	2.7
Pregnancy after sterilization	2.5
Electrical complications	2.2
Infection	1.4
Bowel burns	0.5
Cardiac arrest	0.3

Table 8.3: Incidence of complications of laparoscopy (from Phillips)[1].

Haemorrhage

Establishing an adequate pneumoperitoneum is paramount for the safe and successful performance of any laparoscopic procedure. There are many reported cases of serious and/or fatal complications that stem from this seemingly simple step[1-3].

Author	Age of patient	Indication	Offending instrument	Vessel injured	Operation	Outcome
Shin (1982)	23	Diagnostic	P-needle	Aorta	Suture	Survived
Katz (1979)	?	Sterilization	P-needle	Aorta	Suture	Survived
	?	?	Trocar	Common iliac artery & vein	Suture, ligature	Survived
Madrigal (1977)	?	Sterilization	P-needle	Aorta	Suture	Survived
Lynn (1982)	40	Sterilization	Trocar	Aorta	Suture	Survived
McDonald (1978)	32	Sterilization	P-needle	Aorta	Suture	Survived
	21	Diagnostic	P-needle	Aorta, vena cava, common iliac artery		
Heinrich (1985)	?	?	P-needle	Common iliac artery	?	Survived
Lignitz (1985)	29	Diagnostic	P-needle	External iliac artery	Suture	Died
Bisler (1980)	44	Sterilization	?	Common iliac artery & vein	Vein patch	Survived
	42	Sterilization	P-needle	Aorta	Suture	Survived
	36	Sterilization	?	Aorta	Suture	Survived
Rust (1980)	36	Sterilization	P-needle	Aorta, common iliac artery	Suture	Survived
Ekrath (1979)	30	Diagnostic	P-needle	Aorta	Suture	Died
	39	Sterilization	P-needle	Aorta	Suture	Survived

Table 8.4: Published cases of major vessel injury caused by gynaecological laparoscopy (from Baadsgaard *et al.*)[6]

The proper technique is to place the insufflating needle in the free peritoneal space, so that the tip of the needle does not traverse any hollow viscus or retroperitoneal vessel.

Most laparoscopists favour blind passage of the needle for insufflation because it is fast and convenient. However, the procedure must be followed with meticulous care in order to avoid mishaps.

Haemorrhage is the most dreaded complication related to insertion of the insufflating needle or trocar[4-6]. It usually results from perforation or laceration of the aorta or its principal branches, the iliac arteries. The likely mechanism of injury is the insertion of the needle at a near-perpendicular angle to the retroperitoneum. The resulting perforation can be extended to become a laceration by the operator's rocking of the needle shaft. Lacerations no larger than 2–3 mm long can result in rapid and life-threatening bleeding which is poorly contained by the loose tissue surrounding the injured vessel.

The diagnosis of vessel injury is usually made by the patient's rapidly deteriorating vital signs. If a trocar has been inserted, free blood or an enlarging haematoma in the area of the perforation is seen. Once the injury is suspected, an immediate laparotomy should be performed; the vessels proximal and distal to the injury should be exposed, digital pressure should be applied to the perforation and vascular clamps applied to control the haemorrhage (Figure 8.1).

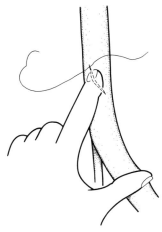

Figure 8.1: Digital control of bleeding vessel. (Reprinted by permission of Williams and Wilkins Co.)[7].

Most injuries caused by needles can be repaired by primary suture[4,6]. Proper vascular technique dictates that the vessel ends should be approximated without tension, while the intimal layers are accurately opposed and securely sutured to prevent dissection and thrombosis of the anastomosis after blood flow has been re-established. Monofilament suture of 4-0 or 5-0 polypropylene is adequate to perform the repair (Figures 8.2–8.4).

If the injury results in significant loss of length of vessel wall, the damaged segment should be resected to healthy tissue and the continuity restored with the appropriate length of autogenous reversed saphenous vein. Care should be taken to handle the vessel wall with fine vascular tissue forceps to avoid intimal damage.

Larger vessels such as the common or external iliac arteries can be repaired with synthetic graft material. Knitted Dacron or expanded polytetrafluoro-ethylene (PTFE) vascular prostheses are used for reconstruction if there is no peritoneal soilage from an associated bowel injury or intra-abdominal abscess (Figure 8.5). Prosthetic materials should not be used if significant contamina-tion of the peritoneal cavity has taken place. In these cases, it may be necessary to ligate the vessel and re-establish blood flow by an extra-anatomical route such as a subcutaneous femoro–femoral crossover graft.

Venous injuries should be repaired primarily whenever possible. However, if the patient's condition is tenuous due to shock of associated conditions, ligation is appropriate. This includes the inferior vena cava below the junctions of the renal veins.

Perforation of the epigastric arteries can be encountered when the needle is inserted lateral to the linea alba. This results in haematoma formation which is usually self-limiting. If persistent bleeding from these vessels is encountered, haemostasis can be obtained by extending the incision enough to expose the artery to ligate it. Alternatively, the bleeding trocar site can be tamponaded by placing a balloon-tip urinary catheter through the sleeve and inflating the balloon. Traction is then applied by pulling the balloon snugly against the

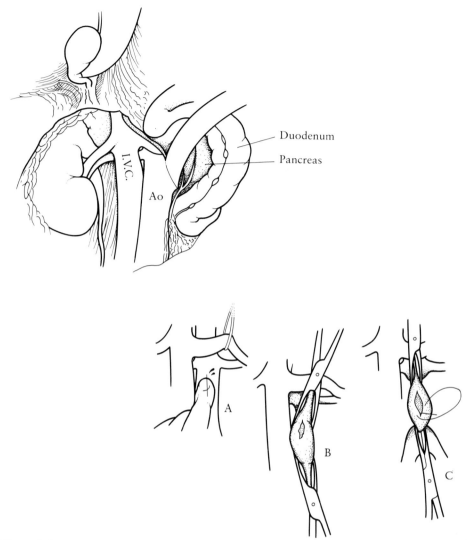

Duodenum

Pancreas

I.V.C.

Ao

A

B

C

Figure 8.2: Primary suture repair of major vascular injury. (Reprinted by permission of Thieme-Stratton Inc.)[8].

abdominal wall. Traction is maintained for eight hours and then removed (Figure 8.6).

Bowel insufflation

It is of the utmost importance that the insufflating needle be aspirated prior to instituting CO_2 flow. If blood or intestinal contents are aspirated, the needle should be withdrawn and repositioned.

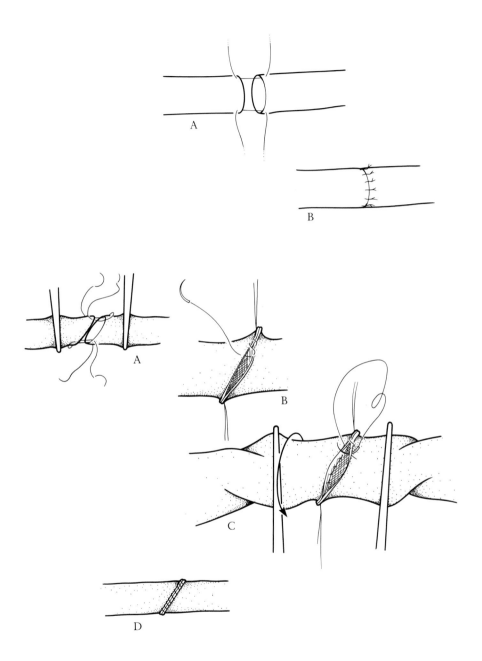

Figure 8.3: Primary interrupted anastomosis, used in repair of smaller vessels to minimize narrowing of the suture line. (Reprinted by permission of Thieme-Stratton Inc.)[8].

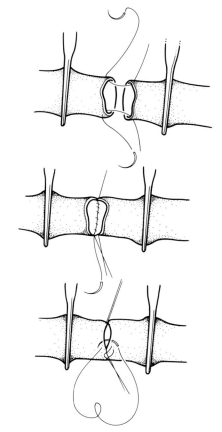

Figure 8.4: Anastomosis of larger vessel with continuous suture. (Reprinted by permission of Thieme-Stratton Inc.)[8].

Insufflation of the bowel can occur if the position of the needle is not tested by aspiration prior to initiating insufflation. If asymmetrical distension of the abdomen is not observed, one should suspect misplacement of the needle into the bowel lumen, and insufflation should be stopped. If the intestine is not insufflated excessively, it may not result in serious injury[9].

Gas embolus

Carbon dioxide gas is less likely to cause fatal embolism than air when it enters the vascular space. This characteristic renders it a safer medium for insufflation, but if too much is injected into the vascular space, the same consequences result as with air embolus[10].

Direct insufflation of gas into the vascular space has been reported, and can lead to severe or even fatal cardiovascular collapse. This complication results from inadvertent introduction of the insufflating needle into a major retroperitoneal vein. If gas embolism is suspected, the insufflator must be

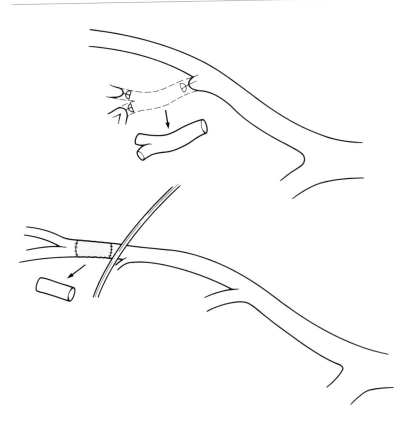

Figure 8.5: Repair of segmental loss of vessel with autogenous segment of vessel (internal iliac artery). (Re-printed by permission of Thieme-Stratton Inc.)[8].

disconnected immediately and the patient placed in a steep Trendelenburg position to allow the gas bubble to float away from the right ventricular outflow tract.

There have been rare cases of insufflation of CO_2 into the portal circulation which have resulted in death due to cardiovascular collapse[11].

Bowel perforation

Any procedure which requires the lysis of adhesions or extensive dissection carries the risk of inadvertent bowel perforation. For this reason it seems reasonable to prepare the patient's bowel preoperatively so that contamination of the surgical field is minimized in the event of perforation.

An adequate bowel preparation can be obtained by the administration of oral polyethylene glycol solution 12 hours prior to the operation. Complete cleansing of the small and large bowel can usually be accomplished with four litres of solution.

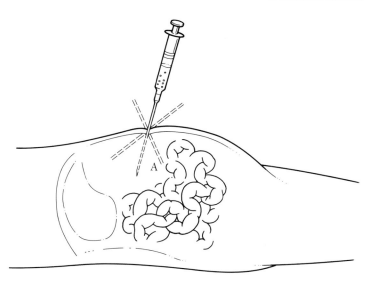

Figure 8.6: Verres needle sounding after insufflation with attached syringe containing saline solution. Detection of gas bubbles indicates that the tip is in the free peritoneal space. (Reprinted by permission of Thieme-Stratton Inc.)[8].

Bowel perforation can also occur from placement of the needle into an area of adhesions. This is more likely if the patient has had previous abdominal surgery or peritonitis. It is a good idea to place the insufflating needle away from scars and instead insufflate the patient in any abdominal quadrant which has not been involved in a previous surgical procedure (Figures 8.7–8.10).

Most bowel perforations due to percutaneous placement of Verres needle do not seem to result in spillage of intestinal contents severe enough to cause peritonitis, but the complication has been described. If the operator suspects that a loop of bowel has been punctured, the area should be inspected for leakage of bowel contents. Then, if a leak is found, the hole can be repaired by endoscopic suture repair or by the creation of a laparotomy incision large enough to eviscerate the loop for direct suture repair. This applies to small as well as large bowel punctures.

Full-thickness, single-layer closure of the repair with a continuous or interrupted 4-0 monofilament suture on an atraumatic intestinal needle is adequate if the repair is watertight (Figure 8.11).

Injuries of the colon which result in significant spillage of faecal matter are best managed by exteriorization of the injury with or without repair and by a proximal diverting colostomy. If the repair breaks down after exteriorization, it simply becomes a loop colostomy. A colostomy closure can be performed four to six weeks later (Figure 8.12).

If the damage to the colonic wall is extensive, it should be resected and the ends re-anastomosed or brought out to the surface of the anterior abdominal wall as a proximal colostomy and mucus fistula (Figures 8.13 and 8.14).

Sigmoid colon injuries can be resected and the proximal end brought out as a left-sided colostomy. The distal rectum is oversewn as a Hartman Pouch.

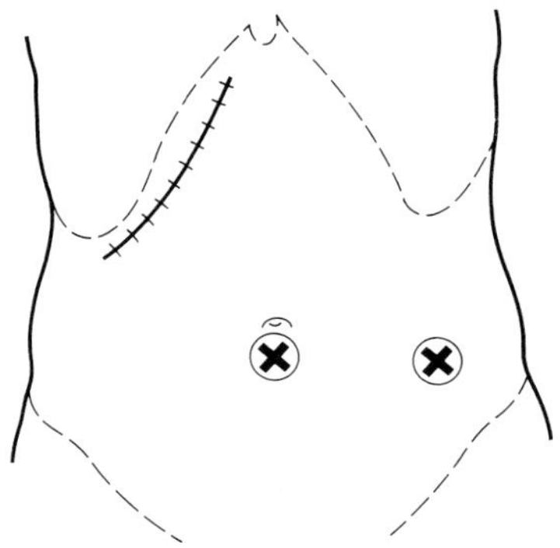

Figure 8.7: Insufflating sites for right upper quadrant scar. (Reprinted by permission of Baillière Tindall)[9].

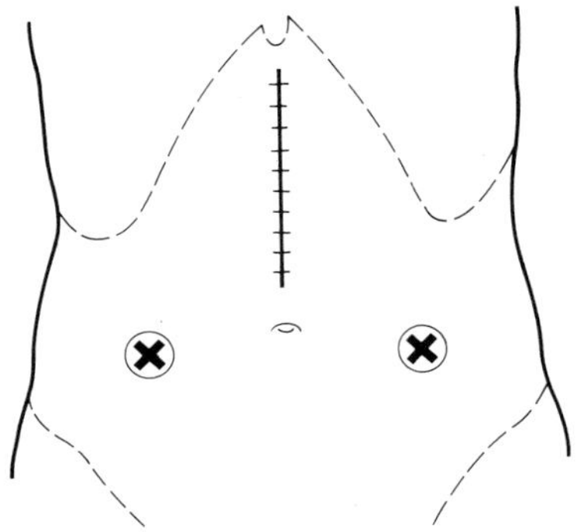

Figure 8.8: Insufflating sites for upper midline scar. (Reprinted by permission of Baillière Tindall)[9].

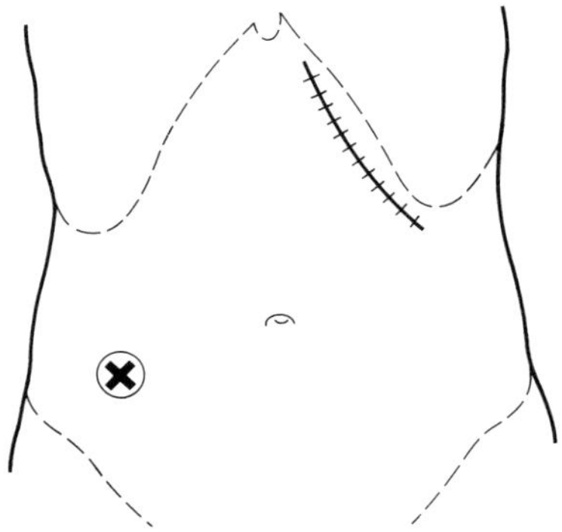

Figure 8.9: Insufflating site for upper left quadrant scar. (Reprinted by permission of Baillière Tindall)[9].

Re-anastomosis is performed several weeks later (Figure 8.15).

Broad-spectrum antibiotics with anaerobic bacterial spectrum should be instituted for one week to minimize the formation of intra-abdominal abscess or disruption of the repair[1,2,12,13].

Over-insufflation

Over-insufflation of the abdominal cavity may occur if the pressure settings of the insufflator have not been checked prior to commencing the procedure. It should be the operator's responsibility to instruct the circulating nurse to set

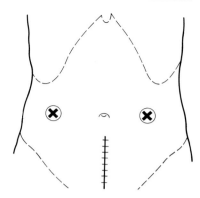

Figure 8.10: Insufflating sites for lower midline scar. (Reprinted by permission of Baillière Tindall)[9]

the desired maximum pressure and the initial rate of insufflation to avoid interference of venous return, which will reduce the cardiac output and make assisted ventilation difficult. This detail is particularly important if the laparoscopy is being conducted with the patient under local anaesthesia.

Most laparoscopists agree that intra-abdominal pressure should be maintained between 15 and 20 mmHg to avoid overdistension. Some patients may respond adversely to this range of pressure, so the procedure may have to be done with the lowest pressure which will still afford adequate exposure.

Numerous reports have appeared in the literature describing the physiological changes that the patient undergoes as a result of an increase of arterial PCO_2. These include hyperventilation, rise in the mean central venous pressure, decrease in the cardiac output and cardiac arrhythmias[14,18].

These changes are well tolerated by otherwise healthy individuals, and when they occur the anaesthesiologist can compensate by controlling the respiratory rate. It should be noted, however, that in elderly patients with pre-existing impairment of cardiac or pulmonary functions, these effects may have serious consequences. For this reason, it is wise to monitor these patients very closely by means of indwelling central venous catheter, arterial blood gases, expiratory CO_2 content and electrocardiography.

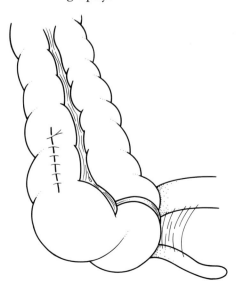

Figure 8.11: Primary suture repair of colon injury. (Reprinted by permission of Thieme-Stratton Inc.)[8].

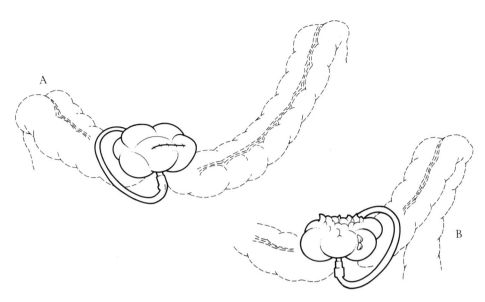

Figure 8.12: Exteriorization of colonic injury, showing site of primary closure (A). (Reprinted by permission of Thieme-Stratton Inc.)[8].

Patients with conditions which result in a reduced intravascular volume, such as intra-abdominal sepsis, are particularly sensitive to decreases in venous return and should be prepared preoperatively with adequate volume replacement.

It is important that there is clear communication between the surgeon and the anaesthesiologist so that any significant changes in the parameters being monitored can be recognized and discussed, and appropriate action taken to correct any abnormality.

Solid visceral injuries

The likelihood of encountering injury to a solid viscus is quite remote (Table 8.2). Tears of the hepatic or splenic capsules from traction on an adhesion usually result in some bleeding which can be controlled by application of fulgurating electrosurgical current or defocused laser beam. If the bleeding is not controlled in this manner, direct application of haemostatis agents such as Avitine®, Gelfoam® or Surgicel® can be applied to the area to promote platelet adhesion.

Larger or deeper tears, particularly of the spleen, will require suture ligation with large U stitches of no. 0 or 1 absorbable suture material. If this fails to stop the bleeding, laparotomy may be required.

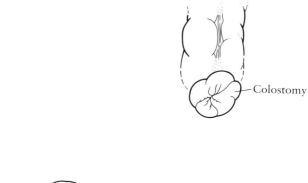

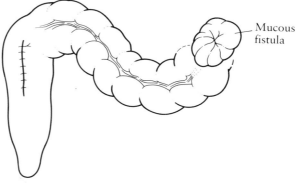

Figure 8.13: Proximal colostomy and mucus fistula after resection of injured sigmoid colon. (Reprinted by permission of Thieme-Stratton Inc.)[8].

Diaphragmatic perforation

Inadvertent perforations of the diaphragm will result in collapse of the corresponding lung and some degree of tension pneumothorax.

A closed chest tube thoracotomy placed through the second intercostal space and the mid-axillary line will promptly correct the situation. The perforation, if accessible laparoscopically, can be repaired with non-absorbable horizontal mattress suture (size 2-0 or 3-0). If the location of the injury is inaccessible endoscopically, then laparotomy will be required.

Open laparoscopy

The many reports of iatrogenic injuries related to percutaneous insufflation prompted the development of alternative methods of introducing gas into the peritoneal cavity. The most widely used has been the Hasson cannula[19–21]. This technique enables the surgeon to enter the abdominal cavity by direct

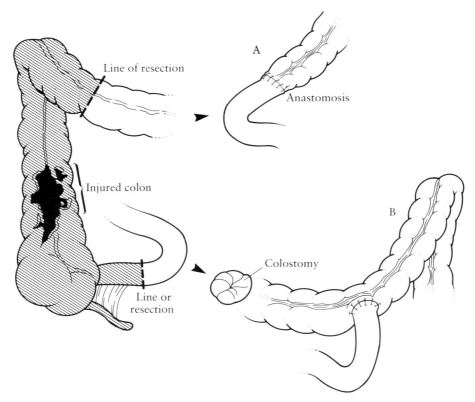

Figure 8.14: Extensive laceration of ascending colon treated by resection and primary anastomosis (A). Iliocolic anastomosis with a 'venting' colostomy (B). (Reprinted by permission of Thieme-Stratton Inc.)[8].

incision and to place a blunt-tip cannula in a place free of adhesions or bowel. Vascular injuries due to introduction of the Hasson cannula are virtually non-existent.

Open laparoscopy can result in bowel perforation if the site chosen for the incision has an adherent bowel loop. However, careful dissection of the fascia and pre-peritoneal area, as well as adequate exposure can minimize the risk of this happening. In addition, the surgeon is usually well aware that the bowel has been entered, and the damage can be repaired quickly and with minimal consequences. For these reasons, the author has adopted this technique in most laparoscopic procedures, and resorts to percutaneous Verres needle insufflation only when the patient is extremely obese and the dissection results in a very deep hole. In these cases a cutdown to the fascia is done and the needle is placed at this deeper level, which makes it easier to know when the peritoneum has been entered.

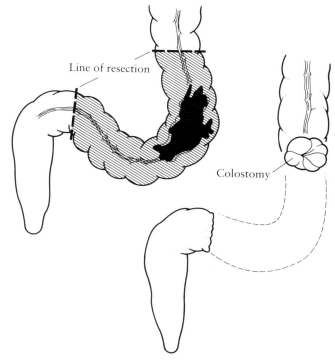

Line of resection

Colostomy

Figure 8.15: Resection of extensively damaged sigmoid colon with a proximal colostomy and distal Hartman's pouch. (Reprinted by permission of Thieme-Stratton Inc.)[8].

Trocar placement

Once the peritoneum has been adequately insufflated, the introduction of trocars presents further risks of complications. Trocar injuries that involve hollow viscera or blood vessels are similar to those already discussed above. The severity of these injuries, however, is usually greater, especially those involving retroperitoneal vessels.

The correct insertion technique should keep these accidents to a minimum. Great attention should be placed when making a skin incision which will be just long enough to allow the sleeve of the cannula to enter the subcutaneous tissue, so that the force needed to penetrate the abdominal wall is slight and the introduction is carried out in one smooth and controlled movement. If the operator finds that moderate force is needed to enter the abdomen, the result is that the abdominal wall is pressed dangerously close to the peritoneal structures. The presence of a retractable safety shield as found in most disposable trocars, does not prevent the vessels from harm because the sharp tip is not covered until the tip of the sleeve is free in the peritoneal cavity. The distance between the anterior abdominal wall and the aorta at the level of the umbilicus is surprisingly short, especially in thin individuals.

Lacerations of the epigastric vessels by the trocar tip can be avoided by first transilluminating the abdominal wall and placing the trocars lateral to the rectus sheath.

If blood is obtained from the cannula after the trocar is removed, indicating a possible vascular injury, it should not be withdrawn and instead the area should be inspected laparoscopically to rule out a major vascular injury. If the mishap occurs on the placement of the first trocar, as is often the case, and there is a significant amount of blood, an immediate laparotomy should be performed to avoid significant blood loss.

Bowel penetration by trocars is usually made evident by the presence of bowel contents emanating from the sleeve or being found free in the peritoneal cavity at the commencement of the exploratory phase of the operation. The management is similar to the one described previously. Always look for paired perforations, as these injuries may be through-and-through wounds.

Dissection

Once the operative field has been established and the cannulae are in place, the mobilization of the viscera and lysis of adhesions has to be performed. Some form of energy source is required, from mechanical disruption of tissue planes with dissectors or scissors to monopolar and bipolar electrosurgical instruments and lasers. Each has its applications, benefits and hazards.

Blunt dissection

This technique is familiar to all trained surgeons, and if performed properly should provide easy and relatively bloodless mobilization of structures. It does require a working knowledge of tissue planes and anatomical landmarks which should be familiar to all from experience gained in open surgery. Visual clues such as anatomical landmarks are relied upon more heavily, because tactile feedback such as palpating a pulse through the instruments is greatly impaired in these procedures.

Electrosurgery

The use of monopolar instrumentation has proliferated during the last few years. This system has been applied to scissors, graspers, and varied configurations of cutting and coagulating tools. Monopolar current uses the patient, who is connected to a return electrode pad, as part of the electrical circuit.

A number of mishaps have been described, from accidental burns to intra-abdominal structures by monopolar instruments[22–24]. There are many situations which can lead to these complications. Inadvertent grounding of the current away from the target tissue and through a loop of bowel may cause a full-thickness burn of the wall. This can happen if the insulating sheath on the instrument shaft is defective, or if the prolonged application of coagulating current desiccates the tissue and increases the resistance to electron flow, creating aberrant return pathways.

The operator must be constantly aware of the location of the active electrode tip, to apply the current accurately and at the minimum wattage needed to obtain the desired tissue effect. Only the surgeon should have the ability to activate the current by hand- or foot-switches.

Bowel perforations due to electrical burns are typically not noted at the time of the original operation. Patients will present with signs and symptoms of peritoneal irritation a day or so after the incident. The initial tissue changes are those of coagulation, which subsequently leads to tissue necrosis and breakdown. This progression has been well documented in the experimental animal[12].

In repairing these injuries, it is necessary to excise the injured segment of bowel with a reanastomosis rather than simply suturing the perforation. The latter approach may lead to breakdown of the repair because of unsuspected ongoing necrosis of the edges of the defect which will not heal primarily.

During the early part of this decade gynaecologists began to abandon monopolar instrumentation in favour of bipolar technology. Bipolar current does not rely on the patient being part of the electrical circuit. The energy flow is controlled more predictably by providing a return pathway close to the active electrode. Kleppinger pioneered the use of coagulating forceps for sterilization[25]. Similar instruments are now available to cut and coagulate tissue. The increased safety of these instruments has still not been fully documented.

Many of the bowel injuries reported in the literature used to be attributed to electrical burns. However, because of the typical histological features of these injuries, many of these incidents were restudied and Levy et al.[10] concluded that many of these injuries were caused by needles, trocars or other instruments.

Infection

Infections of the trocar sites have been described. Most are transient episodes of cellulitis, which is selflimiting, or require simple drainage and a short course of oral antibiotics to cure them.

Occasionally a more serious form of infection can develop. Synergistic infections caused by mixed bacteria of gram-positive and gram-negative anaerobic organisms have been encountered[26]. The typical presentation is that of a rapidly spreading area of cellulitis and subcutaneous crepitus which appears surprisingly soon after the procedure. A sero-sanguineous wound discharge may also be present which, on gram stain, shows the mixed nature of the infection. The patient is severely toxic and has a high fever.

These infections must be treated aggressively by wide debridement of the involved skin, fascia and muscle, which may have to be carried out as frequently as every 8–12 hours. Broad-spectrum antibiotics with good gram-positive and anaerobic coverage should also be instituted.

Hernia

Abdominal wall hernias at the site of trocar insertions are not common, although there have been anecdotal accounts of an increased incidence of hernia associated with the larger trocars (12 mm or greater). Therefore it seems wise to attempt to repair the fascia at these sites to prevent herniation.

Some of these hernias can be associated with bowel incarceration, in which only part of the bowel wall is trapped in the sac leading to necrosis and perforation of the bowel.

Conclusion

Operative laparoscopy is a safe and effective technique for performing previously painful therapeutic procedures. However, it does present the surgeon with many challenges which must be understood and met, so that the complication rate of these operations is kept to an acceptable minimum, comparable or preferably lower than the traditional method. A clear understanding of the anatomy, the techniques and the instrumentation is crucial to attain this goal.

References

1   Phillips JM (1977) Complications in laparoscopy. *International Journal of Gynaecology and Obstetrics*. **15**:157–62.

2   Kane MG and Krejs GJ (1984) Complications of diagnostic laparoscopy in Dallas: a 7-year prospective study. *Gastrointestinal Endoscopy*. **30**:237–40.

3   Peterson HB *et al.* (1990) American Association of Gynecologic Laparoscopists' 1988 member survey on operative laparoscopy. *Journal of Reproductive Medicine*. **35**: 587–90.

4   Yuzpe, AA (1990) Pneumoperitoneum needle and trocar injuries in laparoscopy. *Journal of Reproductive Medicine*. **35**: 485–90.

5   McDonald PT *et al.* (1978) Vascular trauma secondary to diagnostic and therapeutic procedures: laparoscopy. *American Journal of Surgery*. **135**:651–5.

6   Baadsgaard SE *et al.* (1989) Case report, major vascular injury during gynecologic laparoscopy. *Acta Obstetrica et Gynecologica Scandinavica*. **68**:283–5.

7   Perry MO (1981) *The management of acute vascular injuries*. Williams and Williams, Baltimore.

8   Blaisdell FW and Trunkey DD (1982) *Trauma management, vol. 1: abdominal trauma.* Thieme-Stratton, New York.

9   Berci G and Cuschieri A (1986) *Practical Laparoscopy.* Baillière Tindall, London. p. 172.

10   Graff TD *et al.* (1959) Gas embolism: a comparative study of air and carbon dioxide as embolic agents in the systemic venous system. *American Journal of Obstetrics and Gyneocology.* **78**: 259–65.

11   Root B *et al.* (1978) Gas embolism death after laparoscopy delayed by 'trapping' in portal circulation. *Anesthesia and Analgesia.* **57**: 232–7.

12   Levy BS *et al.* (1985) Bowel injuries during laparoscopy. *Journal of Reproductive Medicine.* **30**: 168–72.

13   Ivatury RR *et al.* (1993) Definitive treatment of colon injuries: a prospective study. *American Surgeon.* **59**: 43–9.

14   Hodgson C *et al.* (1970) Some effects of the peritoneal insufflation of carbon dioxide at laparoscopy. *Anaesthesia.* **25**: 382–90.

15   Versichelen L *et al.* (1984) Physiopathologic changes during anaesthesia administration for gynecologic laparoscopy. *Journal of Reproductive Medicine.* **29**: 697–700.

16   Puri GD and Singh H (1992) Ventilatory effects of lap under general anaesthesia. *British Journal of Anaesthesia.* **68**: 211–13.

17   Scott DB and Julian DG (1972) Observations on cardiac arrythmias during laparoscopy. *British Medical Journal.* **1**: 411–13.

18   Motew M *et al.* (1973) Cardiovascular effects and acid-base and blood gas changes during laparoscopy. *American Journal of Obstetrics and Gynecology.* **115**: 1002–12.

19   Penfield AJ (1985) How to prevent complications of open laparoscopy. *Journal of Reproductive Medicine.* **30**: 660–3.

20   Baggish M (1979) Complications of laparoscopic sterilization. *Obstetrics and Gynecology.* **54**: 54.

21   Mintz M (1977) Risks and prophylaxis in laparoscopy: a survey of 100,000 cases. *Journal of Reproductive Medicine.* **18**: 269.

22   Peterson HB *et al.* (1981) Deaths associated with laparoscopic sterilization by unipolar electrocoagulating devices, 1978/1979. *American Journal of Obstetrics and Gynecology.* **139**: 141–3.

23   Neufeld GR *et al.* (1973) Electrical burns during laparoscopy. *Journal of the American Medical Association.* **226**: 1465.

24 Maudsley RF and Qizilbash AH (1979) Thermal injury to the bowel as a complication of laparoscopic sterilization. *Canadian Journal of Surgery.* **22**:232.

25 Kleppinger RK (1977) Laparoscopy at a community hospital: an analysis of 4300 cases. *Journal of Reproductive Medicine.* **19**: 353–63.

26 Sotrel G *et al.* (1983) Necrotizing fasciitis following diagnostic laparoscopy. *Obstetrics and Gynecology* (Suppl.). **62**: 675–95.

27 Brühl W (1966) Zwischenfälle und komplikationen bei der Laparoskopie und gezielten Leberpunktion. *Deutsch Med. Wochenschr.* **51**: 2297–9.

9

Appendectomy

MICHAEL S. KAVIC

Historical introduction

The appendix has been characterized as an individual organ since ancient times. The Egyptians, for example, used coptic jars to store abdominal viscera during the ritual of mummification. Some of these coptic jars have inscriptions that refer to the appendix as the 'worm' of the bowel[1].

Neither Aristotle nor Galen recognized the appendix as a distinct organ because they dissected only the bodies of lower animals. In their particular animal studies, the appendix was absent. Andreas Vesalius published the first illustration of the appendix in the fifth volume of his work *De Humani Corporis Fabrica*, in 1543[1].

Though many physicians of the middle ages noted the appendix, few understood its significance. In the early 19th century, the leading physician in Paris, Baron Guillaume Dupuytren, did not believe the appendix was a source of abdominal pathology. Instead, he felt that disease in the appendix actually began in the caecum, which was termed typhlitis. Dupuytren's opinions were highly regarded in France, and his opposition to considering an appendiceal origin of this disease retarded the diagnosis and treatment of appendicitis for decades[1].

The first surgical removal of the appendix took place in 1735[2]. Claudius Amyand, a surgeon to King George II, operated on an 11-year-old boy who presented with a scrotal hernia and faecal fistula. Amyand opened the hernia via a scrotal incision and removed a perforated appendix and omentum. The child survived.

Many outstanding surgeons of the late 19th century reported on isolated incidents of appendectomy. In the USA, the Harvard pathologist Reginald Fitz alerted the medical profession to the importance of the appendix and inflammatory disease. Fitz described the signs and symptoms of acute appendicitis and advocated surgical intervention, coining the term appendectomy[3]. Charles McBurney, a US surgeon and contemporary of Fitz, described the point of abdominal tenderness due to appendicitis that bears his name[4]. McBurney and Fitz were strong advocates of early operative intervention.

The acceptance of appendectomy was stimulated by events surrounding the coronation of King Edward VII. In 1902, Edward experienced an episode of severe abdominal pain, which became so intense that his coronation had to be postponed. Sir Fredrick Treves was summoned and performed an exploration on the king at Buckingham Palace. Treves evacuated an appendiceal abscess, but did not remove the appendix. The king made a full recovery and appendicitis thereafter became a 'fashionable' disease[1].

Incidence

Acute appendicitis is one of the most common surgical emergencies. It occurs at all ages, with a peak incidence in young adults.

Epidemiological data derived from the United States National Hospital Discharge Survey Data, from the years 1979 to 1984, suggest that approximately 250 000 cases of appendicitis occur annually[5]. The highest incidence of appendicitis was found in persons aged 10 to 19 years. Males had a higher rate of appendicitis than females for all age groups.

Life table models demonstrate that the lifetime risk for appendicitis is 8.6% for males and 6.7% for females. The peak incidence for males occurs between 10 and 14 years, and the peak incidence for females between 15 and 19 years. Interestingly, the incidence of appendicitis decreased by 14.6% during 1979–84. The reason is not known, but may include factors such as changing dietary habits, better nutrition, and perhaps the widespread use of antibiotics.

Aetiology and pathogenesis

Obstruction of the appendiceal lumen is the principal reason for the production of acute appendicitis[6]. Common causes for appendiceal obstruction include faecalith, hypertrophy of submucosal lymphoid tissue, and kinking of the wall. Less common reasons for obstruction include blockage secondary to vegetable seeds, foreign bodies and intestinal worms.

The proximal blockage of the appendiceal lumen produces a closed loop obstruction. Acute inflammation of the mucosa is followed by ulceration and inflammation of the entire wall. Stagnation distal to the obstruction permits growth of colonic bacterial flora including pathogens such as *Escherichia coli*, *Streptococcus fecalis* and anaerobic bacteria.

Progressive distension of the appendix leads to occlusion of the vascular supply and infarction of the antimesenteric border. Perforation can occur with frank peritonitis.

Clinically patients present with abdominal pain, fever or vomiting[7]. Abdominal pain frequently starts in the periumbilical area, but eventually localizes in the right lower quadrant. Leukocytosis of 11 000 to 18 000

WBC mm^{-3} is common. CAT scan of the abdomen may reveal a right lower quadrant abdominal mass or phlegmon.

Appendectomy

Until recently, laparotomy was the only option available for removal of the inflamed, noninflamed or perforated appendix. Kurt Semm performed the first laparoscopic appendectomy in 1982[8]. Other gynaecologists soon followed Semm's pioneering efforts[9].

There are several large series of laparoscopic appendectomy in the medical literature[10,11]. Pier and colleagues reported on a series of 997 patients with appendicitis, in whom 915 appendectomies were performed laparoscopically[12]. In this series, 6.4% of the cases were performed in an open fashion. Of the 933 cases attempted laparoscopically, 2% required conversion to open exploration.

Advantages attributed to the laparoscopic approach include improved diagnostic accuracy, minimal postoperative pain, decreased ileus and rapid return to full activity. Initial evidence also suggests that there is decreased adhesion formation following laparoscopy, and cosmesis is excellent.

In those cases of vague abdominal pain or marked obesity, laparoscopic visualization can improve diagnostic capability without exposing the patient to the risk of an open procedure.

Technique

Preparations for surgery

The appendix is an end organ, and its removal can easily be accomplished utilizing laparoscopic techniques. As with open surgery, exposure of the organ and control of its blood supply are the principal steps in a laparoscopic procedure.

After appropriate investigation, the patient is brought to the operating theatre equipped for laparoscopic surgery (Figure 9.1). The urinary bladder is catheterized and a nasogastric tube is inserted into the stomach. Typically, cefoxitin (1 g i.v) is given preoperatively.

The abdominal wall is carefully prepared for surgery in the standard manner and a transumbilical puncture with a Verres needle is used to initiate the pneumoperitoneum. In patients with previous abdominal surgery, the Hasson open technique may be used or an alternative access site selected.

Alternative access sites may be anywhere on the abdominal wall; however, the most desirable site is the subcostal midclavicular line of the right or left upper quadrant. The technique of alternative access Verres needle insertion is similar to that of needle liver biopsy. A distinct 'pop' can be felt as the needle traverses the different fascial layers and peritoneum.

The intra-abdominal position of the Verres needle can be ascertained with the water drop test. Pneumoperitoneum is established with a maximum

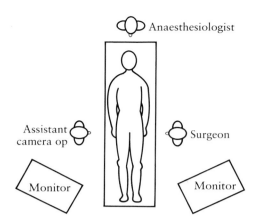

Figure 9.1: Operating room positions.

insufflation of 12–15 mmHg. A 10 mm cannula and laparoscope are inserted in the infraumbilical position for diagnostic survey. If an alternative access site is selected, a 5 mm laparoscope typically is introduced via the midclavicular line cannula to evaluate the status of adhesions and the abdominal viscera.

Acute appendicitis

In cases of acute appendicitis, three other cannula are utilized (Figure 9.2): a 5 mm cannula is positioned in the midclavicular line of the right upper quadrant, lateral to the rectus sheath. A second 5 mm cannula is placed in the right lower quadrant, lateral to the rectus sheath and inferior to the level of the iliac crest. A third 12 mm cannula is placed in the left lower quadrant lateral to the rectus sheath midway between the symphysis pubis and umbilicus. Free fluid within the peritoneal cavity may be aspirated and collected in a Chieftain Lukens tube (Baxter Health Corp., Illinois, USA) for appropriate study.

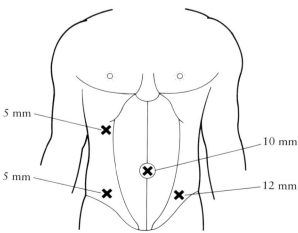

Figure 9.2: Appendectomy trocar sites.

Dissection

The appendix is identified, and after preliminary mobilization (Figure 9.3), the tip is secured with a pre-tied Roeders loop (Figure 9.4). Cutting the tail of the loop with ample excess provides a traction point, so that the appendix can be manipulated with little fear of tear or rupture.

Dissection is performed about the base of the appendix. It may be necessary to divide the fascia fusion line to mobilize the caecum and visualize a retrocaecal appendix. The mesoappendix is defined and the vessels in the mesoappendix serially clipped with an endoclip device or sutured with intracorporeal suture tied in an extracorporeal manner (Figure 9.5).

The laparoscopic Endo-GIA stapler (USSC, Norwalk, CT, USA) provides a very efficient way to secure the mesoappendix. This laparoscopic stapler is introduced through the left lower quadrant 12 mm cannula and positioned on the mesoappendix. The Endo-GIA fires a triple row of haemostatic staples 30 mm long on either side of its cutting blade (Figure 9.6). One or two firings of the stapler will skeletonize the appendix (Figure 9.7).

The base of the appendix can be secured with three loops of pre-tied chromic catgut and divided (Figures 9.8 and 9.9). It can also be divided with the Endo-GIA stapler (Figures 9.10 and 9.11). It is my preference first to secure the base of the appendix with a pretied loop of catgut and then divide it with the Endo-GIA stapler, to secure the stump more completely (Figure 9.12). The stump need not be inverted[13].

Bagging the appendix

The appendix is contained by using a commercially available extraction bag or the cut finger of a sterile surgical glove (Figure 9.13). By isolating the appendix, prior to removal, the risk of contaminating other structures and the abdominal wall is lessened. Once the appendix has been amputated and bagged, it is extracted through the 12 mm port (Figures 9.14 and 9.15).

Irrigation of the appendiceal fossa is performed with a normal saline solution containing 5000 units of heparin per litre and 1 g of cefoxitin (Figure 9.16).

Closing the sites

The fascia of the 12 mm port and umbilical fascia are closed with absorbable sutures of 2–0 Polydioxanone (PDS, Ethicon, USA). The 5 mm sites are closed with plain catgut suture. Steri-strip tapes (3M, St Paul, MN, USA) complete the skin closure.

The puncture sites are usually infiltrated with 0.25% bupivacaine hydrochloride solution, and the adult patient given 60 mg of ketorolac tromethamine IM, to lessen postoperative discomfort.

The urinary catheter and nasogastric tube are removed prior to transfer to the recovery room. Intravenous antibiotics are given depending on the clinical status of the patient at the time of appendectomy.

Clear liquids are initiated post-anaesthetic and diet is progressed as ileus resolves.

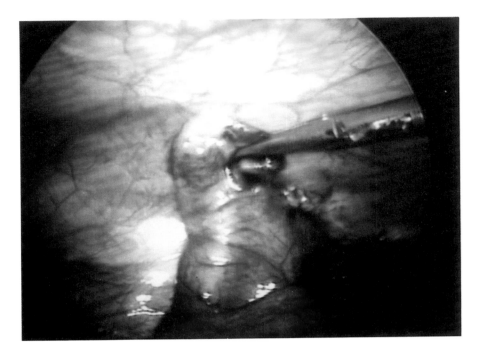

Figure 9.3: Tip of appendix.

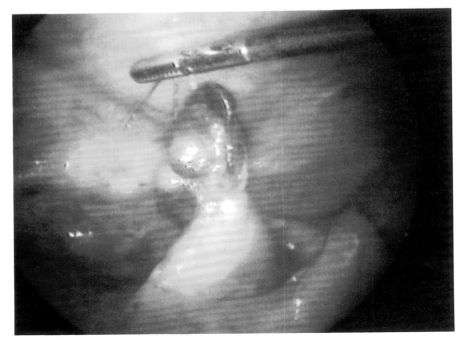

Figure 9.4: Tip secured with pre-tied Roeders loop.

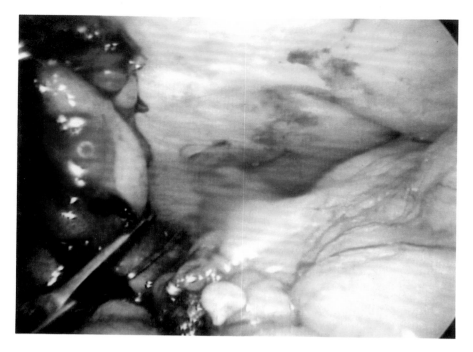

Figure 9.5: Mesoappendix secured with Endoclips.

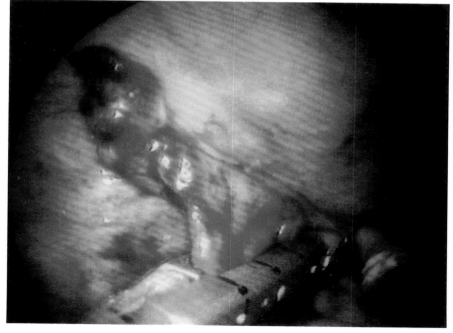

Figure 9.6: Mesoappendix secured with Endo-GIA.

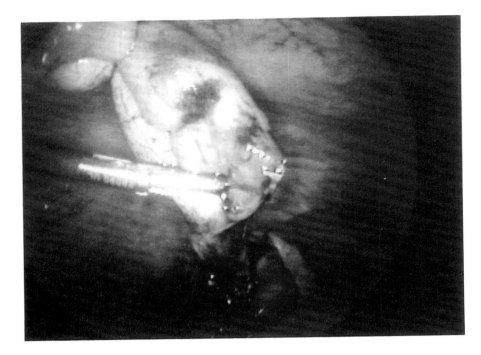

Figure 9.7: Skeletonized appendix.

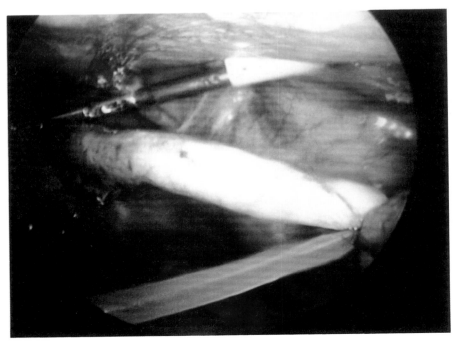

Figure 9.8: Base of appendix secured with Endoloop.

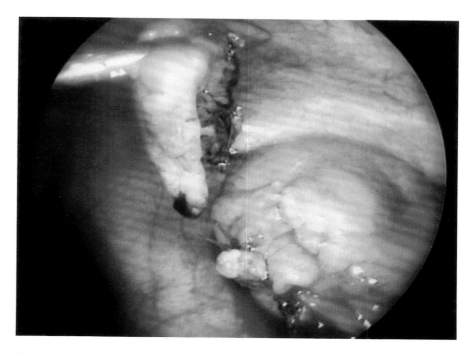

Figure 9.9: Endoloop-secured stump of appendix.

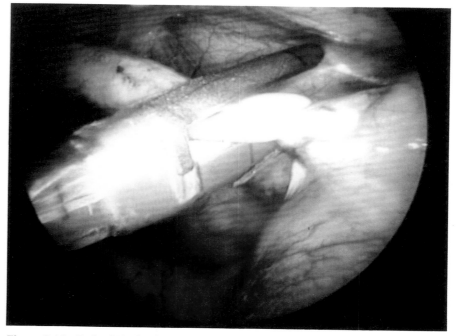

Figure 9.10: Endo-GIA dividing base of appendix.

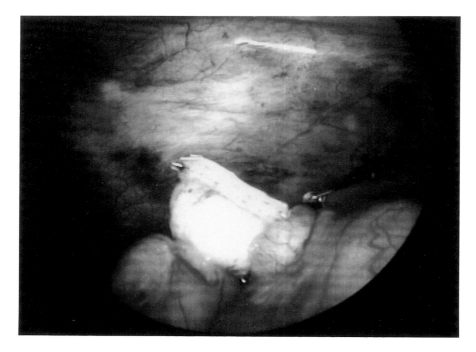

Figure 9.11: Stapled stump of appendix.

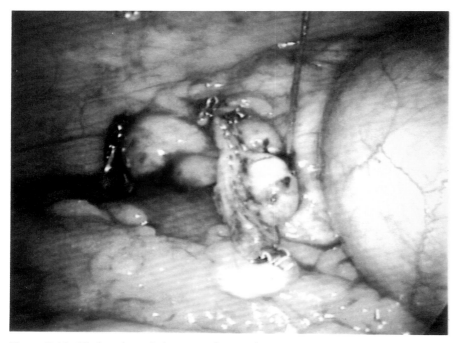

Figure 9.12: Tied and stapled stump of appendix.

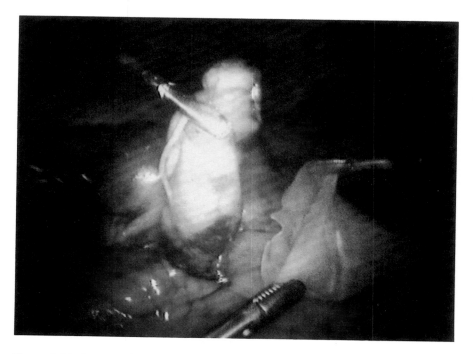

Figure 9.13: Bagging the appendix.

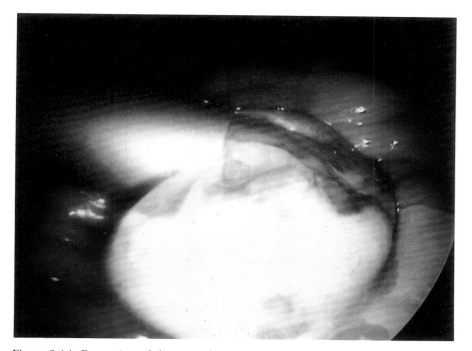

Figure 9.14: Extraction of the appendix.

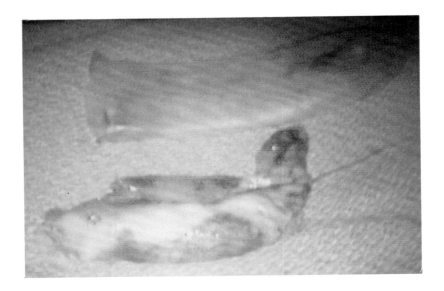

Figure 9.15: Delivered appendix.

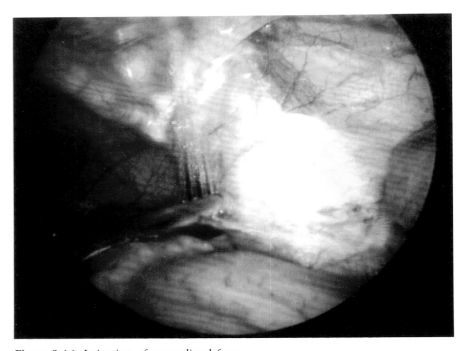

Figure 9.16: Irrigation of appendiceal fossa.

Discussion

Laparoscopic surgery has added a new dimension in diagnostic practice, permitting discovery of unsuspected abdominal pathology. The superior visibility afforded by the laparoscope makes it useful for determining the cause of abdominal pain[14]. In those patients with conditions such as ruptured ovarian cyst or endometriosis, the primary disease can usually be managed laparoscopically. Removal of the appendix under these circumstances alleviates the dilemma of determining the cause of lower abdominal pain post laparoscopy.

The diagnostic capabilities of the laparoscope is especially important in obese patients or in cases of abnormal anatomy. In these instances, an extensive abdominal incision would be necessary to secure adequate visualization. The small scars of laparoscopic access permit superior visualization and provide excellent cosmesis.

Before surgeons become experienced in this technique, they must be prepared to convert to an open exploration at the first signs of complications. As experience is gained, however, fewer cases will require conversion to the open approach. Acute pain in the female patient provides a rich opportunity for cooperation between the laparoscopic general surgeon and the gynaecologist.

Conclusion

Although current data are limited, laparoscopic appendectomy appears to be a safe and effective alternative to open appendectomy[11,12,15,16]. The laparoscopic approach can be applied to almost all patients with suspected appendicitis. Controlled randomized trials will also be required to make proper comparisons between the laparoscopic approach and traditional open appendectomy.

References

1   Herrington JL,Jr (1991) The veriform appendix: its surgical history. *Contemporary Surgery*. **39**:36–43.

2   Amyand C (1736) Of an inguinal rupture with a pin in the appendix coeci, incrusted with stone and some observation on wounds in the gut. *Philosophical Transactions of the Royal Society, London*. **39**:329.

3   Fitz RH (1886) Perforating inflammation of the vermiform appendix with special reference to its early diagnosis and treatment. *Transactions of the Association of American Physicians*. **1**:107–44.

4   McBurney C (1894) The incision made in the abdominal wall in cases of appendicitis with a description of a new method of operating. *Annals of Surgery*. **20**:38.

5   Addis DG *et al.* (1990) The epidemiology of appendicitis and appendectomy in the United States. *American Journal of Epidemiology.* **132**:910–25.

6   Chandrasoma P and Taylor C (1991) *Concise pathology.* Appleton & Lange, London. pp.605–6.

7   Swartz S *et al.* (1969) *Principles of Surgery.* McGraw-Hill, New York. pp.1020–30.

8   Semm K (1983) Endoscopic appendectomy. *Endoscopy.* **15**:59–64.

9   Schreiber JH (1990) Laparoscopic appendectomy in pregnancy. *Surgical Endoscopy.* **4**:100–2.

10 Spirtos NM *et al.* (1987) Laparoscopy – diagnostic aid in cases of suspected appendicitis. *American Journal of Obstetrics and Gynecology.* **156**:90–4.

11 Valla JS *et al.* (1991) Laparoscopic appendectomy in children: report of 465 cases. *Surgical Laparoscopy and Endoscopy.* **1**:166–72.

12 Pier A *et al.* (1993) Laparoscopic appendectomy. *World Journal of Surgery.* **17**:29–33.

13 Engstrom L and Fenyo G (1985) Appendicectomy: assessment of stump invagination versus simple ligation: a prospective, randomized trial. *British Journal of Surgery.* **72**:971–2.

14 Sugarbaker PH *et al.* (1975) Preoperative laparoscopy in diagnosis of acute abdominal pain. *Lancet.* **22**:442–4.

15 Geis WP *et al.* (1992) Laparoscopic appendectomy for acute appendicitis: rationale and technical aspects. *Contemporary Surgery.* **40**:13–19.

16 Schirmer BD *et al.* (1993) Laparoscopic versus traditional appendectomy for suspected appendicitis. *American Journal of Surgery.* **165**:670–5.

10

Urological Considerations and Complications of Operative Endoscopy

MARTIN R. CURLIK

Introduction

Surgeons who claim never to encounter complications either do not operate, or have not done a sufficient number of surgical cases to have experienced them. No matter how competent a surgeon may be, increasing numbers of cases will also increase the likelihood of encountering complications. The hope is, however, that this growing experience will also increase our expertise and ability to overcome these complications, and to keep morbidity to a minimum.

With the advent of interventional endoscopy, the complications related to urology have recently increased very rapidly. This is partly because, as in any field, the number of new practitioners involved means that larger numbers lack experience. The urologist who is supposed to be an expert in pelvic urologic anatomy may experience a high morbidity in the performance of endoscopic pelvic lymph-node dissections for the staging of prostatic malignancy. This morbidity certainly decreases with experience. Ureteral ligations, transsections and bladder perforations have frequently been reported in the early stages. Such complications have occurred within the community practice of urology at a much higher rate than reported in the urological literature.

The purpose of this chapter is to define the urological anatomy in relation to the female pelvic organs, in an attempt to prevent urological injuries. Troublespots for the gynaecologist will be noted and preventative urological measures will be explained in detail to guide the interventional endoscopist. Finally, endoscopic surgical management of the stated injuries will be explained. I am convinced that endoscopic management can be accomplished in the majority of cases without the need for open surgical repair. This can be gained by proper patient preparation and surgical planning. Although endoscopic instrumentation may be limited in certain instances, the surgeon must be prepared to innovate in order to keep morbidity to a minimum. The techniques to repair urological injuries have specific indications and contraindications; their advantages and disadvantages are discussed below.

Anatomy

The adrenal system, kidney, ureter and bladder are retroperitoneal structures. The operating surgeon must be familiar with these structures and their precise anatomy in relation to other pelvic organs in order to prevent urological injuries. In addition, the uterus and lower vagina are considered retroperitoneal structures.

Kidneys

The kidneys are usually embedded and well protected by the retroperitoneal fat pad in the lumbar fossa. The lower pole of the right kidney reaches approximately the lower third lumbar vertebra; the left lower pole is somewhat higher. The vascular supply to the renal hilum is located at approximately the first lumbar vertebra. 10% of kidneys have accessory renal vessels which are end arteries and must be spared during renal dissections in order to preserve renal parenchyma. Due to this high retroperitoneal position the renal units are not usually a consideration for the pelviscopists.

Occasionally a pelvic kidney will be encountered. This may be picked up on preoperative physical exam or preoperative pelvic sonography. A pelvic kidney does not usually interfere with interventional laparoscopy since it is a retroperitoneal structure. The renal vessels usually have their origins along the major intra-abdominal vasculature. The ureter usually maintains its normal length and can be redundant within the pelvis. The renal pelvis maintains a position anterior to the pelvic kidney. Anomalies of ascent occur in 1 : 990 cases. The horseshoe kidney, which may extend down into the pelvis, occurs in 1 : 250 cases. A preoperative ureteral catheter can be placed to help ureteral identification. With a pelvic kidney, of course, especial care must be taken for the establishment of the pneumoperitoneum and for trocar placement. The Hasson technique should be utilized in such cases. Occasionally a pelvic kidney may be initially mistaken as a pelvic mass. It should be realized that 10% of pelvic kidneys are solitary.

Ureters

The ureters are anatomically divided into upper, middle and lower segments. The upper ureter extends from the renal pelvis to the upper sacrum; the mid-ureter extends from the upper sacral border to the lower sacrum; and the lower ureter extends from the lower sacral border to its insertion into the bladder. The lower half of the ureter is below an arbitrary line at the pelvic rim. The ureteral length varies between 22 and 25 cm. The ureter can be found immediately lateral to the transverse processes of the vertebral column above the pelvis. At the level of the common iliac vessels it crosses anteriorly and medially into the hollow of the pelvis. The ureters cross over into the pelvis immediately above the bificuration of the internal and external iliac vessels on the right and at the common iliac vessel on the left. This is where the ureter can most commonly be located when trying to expose it during the surgical dissection. The ureter is located on the posterior peritoneal surface in the retroperitoneum. The ureters follow the concave pelvic wall as they continue their descent into the female pelvis. They are medial to the vesical artery, obturator nerve and vessels. The ureter is posterior to the ovary and lateral to the infundibulo-pelvic ligament. It enters the broad ligament and courses lateral to the uterus, and then crosses the vesico–vaginal space to enter the bladder. At this point the uterine artery crosses superiorly and anteriorly to the ureter to enter the cervix. The ovarian artery and vein cross anteriorly and obliquely to the ureter at the level of the fourth or fifth lumbar vertebra.

Due to the intimate relationship of the ovarian and uterine vessels to the ureter, injuries can easily occur. A third site of injury is where the ureter courses through the broad ligament. Ureteral injuries also occur at the time of reperitonealization (Figure 10.1).

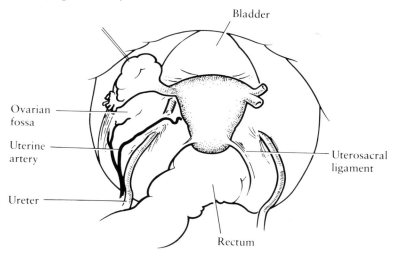

Figure 10.1: Anatomy of the female pelvis.

The main blood supply to the ureter is from a branch of the renal artery. The arterial supply courses along the medial aspect of the ureter and picks up additional arterial feeders from the abdominal aorta, common iliac and ovarian arteries. In the pelvis the blood supply enters from the lateral pelvic wall and is supplied from a branch of the inferior vesical artery (Figure 10.2).

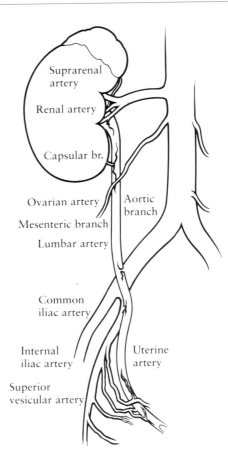

Figure 10.2: Ureteral blood supply (arterial).

Bladder

The bladder is in a retropubic position and the posterior wall is in continuity with the anterior vaginal cuff and uterus. As the uterine isthmus meets the bladder, the peritoneal surface reflects from the dome of the bladder onto the uterus. The bladder is enclosed within the endopelvic fascia. The bladder arterial blood supply is from the superior vesical artery which has three branches. A wisp of the vesical artery supplies the distal ureteral segment. This is an important factor in the repair of distal ureteral injuries.

Assessment

All informed consents for interventional pelvic endoscopy should include the possibility of urological injury. Although the possibility is small, aggressive interventional procedures carry an increased risk of urological injury, especially when performed by the novice endoscopist. If such an injury occurs, and it is immediately recognized and corrected at the time of the surgical procedure, it will save the surgeon a great deal of trouble if properly informed consent has already been obtained.

The most common intraoperative urological injury is to the ureter. Unfortunately, gynaecological surgery accounts for the largest percentage of such injuries. As previously stated, it is probably the intimate relationship between the ureter and the ovarian vessels, broad ligament and the uterine artery which allows these injuries to occur. In benign gynaecological surgical procedures, the incidence of ureteral injury is from 0.3 to 3%[1]. This rate is clearly higher when malignancies are present.

History

Once a urological injury has occurred, a complete assessment of the genito-urinary system must be performed intraoperatively. The surgeon must be aware of the patient's renal function and the presence or absence of functioning kidneys. The presence of sterile or infected urine should also be identified. A history of previous urological visits for infections, stone or urological manipulations should be sought. These factors play an important role in the intraoperative management of the injury. The patient's preoperative X-rays should also be reviewed. Previously performed radiographs within the patient's X-ray packet may provide valuable information. Patients with a history of intra-abdominal malignancies, urinary stones or recurrent urinary tract infections may have limited surgical management options. Present-day management methods are aimed strongly at renal salvage, although each case must be managed individually. Renal loss is fortunately rare if the injury is appropriately recognized and managed.

Intravenous urogram

Occasionally, if it is absolutely mandatory to identify the presence of two functioning renal units, an intravenous urogram can be performed on the operating room table. A contrast bolus or drip technique may be utilized depending on the contrast agent used. Usually a flat plate of the abdomen taken 1 and 15 minutes after the injection of contrast is sufficient to define the functioning renal units and their intrarenal collection systems. In the presence of hypovolemia, delayed films may be required to obtain visualization. A preoperative intravenous urogram should be performed when a difficult case presents itself. The study can be used as a road map for identification of the ureter intraoperatively, and it becomes valuable should an urological injury occur.

Intravenous dyes

There are several manoeuvres which can aid the surgeon when urological injury is suspected. Sometimes it appears that urine may be within the surgical field. When irrigation fluids are used it is sometimes very difficult to detect. The intravenous administration of methylene blue or indigo carmine will dye the urine within the wound. Usually 10 cc of the dye is administered intravenously. It may take upwards of 10–15 minutes for the dye to appear in the urine, therefore if there is any question of urological injury the dye should be administered as soon as an injury is suspected. These agents are harmless if your fears of an injury are unproven. The patient should be informed of the persistence of discoloured urine for 24–48 hours postoperatively since it may cause some anxiety, especially when administered in an outpatient or ambulatory setting. Most importantly, the administration of a methylene blue will alter the signals received from the pulse oximeter. The pulse oximeter reads the arterial saturation on a colorimetric basis, and methylene blue will alter oxygen measurement, giving an incorrect reading. If the anaesthesiologist is unaware of this alteration a moment of anxiety will ensue as the pulse oximeter signals a reading of hypoxia. Recalibration occurs within several minutes and oxygen levels return to normal.

Furosemide, a loop diuretic, can also be administered along with the dye to ensure a brisk diuresis and a prompt visualization in the urine. Approximately 10–20 mg of furosemide is administered intravenously along with a fluid challenge of 250–500 cc isotonic intravenous fluids.

When bladder injuries occur, the bladder can be distended with 250–500 cc isotonic fluids through the Foley catheter to identify the site of injury. One ampule of dye may also be added to the irrigation to confirm the presence of urine within the operative field.

Samples

A specimen of intra-abdominal fluid suspected to be urine may be sent for a BUN and creatine to confirm or deny its presence within the wound, but this is time-consuming and not routinely performed intraoperatively. A simultaneous serum sample must also be sent to use as a comparison. In urine the blood urea nitrogen (BUN) and creatine are elevated in relation to that of serum. Most importantly, this test is accurate in the determination of a delayed diagnosis if a drain has been placed. A sample of drainage may be sent for analysis. Clear drainage from a wound or drain site may also represent lymph fluid and not urine if a large retroperitoneal dissection has been accomplished. Methylene blue may also be helpful in this instance to dye the abdominal dressings and confirm the urinary leak.

Clear drainage from a wound in the postoperative period at times may be difficult to diagnose. Bowel involvement should always be ruled out. Gastrografin given orally or through an enema may also be needed in complex cases to rule out simultaneous bowel injury.

Postoperative assessment

I currently believe that, after an interventional pelvic procedure, a brief survey of the urinary system should be undertaken prior to the removal of the abdominal trocars. If a large amount of ureteral dissection has been performed, methylene blue can be administered intravenously to ensure that there is no evidence of ureteral injury before the termination of the procedure. The bladder may also be filled and emptied under laparoscopic visualization. These manoeuvres should definitely be performed if the surgeon has any suspicion of an injury or is unsure of the anatomical relationships at the end of the procedure. In cases of endometriosis, large surgical dissection or pelvic adhesions, it may be difficult to identify an injury, but the possibility of injury should not be ignored. Early diagnosis will prevent a return to the operating room and ensure a more successful outcome if the injury is recognized and repaired immediately.

Removal of the ureteral catheters (placed preoperatively) under direct laparoscopic visualization will help the diagnosis of ureteral entrapment or injury to be made quickly. Ureteral catheters should be removed under direct vision as the last surgical manoeuvre before trocar removal.

Management

Kidney

Due to the high retroperitoneal position of the kidneys, the possibility of renal injury during laparoscopic procedures is very small. Laparoscopic guidance has been utilized for the performance of pericutaneous nephrostomy placement in urinary stone management techniques for pelvic kidneys.

Management techniques for both blunt and penetrating trauma can be utilized through the laparoscope. Blunt trauma via instrumentation or trocar introduction can be observed. Small retroperitoneal haematomas that are not expanding can be followed conservatively. Adequate time should be set aside for surgical observation. The pneumoperitoneum should be released to look for venous bleeding. Penetrating trauma for small lacerations may be controlled with a surgical haemostatic agent such as Avitene or Surgicell. The role of the argon beam coagulator is yet to be defined in the management of surgical bleeding. Surgical lasers (both contact and non-contact) rarely stop haemorrhage from vessels larger than 2 mm. Any major trauma with suspected collecting system penetration should be managed with closure of the collecting system and renal parenchyma. This manoeuvre will usually require open surgical management for vascular control. Urologists have already performed a partial nephrectomy for stone management using a laparoscopic technique (Clayman, personal communications). As in all types of laparoscopic procedures, if there is any question of an imperfect repair, conventional open surgical techniques should be employed. Renal cyst unroofing for pain and obstruction as well as renal biopsy are now easily performed using a laparoscopic technique.

Ureter

Avoiding injury

The ureter is a very delicate organ and should be treated with great respect. It may suffer several types of operative insult or injury. These include entrapments, crush injuries, cautery burns, suture or staple ligations, lacerations, avulsions, devascularizations, transsections and resections of ureter. The following paragraphs will explain how each type of injury should be managed conservatively to accomplish a successful outcome.

Entrapment

During the course of an oopherectomy, surgical bleeding may be encountered from the ovarian veins. Mass suture ligature may entrap or angle the ureter with obstruction but without actual involvement. The ovarian fossa is often a site of ureteral injury due to venous bleeding. Closure of the peritoneum may also cause angulation obstruction. Care must be taken in the Endoloop ligation of the ovarian pedicle to prevent angulation obstruction. If such angulation is noticed intraoperatively the suture must be removed. Difficulty in removing a ureteral stent may signal an angulation or entrapment. Preoperative ureteral stent rigidity may protect the ureter and prevent angulation injuries from occurring.

Obstruction

Obstruction of the urinary tract identified in the postoperative period is usually signalled by back pain and fever. Fever does not necessarily indicate infection. A leukocytosis may also be present. A urine culture should be obtained in all cases of postoperative fever and the patient should not be discharged until a temperature of 99.5° F or below is maintained for a 24-hour period. An unidentified source of fever in the postoperative period may be caused by a silent ureteral obstruction. A hydronephrosis may be identified by a renal ultrasound or intravenous urogram. An intravenous urogram will provide valuable information such as hydronephrosis, identification of the site of the obstruction and urinary extravasation.

Ureteral repair

Delayed recognition of angulation injuries may be conservatively managed by the passage of a double-J ureteral stent. This should allow fixation of the ureter in a more anatomical position as healing occurs, preventing a ureteral stricture or fibrosis. The use of chromic or gut suture material facilitates this process. These sutures break down within two or three weeks and will allow deangulation. Long-lasting suture such as vicryl or PDS may not be as forgiving and may require surgical release. If a ureteral stent cannot be passed, immediate operative intervention should follow. Laparoscopic deligation has been performed. Early repair in the postoperative period will usually give an excellent surgical result. Unrecognized prolonged renal obstruction for more than six weeks can be expected to lead to renal loss and may preclude renal salvage. If renal obstruction is not identified within two weeks of the ureteral injury, delayed repair should be undertaken. Temporary renal preservation and function can be maintained via a pericutaneous nephrostomy if a ureteral stent cannot be passed. After six weeks' healing and scarification, the ureteral repair can be undertaken with good results.

Timing of ureteral repairs is a controversial subject. It is my opinion that repairs performed between two and six weeks are less successful for several reasons. A delayed repair is preferable because (1) the process of wound-healing inhibits surgical dissection, (2) the difficulty of identifying anatomical landmarks, and (3) inflammatory tissue responses prevent adequate suture placement in healthy tissue.

Crush injuries

At times a clamp or haemoclip may be inadvertently applied to the ureter, causing a crush injury. If the manoeuvre is immediately recognized and the offending object is quickly removed, the injury may be observed and followed conservatively. If an indentation remains, the ureter should be checked for leakage with methylene blue. Ureters that maintain a traumatic defect after removal of the insult should be stented with a double-J stent for a six-week period to allow proper healing. After stent removal, the patient should be followed within six weeks for an intravenous urogram (IVU). This will rule out ischaemic strictures after stent removal. Frequent follow-up IVUs should be repeated at three, six and 12 months to ensure an acceptable result. Ureteral strictures may be managed with balloon dilatation, endoscopic ureterotomy or formal operative repair. Severe crush injuries would be more appropriately managed with surgical debridement and primary repair at the time of injury.

Electrocautery injuries

Electrocautery injuries can be conservatively managed with the placement of a double-J internal stent. It is difficult to assess the importance of a coagulation injury in the operative suite since the effect of the burn may not be evident for several days. If there is any doubt, therefore, ureteral debridement and primary repair should be undertaken. An indwelling ureteral stent should remain for six weeks, with a similar radiographic followup as indicated for crush injuries after stent removal. The ureter should not be directly coagulated. Bleeding points should be managed with small haemo-clips placed parallel to the ureter in order not to compromise its lumen or point suture ligatures. Care should be taken with the use of the Endo-coagulator when used around the ureter since it has a much wider field of coagulation.

Davascularization injuries

Extensive ureteral mobilization may cause a devascularization injury. Ureteral mobilization performed as part of a laparoscopic hysterectomy is not recommended. 10–14 days may be necessary for ureteral necrosis to occur. Such injuries may present as uretero–cutaneous fistula, urinoma formation, or with sepsis. Extensively mobilized ureters may be protected by an indwelling ureteral stent for six weeks in the postoperative period. Postoperative urological care should include follow-up IVUs periodically to look for ureteral stricture after stent removal. Stricture formation is a common complication of devascularization injuries.

Sutures

When a suture is placed around the ureter, a simple deligation is all that is necessary. Delayed deligation can be performed laparoscopically if the aetiology of the injury is certain. Even when sutures are placed through the ureter, as long as ureteral continuity is maintained, no further treatment is necessary if the suture is cleanly removed. Small lacerations to the ureter can be managed with simple closure using absorbable sutures (ie chromic or gut) over a double-J stent. Vicryl suture material is not quickly absorbed by the body and is potentially lithogenic. Silk suture material is highly lithogenic and should never be used in the genito–urinary tract. Closure of ureteral lacerations should be done with a full-thickness mucosal-to-mucosal stitch. Whenever ureteral continuity is disrupted, an external drain should be placed.

Drains

Although ideally drains should be placed in a retroperitoneal position, they can also be placed through an existing lateral trocar site intra-abdominally. In addition a drain can be placed extraperitoneally using a trocar technique. After penetration of the fascia, the obturator can be removed and the trocar guided preperitoneally into position to lie next to the repair (but not in continuity with it). Suction drains placed in continuity with ureteral repairs may maintain urinary extravasation by constant suction. I prefer a passive Penrose drain for this reason. Penrose drains can also be placed easily via a trocar cannula. An appendix or tissue extractor may be used to place the drain into the proper position. The drain is backloaded into a tissue extractor prior to placement into the trocar. Once delivered into position, the drain is held in place by another trocar-grasping forceps, while the extractor and trocar are removed simultaneously leaving the drain in situ. Although the ureter is closed in a watertight fashion, urinary leakage should be diverted to prevent urinoma formation. Ureteral repairs close quickly if the ureter has no distal obstruction.

Closure of the ureter

Ureteral stents allow quick closure of repairs and do an excellent job of internal urinary diversion. External drainage via a Penrose or suction drain is still necessary.

Staple closure of the ureter is now possible with endoscopic stapling devices. The Endo-cutter or Endo-GIA stapling devices have an overlapping staple line in three parallel rows. These staples cannot be removed by picking staples out of the previously fired path. Once fired, the staple line must be surgically removed in its entirety to healthy tissue margins. The last three staples at the end of the firing line are not divided. Repair of a ureteral ligation at the end of the fired staple line requires complete debridement and ureteral repair. Ligations which occur proximal to the three end staples will also be divided. The divided staple line will also require complete resection back to healthy tissue margins.

Invasive laparoscopists are frequently utilizing endoscopic stapling devices for vascular control and to take down the uterine supporting structures.

When a ureteral transsection occurs, its repair depends on its location and the blood supply. Upper ureteral repairs can usually be managed by a simple end-to-end anastomosis (Figure 10.3). Distal ureteral repairs rely on a small branch of the vesical artery which supplies the distal third of the ureter. This artery is sometimes inadequate to maintain ureteral blood supply especially after ureteral mobilization prior to repair. The upper ureter has several feeder vessels along its length to maintain blood flow from a medial location. The pelvic wall's blood supply does not usually supply the ureter. Injuries which occur within 5–6 cm of the ureteral vesical junction are therefore best managed by ureteral reimplantation into the bladder.

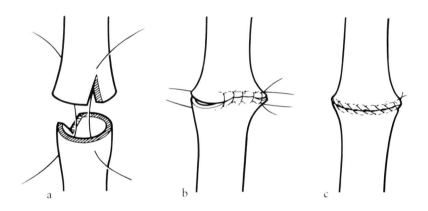

Figure 10.3: End-to-end ureteral anastamosis. a, spatulated ureteral ends; b, ureteral approximation; c, watertight tension-free closure with 4 or 5 absorbable sutures.

There are five important steps to successful ureteral repair:

- the anastomosis must be tension-free
- the ureteral margins must be freshened and viable
- ureteral blood supply must be maintained
- the ureter must be spatulated
- a watertight anastomosis with absorbable sutures must be performed.

Ureteral end-to-end anastomosis has already been accomplished utilizing a complete laparoscopic approach with a successful outcome. When a ureteral transsection occurred in the distal third of the ureter, primary laparoscopic repair was accomplished. The injury occurred during the performance of a laparoscopic hysterectomy. The ureter was entrapped within the distal three staples of an Endo-GIA staple line with complete ligation. The previously placed ureteral stent was secured to the ureter. Complete removal of the staple line was necessary for ureteral deligation. After deligation, the distal segment was not mobilized and it remained in situ, preserving its blood supply. The ligation occurred 4 cm from the uretero–vesical junction. The proximal ureteral blood supply remained intact after mobilization and only then was laparoscopic repair considered. A bleeding proximal ureteral artery was controlled with a haemoclip. A spatulated, tension-free anastomosis was accomplished with four 4–0 chromic sutures tied intracorporally. A pedicle of perivesical fat was used to buttress the repair. A double-J ureteral stent was placed from below and a Penrose drain was placed intra-abdominally. The patient was positioned in the lithotomy position to allow access for cystoscopy. An IVU performed one year postoperatively demonstrates no evidence of obstruction or repair. The injury was recognized in the recovery room when the ureteral stent could not be removed. A supine film of the abdomen confirmed a ureteral stent entrapped within a staple line. A return to the operating room could have been prevented if the ureteral catheters had been removed under direct laparoscopic vision.

Stenting repairs

Most texts on urological injuries and repair indicate that it is debatable whether or not to stent ureteral repairs. Ureteral intubation and stent management are now so simple and basic to urological care that I believe such a controversy no longer exists. All ureteral repairs require placement of ureteral stents. They are relatively well tolerated and protect the anastomosis with continuous diversion of the urine around and through the stent. They allow the repair to close quickly and act as a bridge for ureteral re-epithelization. Most importantly, urinary flow through the repair is necessary to prevent ureteral stricture formation. Strictures are associated with dry anastomoses diverted with nephrostomy tube drainage alone. Stents of 4–5 F are ideal for the narrow lumen of the ureter (Figure 10.4).

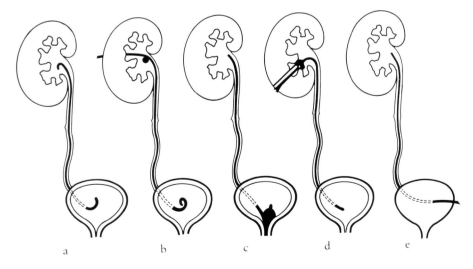

Figure 10.4: Ureteral stents. a, double-J; b, nephrostent; c, simple transurethral stent; d, nephrostomy tube and antegrade simple stent; e, simple retrograde stent department from bladder.

Long ureteral defects or strictures are occasionally managed with indwelling ureteral stents without primary repair. The ureteral defect is left open to heal by secondary intention. A portion of ureteral continuity must be maintained for a successful outcome. Ideally the ureteral mucosa will re-epithealize to cover the defect along the stent. The indications for this Davis intubated ureterotomy are fortunately few. This technique is presently being utilized for endoscopic ureteral stricture incisions from both a retrograde and antegrade endoscopic approach. It has a limited role in acute ureteral injuries (Figure 10.5).

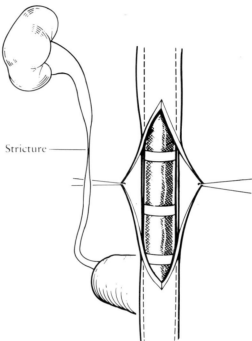

Stricture

Figure 10.5: Davis intubated **ureterotomy.**

Reimplantation

When ureteral injuries occur within 5–6 cm of the bladder, ureteral reimplantation has the best chance of success. A ureteral reimplantation is best performed using a non-refluxing technique. The ureter is reimplanted into the bladder through a submucosal tunnel. This technique requires a submucosal tunnel two-thirds longer than the ureteral diameter. The ureter is secured at the mucosal and serosal margins with absorbable suture. Uretero–vesical reflux in the presence of infection can cause renal damage from pyelonephritis. It is especially harmful in the developing kidney of infants and children. Laparoscopic ureteral reimplantation has already been performed using a simple free anastomotic technique. A stent protects the healing anastomosis. At present there has been limited experience with reimplantation using laparoscopic techniques. Open ureteroneocystostomy has little morbidity and an excellent success rate (Figure 10.6).

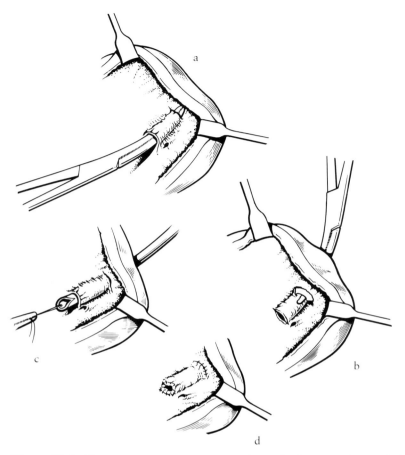

Figure 10.6: Ureteroneocystostomy. a, creation of sub-mucosal tunnel; b, creation of bladder hiatus; c, ureter placed into bladder and sub-mucosal tunnel; d, absorbable suture closure at mucosa hiatus.

In order to obtain a tension-free anastomosis, additional mobilization of the bladder and ureter may be necessary. The bladder may be fixed to the lateral pelvic wall using a non-absorbable suture. This psoas hitch allows added length to reach the ureter for tension-free anastomosis. Mobilization of the opposite side of the bladder is usually required to give added mobility for the psoas hitch (Figure 10.7).

When a psoas hitch is inadequate to reach the injured ureter, a Boari flap may be used. This allows bladder mobilization to the pelvic brim. A tongue of bladder is developed using the base of the bladder as a pedicle flap. A branch of the superior vesicle artery is used to supply blood to the pedicle. The tongue of bladder is then rolled into a tube and closed after a ureteral reimplantation has been accomplished. The anterior bladder surface is then closed with absorbable sutures. This manoeuvre allows management of long distal ureteral defects (Figure 10.8).

At times long segments of ureter are removed with tissue specimens, and urological management may be complicated and difficult. Renal mobilization

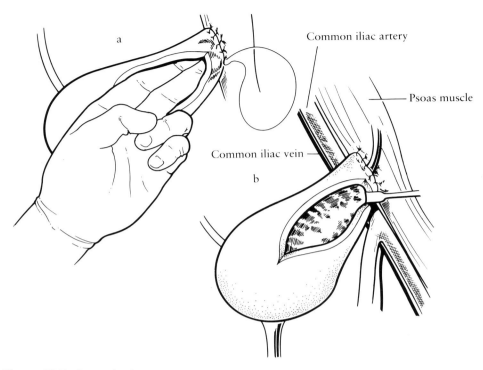

Figure 10.7: Psoas hitch. a, mobilized bladder attached to psoas muscle with non-absorbable suture; b, non-refluxing ureteroneocystostomy.

may give sufficient length to allow a Boari flap reimplantation. The renal unit then must resuture into its new position to maintain and protect the ureteral anastomosis. Renal mobilization may add an additional 2–3 cm of ureteral length.

Contraindications

Occasionally sufficient ureteral length is maintained to swing the injured ureter in a retro-colic position over to the opposite healthy ureter. A patient with a history of stone disease is a relative contraindication to transuretero-ureterostomy. Stone management although possible would be more complicated with this Y connection. Malignancy is a strong contraindication along with the presence of infection, poor blood supply, radiation, fibrosis, and non-urological infections such as pelvic inflammatory disease and diverticulosis. Successful management should not compromise the healthy renal unit. This choice of management is suitable when a small capacity or non-distendible bladder is present. It is used only when other methods previously described are not available (Figure 10.9).

When long defects are encountered, a ureteral substitution with an ileal segment may be performed. The ileal segment can bridge defects from the renal pelvis to bladder. Large amounts of mucus production may make voiding difficult for male patients due to the prostate and a long narrow

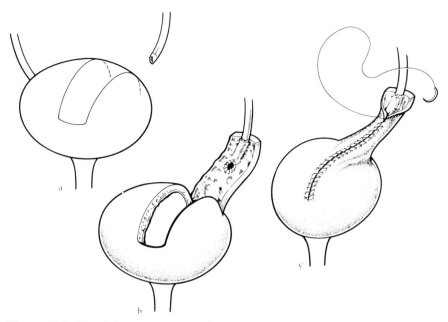

Figure 10.8: Boari flap. a, posterior based pedicle flap supplied by the vesical artery; b, non-refluxing ureteroneocystostomy; c, bladder closure.

urethra. Electrolyte imbalances due to acidbase changes associated with urinary diversions may also be difficult to manage. Laparoscopic ileal conduit diversions have already been performed. Laparoscopic techniques for the management of such complications are on the horizon. Patients considered as candidates for intestinal substitution require an uncontaminated operative field, good renal function and no evidence of bladder outlet obstruction (Figure 10.10).

Cutaneous ureterostomy

Cutaneous ureterostomy is a poor management choice. Almost all fail due to stenosis at the skin margin. There is no acceptable urinary collection appliance for a cutaneous ureterostomy. It can be sometimes used as a temporary measure to maintain renal function. Most renal units lose function due to obstruction when this technique is utilized over time.

Ureteral ligation

Ureteral ligation with a normal functioning kidney is not usually acceptable. Necrosis of the ureteral stump will usually lead to urinary extravasation and sepsis or urinoma formation. Ureteral ligation will usually lead to immediate renal colic with associated fever. Pericutaneous nephrostomy diversion at the time of ureteral ligation may allow renal salvage at a later date after a plan of management can be formulated. The technique of ureteral ligation may be employed in cases of poorly functioning renal units. The risk of ureteral ligation includes uretero-cutaneous fistula, infection, colic and the need for a secondary nephrectomy.

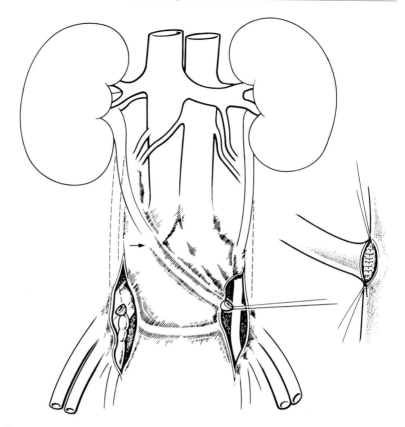

Figure 10.9: Transuretero-ureterostomy (right to left).

Nephrectomy

Nephrectomy is acceptable only in cases of a healthy second kidney, and is usually performed in the very ill or elderly patient. At present it is rarely utilized. An important point to remember is that pericutaneous nephrostomy tube drainage is an excellent method to temporize almost any case of ureteral injury and allow delayed ureteral repairs.

Bladder

Bladder injuries are less common than ureteral injuries. They are easy to manage and probably go unreported most of the time. The bladder is a forgiving organ and easy to repair. Even small holes in the bladder will self-heal and heal within several days without a Foley catheter. Retroperitoneal injuries, even with larger holes, can certainly be managed with catheter drainage alone. Intra-abdominal injuries, however, are different: urinary leakage into the peritoneal cavity is unacceptable and is a source of urinary ascites and sepsis.

Injuries incurred as part of laparoscopic procedures are easily repaired. Small holes may be closed with an Endoloop knot over the defect for

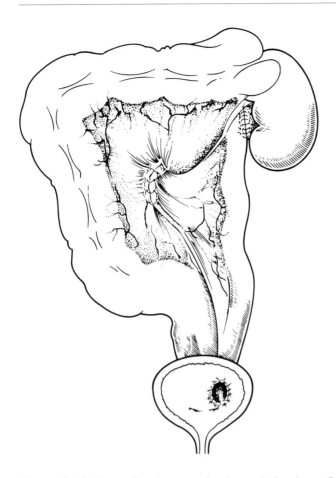

Figure 10.10: Ureteral replacement by ileum. Left colon reflected medially; ileal segment brought through mesentery.

watertight closure. A second purse-string or figure-of-eight stitch may be utilized to bury the first knot for a two-layer closure of absorbable suture. The bladder may then be filled to assess the water tightness of the closure. A small Penrose drain may be placed along the site of closure for 24–48 h. In female patients, if there is no drainage, the Foley catheter may be removed in five to seven days. Larger defects may be closed with running chromic or gut suture for a two-layer closure utilizing endoscopic suture techniques. In addition an endoscopic Endo-GIA or Endo-cutter can close long defects in a watertight fashion using vascular staples without the need for catheter drainage. A staple line within the bladder may be lithogenic and further follow-up will be necessary. Several patients have undergone bladder stapling, but we await follow-up reports. In my own experience the bladder mucosa always overgrows the staple line and causes no problems.

When in doubt, for difficult closures, a Foley may remain for 10–14 days. A cystogram should be performed prior to catheter removal when complicating factors arise (ie poor wound-healing or infection). Prolonged catheter drainage is usually unnecessary. With all bladder closures the position of the ureteral orifices must be kept in mind, and injuries prevented. Urinary antibiotics can be used to prevent urinary tract infections during the healing period. Suppressive antibiotic therapy can be used when indwelling stents or Foley catheters are present.

Preventive urological measures and patient preparation

Several of the following comments may seem inappropriate to experienced surgeons but all are realistic and apply to many of the case histories of the author and his colleagues in academic and community practice.

Positioning

Patient positioning is an important aspect of operative endoscopy — especially for the management of urological complications, should they arise. The lithotomy position is not always employed for operative endoscopy but can be a very useful tool in the management of pelvic injury and for the manipulation of the pelvic organs. The lithotomy position allows immediate access to the genitourinary tract should manipulation be necessary. In cases of simple diagnostic laparoscopy or tubal ligation, the supine position may limit access to the urologic and pelvic organs. The lithotomy position may take a few extra minutes to set up, but it is well worth the time in patient preparation should any problem arise.

In the male patient, the penis should always be prepared in the operative field. Access to the urinary tract can be gained with the use of a flexible cystoscope. In cases of planned urological surgery, the male patient can also be placed in the lithotomy position to allow rigid cystoscopy. Moderate haematuria during an operative endoscopy can be difficult to handle with the small irrigation ports of the flexible cystoscope, and is best managed with rigid cystoscopy. The same applies to female patients.

Proper drainage of the bladder is necessary in operative endoscopy for several reasons. Again, patient preparation is the key to a successful surgical outcome with minimal morbidity. Simple bladder drainage prior to endoscopy via a hollow urethral sound or simple red rubber catheterization may not be adequate for several reasons. Occasionally, simple sound drainage may not adequately empty the bladder when impatient hands are applied. The author has already dealt with a bladder trocar injury from an inadequately emptied bladder using this technique. Large cystoceles, uterine descent or obstruction of the bladder neck by a large fibroid uterus may preclude complete emptying on straight catheterization. A Foley catheter placed to allow gravity drainage has several advantages. With gravity drainage the tubing and drainage bag are placed below the level of the bladder. A tubing and drainage bag placed next to the thigh in the lithotomy position may not allow adequate bladder drainage, especially after the patient is placed in this position. A brisk diuresis during operative endoscopy, and the Trendelenberg position, may allow bladder filling during the procedure which may interfere with the case. For prolonged operative endoscopy, catheter drainage usually provides an accurate measurement of urinary output and assists in the fluid management of the patient. This is important for our increasingly elderly patient population now undergoing operative endoscopy. Elderly women undergoing laparoscopic hysterectomies or fibroid removal are subject to increased cardiac risk and large blood volume losses. I specifically note that due to the Trendelenberg positioning and pneumoperitoneum of greater than 15 mmHg pressure, urinary output may actually decrease during the operative endoscopy in spite of fluid challenges during the procedure. Returning the patient to a level position and decreasing the intra-abdominal pressure allows a brisk diuresis to ensue in all cases of normal volemic patients. When urinary output is decreased obviously other causes for low urinary volumes should be sought (ie ureteral ligation, transsections or hypovolemia). Haematuria can be picked up early when there is continued catheter drainage and may signal ureteral or bladder injury. Pelvic organ manipulation itself may cause haematuria with bladder manipulation. Several diagnostic manoeuvres may aid in the identification of urinary tract injuries and are covered in the assessment portion of this chapter.

Placement of catheters

There can be no substitute for knowledge of our ureteral anatomy. Preoperative ureteral catheters at times can be used for the prevention of ureteral injuries. Cystoscopy and placement of ureteral catheters is a simple procedure and can be learned easily by a gynaecologist interested in operative endoscopy. Passage of ureteral catheters in the female patient has little or no morbidity once the technique is learned. Instrumentation of the male urinary tract is much more difficult. The long pendulous and prostatic urethra can be an obstacle to ureteral intubation, especially when prostatic enlargement is encountered, therefore male ureteral catheterization should be left to a urological surgeon. Improper uretheral instrumentation carries a higher morbidity in the male patient.

Often ureteral catheters do not actually prevent injury but allow us to identify a major injury when it occurs. Ureteral injuries that are recognized immediately can be repaired easily without significant morbidity. A delayed diagnosis of ureteral injury significantly increases the complication rate and may lead to loss of the renal unit. During operative endoscopy, ureteral palpation is not possible: although, once located, a ureter may be palpable with smooth grasping forceps when a ureteral stent is in place. Ureters are delicate structures and should be treated atraumatically.

Diagnostic endoscopy

Ureteral catheters are not necessary for diagnostic endoscopy. When significant pelvic pathology is expected with a planned operative endoscopy, ureteral catheters may provide a sense of security and protection. Simple ureteral catheters (5 or 6 fg) can be passed easily in most cases even with significant pelvic pathology. Extrinsic ureteral compression does not preclude simple ureteral catheter passage. Open-ended or side-port catheters allow continued urinary flow through the catheter lumen as well as around the catheter. They are non-obstructing and relatively atraumatic.

Operative endoscopy

Movement of the catheter at the urethral meatus during operative endoscopy can easily identify the intra-abdominal position or near location of the ureter when pelvic adhesions are present. Disposable ones are stocked in most cysto suites and are relatively inexpensive. Bilateral ureteral catheters are simply passed on cystoscopy. Unilateral placement can be performed but it may be a self-limiting step since a majority of pelvic pathology may involve both pelvic walls. The sigmoid colon offers a large amount of protection to the left ureter deep within the pelvis. Ureteral catheterization may not be necessary for left-sided pathology.

Ureteral catheters are ideally placed for transsections of the uretero-sacral ligaments when used in the treatment of chronic pelvic pain. The ureters are millimetres away in a lateral position. Although ureteral injury is uncommon with uretero-sacral division, laparoscopic visualization of the ureters shows them in close proximity to the uretero-sacral ligaments.

Urological assistance

In cases where pathology involves the ureter, urological assistance may be warranted. At times of difficult ureteral intubation a ureteral guide wire may be necessary to assist in the passage of ureteral catheters. If a planned endoscopy involves the urinary tract, a preoperative ureteral stent may be placed which can remain on a long-term basis. Several specialty catheters have been designed to remain within the urinary tract for up to six months to allow healing of any manipulation or injury. These soft flexible catheters provide maximum comfort. A preoperative intravenous urogram can be obtained to define the ureteral anatomy and determine whether pelvic pathology involves the genito-urinary tract.

Illumination

Ureteral illumination can be advocated as a measure in the prevention of ureteral injuries. Several types of illuminated ureteral catheters can be employed. Karl Storz (Culver City, CA, USA) manufacture a 6 fg closed-ended ureteral catheter which connects to a high-intensity light source. A Y connector Storz light cable allows both ureteral catheters to be illuminated simultaneously. A high-intensity light source is required for proper illumination. Low-intensity light sources are not sufficient. A second light source, in addition to the abdominal light source being used for laparoscopy, is needed. The xenon light source can provide sufficient intra-abdominal illumination of the ureters even with full endoscopic illumination. Decreasing the intra-abdominal illumination can aid in visualization through dense pelvic adhesions. The disadvantage of these catheters is that sometimes small ureteral orifices will prevent their passage without ureteral orifice dilatation, which can be time-consuming. Closed-ended ureteral catheters may decrease urinary output temporarily during the case. Urinary flow may continue around the catheter and urinary output is usually maintained although at a lesser degree. In addition the Storz catheters have a metal tip which is blunt but has a small bevel at its site of attachment to the plastic catheter. This small bevel tends to cause a small amount of ureteral trauma upon removal. This trauma occasionally precipitates ureteral bleeding and the passage of small clots which act much like a stone and give rise to renal colic. The author has had no hospital admission for postinstrumentation colic, but several patients have required narcotic pain relief at home.

Pilling, a Rusch International company (Fort Washington, PA, USA), has a similar set-up. A 65 cm 5–8 fg soft transparent plastic catheter with a round tip is utilized. Three lateral ports allow urinary drainage. The catheter is X-ray opaque. Two fibreoptic stems are connected to a cold light source. The connector adapts to most cold light sources including ACMI light sources. Two fibreoptic stems are inserted into the two transparent ureteral catheters after positioning into the patient. The ureteral illuminator is supplied as a set comprising one illuminator and two 5 fg ureteral catheters.

Open-ended ureteral catheterization is a simple and inexpensive method for visualization of the ureters on endoscopy and it works very well. Illumination of the ureters is most helpful in the difficult cases where dense adhesion or endometriosis is present. Trying all methods of ureteral identification (illumination and non-illumination) is necessary for the laparoscopic surgeon to become familiar and comfortable with the different techniques.

Since the morbidity and mortality of ureteral injuries are significantly higher when the diagnosis is delayed, ureteral catheters may be advantageous in difficult cases.

At the termination of the procedure, both ureteral catheters can be removed along with the Foley catheter.

Conclusion

Many of the above comments and suggestions are meant to be used merely as a guide to operative endoscopy. A surgeon should be familiar with all the possible ways, so that he can make an educated choice about how to choose to perform his surgical procedures. Knowledge of how and why we proceed in operative laparoscopy allows the surgeon to choose the most acceptable style to suit his practice and better serve his patients.

References

1   Pearse HD *et al.* (1985) Intraoperative consultation for the ureter. In: *Urological clinics of North America*. WB Saunders, Philadelphia.

Suggested reading

Aronson WJ and Ehrlich RM (1992) Complications of ureteral surgery management and prevention. *American Urological Association Update Series*. **11**. 180–5.

Kay R and Straffon RA (1987) Intraoperative urological complications of abdominal surgery. *American Urological Association Update Series*. **6**. 1–7.

Spirnak JP and Resnick MI (1985) Intraoperative consultation for the bladder. In: *Urological Clinics of North America*. WB Saunders, Philadelphia.

Zabbo A and Montie JE (1985) Intraoperative consultation for the kidney. In: *Urological Clinics of North America*. WB Saunders, Philadelphia.

Part III: Laparoscopic Procedures

Management of the Pelvic Mass by Operative Laparoscopy

Laparoscopic Approach to Hysterectomy

Laparoscopic Treatment of Urinary Stress Incontinence

Operative Endoscopy in the Treatment of Infertility

Minimally Invasive Treatment of Endometriosis

Operative Endoscopic Management of Leiomyoma Uteri

Laparoscopic Management of Pelvic Pain

Gynaecological Applications of Optical Catheters (Microhysteroscopy and Microlaparoscopy)

11

Management of the Pelvic Mass by Operative Laparoscopy

WILLIAM H. PARKER and JONATHAN S. BEREK

Introduction

The standard operative approach for the intended removal of a pelvic mass has been via laparotomy. The goal has been to remove a neoplastic lesion before it might compromise the patient, as well as to resect and properly stage ovarian cancer should it be found. However, most adnexal masses are benign. Malignancy is found in only 7–13% of premenopausal and 8–45% of postmenopausal women operated on for the presence of a pelvic mass.

Controversy

It would appear that operative laparoscopic management of a pelvic mass can be accomplished appropriately in most patients, as evidenced by a 1990 survey conducted by the American Association of Gynecologic Laparoscopists[1]. This study reported only 53 cases of laparoscopic management of unsuspected ovarian cancer in 13 739 cases of ovarian cyst surgery, an incidence of 0.04%. A counterpoint to that study comes from a survey of gynaecological oncologists, which found 12 patients with borderline ovarian tumours and 30 patients with invasive ovarian cancers who had been managed initially by laparoscopic excision of the masses[2]. However, the patients in that survey did not have careful preoperative screening, in that many of the masses were complex or solid, and 50% of the patients were found to have advanced stage disease. In addition, many of the patients were inappropriately managed in that they did not have appropriate and timely surgical management when malignancy was found. Staging laparotomy was performed immediately after laparoscopic diagnosis of malignancy in only 17% of cases. In the remaining patients, appropriate surgery was delayed by an average of 4.8 weeks. Thus the delay characterized the poor patient management and not the laparoscopic approach itself.

This same problem was illustrated by a study of patients who had surgical staging of ovarian cancer by laparotomy in the Netherlands[3]. Incomplete surgical staging was done in 95% of the early ovarian cancers studied and 65% of the patients were subjected to a second laparotomy to complete the staging. Frozen section should be done if suspicious areas are noted at the time of laparoscopy, and when invasive cancer is found it is crucial that the surgeon is prepared to proceed with immediate staging laparotomy.

Risks

In the past, laparoscopic drainage or removal of a pelvic mass has been avoided because of the theoretical risk of 'spilling' cancer cells into the peritoneal cavity and the fear of decreasing the patient's chances of survival. This concern, however, resulted from early studies that did not analyse peritoneal washings, omental biopsies, tumour grade, adhesions or ascites. Dembo and colleagues, in a recent multivariate analysis of stage I epithelial ovarian cancer patients, found that the only factors that influenced the rate of relapse in 519 stage I patients were the tumour grade and the presence of dense adhesions and large volume ascites[4]. The rate of relapse and prognosis was not influenced by rupture of the tumour. Thus the potential for tumour dissemination by iatrogenic rupture of a malignant cyst remains conjectural.

Malignancy

Laparoscopic aspiration of an adnexal cyst as an isolated procedure is not recommended. Studies show that 10–66% of aspirates are read as benign when, in fact, malignancy is present[5]. This high false-negative rate indicates the inadequacy of this procedure for definitive diagnosis[6]. Many ovarian cysts also contain functional epithelium and often persist unless removed. Cystectomy allows complete removal of the cyst lining, which provides tissue for pathological analysis and prevents recurrence.

The question of malignant transformation of benign neoplastic cysts is unanswered. The transition from benign to malignant epithelium has been described in histological studies of ovarian tumours. Puls et al. reported epithelial transition in 100% of borderline tumours, and in 100% of grade 1, 67% of grade 2, and 32% of grade 3 epithelial ovarian cancers[7]. They concluded that this transition supports the concept of malignant transformation. However, it is not clear whether epithelial transition represents true transformation or rather the coexistence of benign and malignant epithelium in close proximity.

In one study that used transvaginal ultrasonography to screen patients with a positive family history of ovarian cancer, there was a higher proportion of women who had benign epithelial ovarian tumours than in a previous population-based study[8]. The author stated that this was consistent with the hypothesis of malignant transformation. It is possible, however, that these patients had also inherited a predisposition for benign ovarian neoplasia.

The increased use of ultrasound and CT scans for evaluation of pelvic and abdominal complaints has led to the frequent discovery of ovarian cysts, the majority of which are benign. A recent study evaluated the prevalence of unilocular cysts, as detected by ultrasound, in 149 asymptomatic volunteers aged 50 years and older[9]. Unilocular cysts were found in 22 patients (15%) ranging in size from 0.4 to 4.7 cm. The lifetime incidence of ovarian cancer is only 1.3%. Therefore, even if transformation occurs, it does so rarely. If malignant transformation could be anticipated, then aggressive management and removal of ovarian cysts would be imperative. A more complete understanding of malignant transformation is necessary to answer this important issue.

The appropriate management of borderline ovarian tumours is an important issue. One report examined the recurrence rate and survival of 35 patients with borderline ovarian tumours managed initially by just cystectomy via laparotomy[10]. None of these patients, including those who had 'spillage' of cyst contents, developed evidence of disseminated disease. In addition, all 35 patients were still alive with no evidence of disease an average of 7.5 years after diagnosis. Therefore the prognosis of patients with borderline tumours is not likely to be altered by laparoscopic management.

Reported studies

Dermoid cysts and endometriomas have been managed via laparotomy in order to allow complete resection and thus decrease recurrence. Laparotomy was also felt to allow removal of dermoid cysts with minimum spillage, thus decreasing the potential for chemical peritonitis. There is now extensive literature available on the use of operative laparoscopy for premenopausal women found to have a pelvic mass. Pregnancy rates of 40% have previously been reported for patients who have endometriomas resected via laparotomy[11]. Daniell and colleagues reported a pregnancy rate of 38% (12/32) in patients who had laparoscopic resection of endometriomas[12]. Likewise, Marrs reported that 10 of 23 patients (43%) achieved pregnancy after laparoscopic management of their endometriomas[13]. In that study surgical time averaged 52 minutes, mean postoperative recovery time was five hours and there were no complications. In addition, none of the 10 patients who underwent second-look laparoscopy had adnexal adhesions.

Nezhat and colleagues performed operative laparoscopic cystectomies on nine patients with dermoid cysts ranging from 5–8 cm[14]. Four patients had second-look laparoscopies and one of these patients had mild periovarian adhesions. Mage et al. reported that, of 78 patients who had laparoscopic excision of a dermoid cyst, none had chemical peritonitis following the procedure[15]. They also reported that cystic adnexal masses had been safely approached by laparoscopy in 420 of 481 patients aged nine to 88 years. Laparoscopic management of 433 cysts in these patients included 95 functional cysts, 90 endometriomas, 87 serous cysts, 78 teratomas, 45 mucinous cysts and 58 paraovarian cysts. Indications for laparotomy were suspicion of malignancy in 19 patients and dense pelvic adhesions and/or cysts greater than 10 cm in 42 patients. Inspection of the pelvis and internal cyst wall allowed accurate diagnosis of all five ovarian cancers and all four borderline ovarian tumours. These nine patients had appropriate surgery by laparotomy.

Postmenopausal laparoscopy

The role of operative laparoscopy in postmenopausal women has been even more controversial. We have published a pilot study in which 22 of 25 (88%) carefully selected postmenopausal patients with adnexal masses were successfully managed by operative laparoscopy[16]. With careful preoperative screening, as described below, we have found benign masses in all 44 postmenopausal patients to date. Operative findings included 16 serous cysts, seven serous cystadenomas, seven cystadenofibromas, four hydrosalpinges, five paratubal cysts, and one retroperitoneal paraovarian cyst. Operative time has averaged 63 minutes, average postoperative stay has been 12 hours, and average return to normal activity has taken five days. Only three of the 44 patients (7%) required laparotomy: one for an inconclusive frozen section, one for repair of a bowel injury, and one to remove metastatic breast cancer found incidentally at laparoscopy for a benign paratubal cyst. We are currently conducting a multicentred study to continue to evaluate our selection process and operative approach.

Preoperative evaluation

Careful preoperative evaluation may help select patients likely to have a benign mass who may be considered for operative laparoscopy. The patient's age, clinical exam and ultrasound findings provide information that help determine the operative approach. Tumour markers, specifically CA-125, should be evaluated in postmenopausal women.

Ultrasonography

Ultrasonographic examination of the pelvis is a reliable method for determining the size and consistency of a pelvic mass. Transvaginal ultrasonography is preferred over transabdominal exam because the proximity of the vaginal probe to the pelvic structures allows greater resolution and clarity of image.

With the use of specific ultrasound criteria, Herrmann and colleagues accurately predicted benign masses in 177 of 185 (96%) patients studied[17]. In addition, all 48 purely cystic masses < 10 cm were benign and eight out of 10 stage I ovarian cancers were accurately predicted. In a large study of 94 postmenopausal and 86 menstruating women, Granberg and colleagues found that ultrasonography correctly predicted benign masses in 92% of patients[18]. Other studies have reported similar results[19,20]. A number of authors have suggested observation of cystic masses less than 5 cm based on the low risk of malignancy. Luxman and colleagues, however, reported that two of 33 (6%) simple cysts <5 cm found on transabdominal ultrasonography were malignant[21]. Therefore he encouraged an operative approach for these masses. On ultrasound, the following characteristics suggest a benign mass:

- regular borders
- no papillations
- no solid parts
- no thick septa (>2 mm)
- no ascites or matted bowel.

Dermoids, endometriomas, haemorrhagic cysts, cystadenomas and persistent functional cysts will often have a characteristic appearance on ultrasonography[22]. Along with the clinical picture and other laboratory data, ultrasonography may help in the selection of patients who can be approached by operative laparoscopy.

On ultrasonography, functional cysts are usually unilocular and have regular, thin borders. In premenopausal women the majority of purely cystic masses less than 7 cm will resolve spontaneously. Therefore these cysts may be followed for eight weeks. Most cysts will regress spontaneously and recent evidence shows that oral contraceptive suppression is unnecessary[23]. Haemorrhagic cysts contain internal echoes that can vary in intensity from low to high level and be either focal or diffuse. These cysts characteristically change over time and often regress spontaneously. Cysts that persist, although they appear to be functional or haemorrhagic on ultrasonography, should be removed to rule out neoplasia.

Dermoids have a variable appearance on ultrasound. They may appear as a cystic mass that contains an echogenic mural focus, echogenic material in a nondependant area, or highly echogenic areas suggesting bone or teeth. Endometriomas usually have regular but slightly thickened borders. They often contain low-level and diffuse internal echoes, although fresh haemorrhage may appear more highly echogenic. If the diagnosis of a dermoid, endometrioma, haemorrhagic cyst or persistent functional cyst is based on clinical exam and ultrasonography, then operative laparoscopy may be considered.

The presence of irregular borders, papillations, solid areas, thick septa, ascites or matted bowel should raise concern regarding the possibility of malignancy, and laparotomy should be done.

Colour Doppler sonography

Transvaginal colour Doppler sonography has recently been applied to the preoperative evaluation of pelvic masses. Malignant tumours are associated with the formation of new vessels that possess thin walls and arteriovenous shunts. These vessels have low impedance and therefore high blood flow that may be detected by Doppler imaging. Weiner and colleagues found that

16 of 17 malignant masses had an abnormal Doppler study and 35 of 36 benign masses were accurately predicted. In that study, sensitivity was 94% and specificity was 97%[24]. Fleischer and colleagues found that transvaginal ultrasonography accurately predicted malignancy in seven of 11 masses, while the application of colour Doppler allowed accurate prediction of malignancy in all 11 of the masses[25]. They recommended the use of colour Doppler to distinguish masses that have malignant characteristics on transvaginal ultrasonography, ie irregular walls or echogenic internal material. However, the role of Doppler sonography in the evaluation of pelvic masses is not well established and should at present be considered investigational.

CA-125

CA-125, a tumour-associated antigen, has been studied to determine its value in preoperative differentiation of benign and malignant pelvic masses. Vasilev and colleagues found that 128 of 132 (97%) patients with pelvic masses who had a CA-125 <35 u ml^{-1} had benign masses[26]. Eighty per cent of patients over 50 with elevated CA-125 levels had malignant masses. However, in patients less than 50 years old who had an elevated CA-125 value, 34 of 40 patients (85%) had a benign mass. Endometriosis, leiomyomata, adenomyosis, dermoid cysts, pregnancy and acute or chronic salpingitis may all be associated with elevated levels. Therefore CA-125 values add to the evaluation of the postmenopausal patient, but are not helpful in the premenopausal patient.

In addition, a review article compiling the data from a number of studies, Jacobs and Bast found that only 50% of patients with stage I ovarian cancers had elevated CA-125 values (>35 u ml^{-1})[27]. This test will miss many early cancers and is therefore too insensitive to be used alone for selecting appropriate patients for laparoscopic management.

Many tumour markers have been studied in an effort to increase the sensitivity and specificity in the preoperative determination of ovarian tumours. Gadducci et al. studied CA-125, CA-19.9, CA-15.3, CA-72.4 and TATI in 90 patients with ovarian cancer and 254 patients with benign pelvic masses[28]. The combination of CA-125 and CA-19.9 had a higher sensitivity but lower specificity than CA-125 alone in postmenopausal women. They concluded that CA-125 was the most reliable marker for distinguishing a benign from a malignant pelvic mass. Inoue measured serum sialyl-Tn, sialyl-Lewis Xi, CA-19.9, CA-125, CEA and tissue polypeptide antigen in 65 women with early stage ovarian cancer and 317 women with benign pelvic masses[29]. With the combination of all six markers, 20% of the patients with stage I or II ovarian cancer had false-negative results. They concluded that multimodal approaches (ie clinical exam, imaging and serum assays) would be necessary to detect all malignant masses at an early stage.

Combination of ultrasonography and CA-125

Finkler and colleagues combined the use of clinical impression, CA-125 values, and ultrasonographic findings for the preoperative evaluation of ovarian masses[30]. In 74 premenopausal women, ultrasonography alone had a negative predictive value of 86%, which was not improved by the addition of CA-125 values. Due to the high false-positive rate, the addition of CA-125 values unnecessarily excludes many premenopausal women who would benefit from operative laparoscopy. In premenopausal women, therefore, only clinical and ultrasonographic criteria are used to select patients for laparoscopic management.

For postmenopausal women, ultrasonography had a negative predictive value of 71%, but when combined with CA-125 values all 10 postmenopausal patients predicted to have benign masses were accurately predicted. Likewise, Jacobs *et al.* reported that, of nine postmenopausal patients with adnexal masses with benign ultrasonographic appearances and normal CA-125 values, seven had benign processes and two had a normal pelvis[31]. In our own study, using criteria that included ultrasonographic findings of a cystic mass <10 cm, with distinct borders and no evidence of irregular solid parts, thick septa, ascites or matted bowel, and a normal CA-125 value (<35 u ml^{-1}), we have thus far evaluated 44 postmenopausal patients with adnexal masses and have accurately predicted benign masses in all patients.

In postmenopausal patients, therefore, a combination of criteria of ultrasonography and CA-125 values constitutes a reasonable selection process. A laparoscopic approach may be considered if CA-125 values are less than 35 u ml^{-1}, and if ultrasonography shows

- a cystic mass less than 10 cm in size and with distinct borders
- no irregular solid parts or thick septa
- no evidence of ascites or matted bowel.

General considerations

All patients scheduled for operative laparoscopy should also consent to a possible laparotomy, and the surgeon should be prepared to proceed with staging laparotomy without delay if malignancy is found.

Under general endotracheal anaesthesia, surgery is performed in the low lithotomy position. Foley catheters are used in all patients to avoid bladder injury and prevent overdistension during prolonged cases. A 10 mm laparoscope is used because of the excellent optical acuity, wide field of vision and increased light available. The inferior epigastric vessels may be identified by transilluminating the abdominal wall, but are often seen more clearly from within the peritoneal cavity as they course laterally to the obliterated umbilical ligaments. Taking care to avoid the vessels, 5, 11 or 12 mm trocars are inserted via suprapubic incisions as needed.

The initial inspection of the peritoneal cavity is done prior to attaching the video camera. We feel that this allows a better assessment of the fine detail and colour differentiation. The upper abdomen and pelvis are inspected for obvious carcinoma, excrescences and ascites. Pelvic and abdominal washings are done for staging in case a carcinoma is subsequently found. If excrescences are noted, they are biopsied with a 5 mm biopsy forceps and sent for frozen section. (Biopsies should be large enough for the pathologist to interpret.) If obvious carcinoma, ascites or a positive frozen section is found, then we proceed with immediate staging laparotomy. The following is a checklist of surgical considerations:

1   obtain consent for laparoscopy and laparotomy
2   perform general endotracheal anaesthesia
3   put Foley catheter in place
4   make intraoperative assessment of abdomen and pelvis
5   perform pelvic and abdominal washings
6   biopsy and make immediate frozen section of suspicious areas
7   perform immediate staging laparotomy if cancer found.

Although frozen section has been shown to be very accurate, equivocal results should be acted upon according to the patient's age and desire for fertility. We have chosen to proceed with staging laparotomy and hysterectomy in the postmenopausal patient with an equivocal frozen section, but have performed conservative surgery (ie cystectomy or oophorectomy) in premenopausal patients pending the final pathology report.

Once a decision has been made to proceed with operative laparoscopy, the video camera is attached, allowing the assistant and the nurse to participate. The type of procedure is determined by the operative findings.

Procedures

Aspiration and fenestration

Aspiration, as an isolated procedure, is rarely done because it does not allow inspection of the cyst wall or removal of tissue for pathological analysis. Cytological analysis of cyst fluid is associated with a false negative rate that approaches 60% in some studies. Aspiration may also be associated with a recurrence rate approaching 30%. Aspiration may be considered in premenopausal women who are found to have clearly functional ovarian cysts less than 3 cm.

Fenestration has been described as the removal of a window from the cyst wall, thus allowing pathological analysis of a small portion of the cyst wall and providing an opening for continued drainage. Visualization of the entire cyst lining by placing the laparoscope within the cyst allows the surgeon to assess the cyst wall. If excrescences are found, they are biopsied and sent for immediate frozen section. Frank carcinoma or suspicious cells demand immediate staging laparotomy. In most cases of simple cysts we have favoured cystectomy, since this allows removal and complete pathological analysis of the cyst wall.

The ovary is stabilized by grasping the utero-ovarian ligament with an atraumatic grasping forceps. The ligament is rotated laterally in order to bring the ovary into full view. A 1 cm avascular site is chosen on the cyst and the tissue blanched with the point endocoagulator at 120°, thus assuring haemostasis. Using the 5 mm aspirating needle via a suprapubic trocar, the cyst is punctured and the contents aspirated with a syringe and saved for cytology. The cyst wall is incised along the endocoagulated area with the hook scissors. The irrigating instrument is used to fill the cyst with Ringer's lactate. The optics are inserted inside the cyst and the lining is inspected for excrescences or solid parts. If excrescences are found, the entire cyst wall should be removed by cystectomy and sent for frozen section. If the cyst lining is smooth, a 1 cm^2 window of tissue is excised from the ovarian capsule with the hook scissors and the removed tissue is sent for pathological analysis. The cyst lining is endocoagulated with the point endocoagulator which destroys the epithelium, thus decreasing the possibility of recurrence. The edges of the remaining cyst wall are endocoagulated. This will decrease bleeding, eliminate exposed raw surfaces, and thus decrease adhesion formation.

Cystectomy

This technique may be used for removal of dermoids, functional cysts, haemorrhagic cysts and endometriomas. The utero-ovarian ligament is grasped with an atraumatic grasper and rotated laterally to expose the ovary. The antimesenteric portion of the ovarian capsule is endocoagulated in a line approximately one half the length of the cyst. This provides an adequate avascular area through which the cyst may be removed. *See* Figures 11.1–6.

Using the hook scissors, the ovary is incised superficially along the endo-coagulated area exposing the cyst wall below. The edge of the ovarian capsule is grasped with a 5 mm grasping forceps. If it is difficult to develop the plane between the ovarian capsule and the cyst wall, the layers may be separated by injecting Ringer's lactate through an aspirating needle inserted directly under the ovarian capsule. The irrigating instrument, attached either to a pump or a bag of Ringer's lactate within an inflated blood pressure cuff, is inserted between the cyst wall and the ovarian capsule. The high-pressure stream and the blunt edge of the instrument are used to dissect the cyst away from the ovary.

The cyst should be kept intact for as long as possible, since this facilitates dissection. When the cyst is dissected as free as possible, the scissors are used to make a small hole through which the aspirating instrument is placed. It is then emptied of its contents by repeated suction and irrigation until the effluent is clear. The cyst wall is grasped with the 5 mm grasper and teased away from the ovarian capsule. Semm has described a 'hair curler' technique which we have found useful[32]. The cyst is twisted around the grasping instrument repeatedly, which gently pulls the cyst wall away from the ovary. The cyst can then be removed intact from the abdominal cavity through a 5

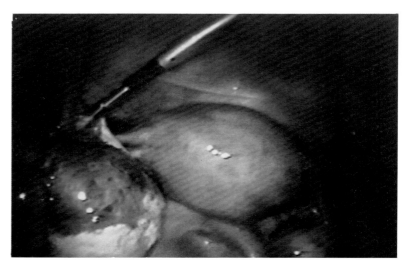

Figure 11.1: Ovarian capsule is incised revealing cyst wall.

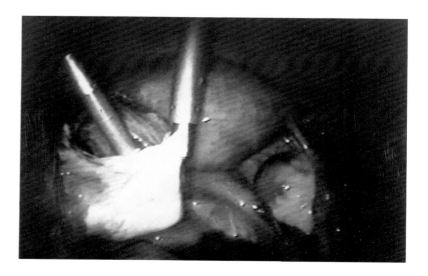

Figure 11.2: Fluid dissection is used to separate the cyst from the ovary.

or 11 mm suprapubic trocar. If necessary, the trocar sleeve may be slid out of the incision, allowing more room for removal. If too large, the cyst may be divided prior to removal. After removal, the cyst should be carefully inspected for papillations, septa or thickening of the wall. If suspicious of malignancy, it should be sent for frozen section; and if malignancy is found, the surgeon should immediately proceed with laparotomy.

The ovary should be inspected and excess ovarian tissue trimmed, allowing the edges of the ovary to approximate each other. The internal portion of the ovary is endocoagualated for haemostasis. Endocoagulating the raw edges

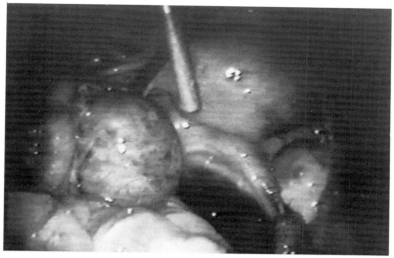

Figure 11.3: The entire cyst has been dissected.

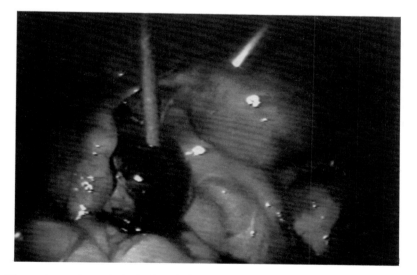

Figure 11.4: The endometrioma is incised and drained with the suction irrigator.

causes them to invert and may decrease adhesion formation. Experimental evidence in an animal model indicates that suturing the ovary increases the likelihood of adhesions[33]. Therefore this is done only when the ovary cannot be reapproximated by endocoagulation alone. We have found the intra-abdominal instrument tie with 4–0 Dexon to be effective, using as few sutures as possible.

The abdomen is copiously irrigated with Ringer's lactate. Suctioning of the sebaceous material found in dermoid cysts is facilitated by warming the solution. This emulsifies the fat, allowing it to flow more freely through the

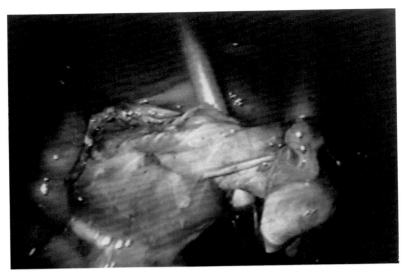

Figure 11.5: The cyst is teased away from the ovary.

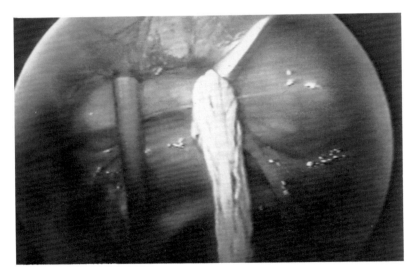

Figure 11.6: The cyst is removed via the 11 mm cannula.

suctioning instrument. Hair and other solid tissue is removed with the 11 mm spoon forceps or placed into an intraperitoneal sac for removal. Care should be taken to irrigate both the upper abdomen and pelvis and to suction with the patient in the reverse trendelenberg position. This avoids leaving debris in the peritoneal cavity that might cause an inflammatory reaction. As much as 5 litres of fluid may be necessary for this final irrigation. We suction the pelvis dry at the end of the case since we see no evidence that either intraperitoneal fluid or dextran reduces adhesion formation.

Some authors have suggested draining the intact cysts via a colpotomy incision, or using an intraperitoneal sac that can be brought partially through the incision to allow removal of the cyst contents. These are reasonable approaches; however, it may be difficult to keep the cyst intact during the course of surgery prior to removal.

Salpingo-oophorectomy

In premenopausal patients, laparoscopic salpingo-oophorectomy may be done in cases where the adnexa is not salvageable. In carefully selected postmenopausal patients with an adnexal mass, using the strict criteria described above, the adnexa should be removed entirely for complete pathological diagnosis. An 11 mm trocar is placed in the midline above the pubis, and a 5 mm trocar is placed laterally on the side of the adnexa to be removed. Pelvic and abdominal washings should be obtained and saved for staging should a malignancy be found. If necessary, lysis of adhesions with the hook scissors, laser or endocoagulator is done to free the adnexa.

If a cyst is present, needle aspiration is done carefully to reduce spillage. The adnexa is grasped with the 11 mm claw forceps and pulled medially to expose the infundibulopelvic ligament. For safety, the ureter should be visualized near the infundibulopelvic ligament. The endoloop is inserted through the lateral 5 mm trocar. The claw is released and passed through the loop, and the adnexa is grasped and pulled medially. The loop is worked around the tube and ovary toward the infundibulopelvic ligament. If necessary, an atraumatic grasping instrument may be inserted through a contralateral 5 mm trocar in order to help position the loop. Following Semm, three endoloops are placed, cinched down and cut. Experimental evidence suggests that two pulls of 10 seconds each give maximum strength to the knot. More pulls fray the suture, resulting in loss of tensile strength.

The adnexa is pulled medially with the 11 mm claw forceps, and the 5 mm hook scissors are passed through the ipsilateral trocar so that the pedicle may be cut at a right angle to the vessels. Care should be taken to remove the entire ovary while leaving enough of a pedicle to prevent slippage of the endoloop. The adnexa is removed via the 11 mm trocar using the claw or spoon forceps. If necessary, it is divided prior to removal. If inspection of the adnexa reveals suspicious areas, immediate frozen section is done. Frozen section is also done in all postmenopausal women. If malignancy is found, the pelvis should be filled with distilled water to lyse malignant cells and an immediate staging laparotomy should be done. In postmenopausal women found to have a benign mass, consideration should be given to removing the other ovary with the same technique.

In some cases, we have chosen to remove tissue through a colpotomy incision. The incision may be made by the standard vaginal approach or intra-abdominally with a laser or electrosurgical instrument. The vagina should be prepped prior to laparoscopic colpotomy. A ring forceps with a moist 4 × 4 gauze is placed in the posterior vaginal fornix and a silicon rectal probe is placed in the rectum. Manipulation of the sponge forceps and rectal probe allows separate identification of the vagina and the rectum. The rectal probe is then removed. This prevents tenting of the rectum toward the vagina and eliminates any confusion as to which area should be incised. The vaginal sponge is pushed cephalad and anterior by the assistant. The laser or electrosurgical instrument is used to incise across the vagina until the sponge is visible. The incision should remain medial to the uterosacral ligaments. Close application of the sponge to the vagina will prevent loss of the pneumoperitoneum.

The adnexa is placed in the cul-de-sac, a weighted speculum is placed in the vagina and the tissue removed with a ring forceps. Intact cysts may be drained through the cul-de-sac prior to removal. The colpotomy is closed with a running 0-vicryl suture. If CO_2 leaks through the suture line, a wet lap sponge may be placed in the vagina to maintain the pneumoperitoneum. The peritoneal cavity is copiously irrigated, suctioned and inspected for bleeding. Haemostasis is obtained as needed.

Oophorectomy

If tubal preservation is desired, or if the fallopian tube has been previously removed, removal of the ovary alone may be accomplished. Three endoloops, as described above, are placed around the mesovarium and tightened. An additional instrument is often needed to hold the tube away from the loop, thus preventing inadvertent tubal injury. The ovary is separated from the pedicle with the hook scissors and morcillated or bisected prior to removal through an 11 mm trocar sleeve.

Salpingectomy

Removal of the fallopian tube is indicated in patients with a large hydrosalpinx, a tubal pregnancy with a diameter greater than 5 cm or a ruptured tubal pregnancy. The proximal portion of the tube, near the cornua, is endocoagulated with the crocodile endocoagulator and cut with the hook scissors. An endoloop is placed in this space, carried around the entire tube and cinched down around the mesosalpinx. The pedicle is incised and the tube is removed through a 5 or 11 mm trocar. *See* Figures 11.7–10.

Paratubal cystectomy

Paratubal cysts, which are benign, are remnants of the Wolffian duct system. Removal may be considered to prevent future torsion. These cysts are usually on a pedicle which can be grasped and endocoagulated with the crocodile endocoagulator. The 5 mm hook scissors are used to cut the pedicle. Aspiration of the cyst fluid with the aspirating needle may be necessary to decompress large cysts and allow removal through a 5 mm trocar.

Retroperitoneal paraovarian cysts

Most commonly found in women of reproductive age, 2% of paraovarian

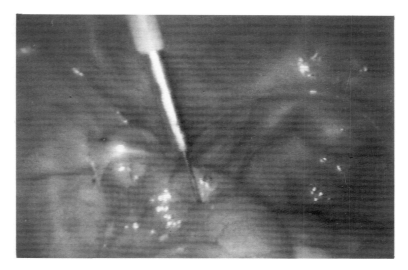

Figure 11.7: The tube is aspirated and decompressed.

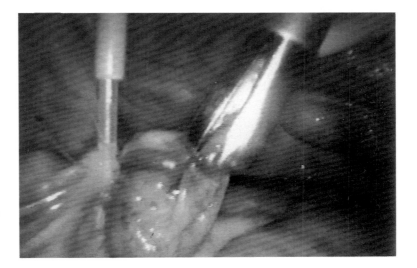

Figure 11.8: Three endoloops are applied.

cysts have been reported to be malignant. Strict ultrasound criteria, as used for ovarian masses, should therefore be applied prior to surgery. The peritoneum over the cyst is endocoagulated until blanched, and incised with a hook scissors. Care is taken to avoid the fimbria of the fallopian tube, thus preventing inadvertent injury and postoperative adhesion formation. Fluid dissection is used to separate the peritoneum from the underlying cyst wall. Aspiration, incision and inspection of the cyst wall are done as described above. The presence of papillations requires frozen section.

The cyst is removed by the hair curler technique. It may be necessary to

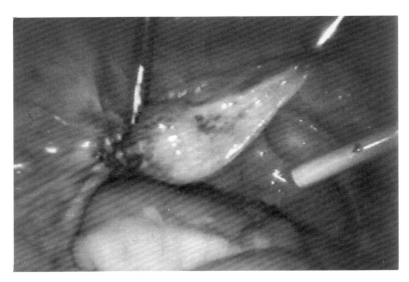

Figure 11.9: The tube is excised at the pedicle.

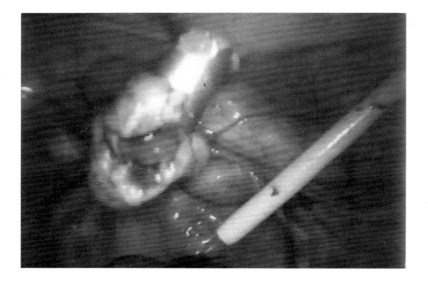

Figure 11.10: The tube is removed via the 11 mm cannula.

endocoagulate and incise adherent tissue near the base of the cyst prior to removal. The cyst is extracted through the 5 mm trocar and inspected. If suspicious areas are seen, the specimen is sent for frozen section. Bleeding areas in the cyst bed are controlled with the endocoagulator. The peritoneal defect is left open.

Management of adnexal torsion

Patients with adnexal torsion will often present with acute pain and the presence of a pelvic mass. Early laparoscopic intervention may offer the opportunity to salvage the adnexa. A probe or grasping forceps may be used to untwist the adnexa. If observation reveals a return of circulation to the tissue, the adnexa may be preserved. Usually torsion is the result of adnexal pathology, ie an ovarian or paratubal cyst, which should be managed by the appropriate surgical procedure. If the utero-ovarian ligament appears too long, it may be shortened with suture. If adequate circulation does not return to the tissue, it should be removed by the endoloop technique described above.

Minilaparotomy

In some cases, difficulty may be encountered during a laparoscopic procedure and it may be prudent to convert the operation to a minilaparotomy. A small lower-abdominal incision, approximately 3–4 cm, will provide enough room in most cases to complete the procedure. This is often best accomplished by extending the suprapubic trocar incision. When done in a limited fashion, minilaparotomy is associated with only slightly greater morbidity and hospital stay than operative laparoscopy.

References

1   Hulka J et al. (1992) American Association of Gynecologic Laparoscopists survey of management of ovarian masses in 1990. *Journal of Reproductive Medicine.* 7:599.

2   Maiman M et al. (1991) Laparoscopic excision of ovarian neoplasms subsequently found to be malignant. *Obstetrics and Gynecology.* 77:563.

3   Trimbos J et al. (1990) Reasons for incomplete staging in early ovarian carcinoma. *Gynecologic Oncology.* 37:374.

4   Dembo A et al. (1990) Prognostic factors in patients with stage I epithelial ovarian cancer. *Obstetrics and Gynecology.* 75:263–72.

5   Kjellgren O et al. (1971) Fine needle aspiration biopsy in diagnosis and classification of ovarian carcinoma. *Cancer.* 28:967.

6   Trope C (1981) The preoperative diagnosis of malignancy in ovarian cysts. *Neoplasia.* 28:117.

7   Puls L et al. (1992) Transition from benign to malignant epithelium in mucinous and serous ovarian tumors. *Gynecologic Oncology.* 47:53–7.

8   Bourne T *et al.* (1991) Ultrasound screening for familial ovarian cancer. *Gynecologic Oncology.* **43**:92–7.

9   Wolf S *et al.* (1991) Prevalence of simple adnexal cysts in postmenopausal women. *Radiology.* **180**:65.

10   Lim-Yan S *et al.* (1988) Ovarian cystectomy for serous borderline tumors: a follow-up study of 35 cases. *Obstetrics and Gynecology.* **72**:775.

11   Buttram V (1979) Conservative surgery for endometriosis in the infertile female: a study of 206 patients with implications for both medical and surgical therapy. *Fertility and Sterility.* **31**:117.

12   Daniell J *et al.* (1991) Laser laparoscopic management of large endometriomas. *Fertility and Sterility.* **55**:692–5.

13   Marrs R (1991) The use of potassium-titanyl-phosphate laser for laparoscopic removal of ovarian endometrioma. *American Journal of Obstetrics and Gynecology.* **164**:1622–8.

14   Nezhat C *et al.* (1989) Laparoscopic removal of dermoid cysts. *Obstetrics and Gynecology.* **73**:278–80.

15   Mage G *et al.* (1990) Laparoscopic management of cystic adnexal masses. *Journal of Gynecological Surgery.* **6**:71–9.

16   Parker W and Berek J (1990) Management of selected cystic adnexal masses in postmenopausal women by operative laparoscopy: a pilot study. *American Journal of Obstetrics and Gynecology.* **163**:1574–7.

17   Herrmann U *et al.* (1987) Sonographic patterns of ovarian tumors: prediction of malignancy. *Obstetrics and Gynecology.* **69**:777–81.

18   Granberg S *et al.* (1990) Tumors in the lower pelvis as imaged by vaginal sonography. *Gynecologic Oncology.* **37**:224–9.

19   Goldstein S *et al.* (1989) The postmenopausal cystic adnexal mass: the potential role of ultrasound in conservative management. *Obstetrics and Gynecology.* **73**:8–10.

20   Rulin M and Preston A (1987) Adnexal masses in postmenopausal women. *Obstetrics and Gynecology.* **70**:578–81.

21   Luxman D *et al.* (1991) The postmenopausal adnexal mass: correlation between ultrasonic and pathologic findings. *Obstetrics and Gynecology.* **77**:726.

22   Neiman H and Mendelson E (1988) Ultrasound evaluation of the ovary. In: Callen P (ed). *Ultrasonography in obstetrics and gynecology.* W.B.Saunders, Philadelphia. pp.423–46.

23   Steinkempf M *et al.* (1993) Hormonal treatment of functional ovarian cysts: a randomized, prospective study. *Fertility and Sterility.* **54**:775–7.

24 Weiner Z et al. (1992) Differentiating malignant from benign ovarian tumors with transvaginal color flow imaging. *Obstetrics and Gynecology.* **79**:159–62

25 Fleischer A et al. (1991) Assessment of ovarian tumorvascularity with transvaginal color doppler sonography. *Journal of Ultrasound Medicine.* **10**:563–8.

26 Vasilev S et al. (1988) Serum CA-125 levels in preoperative evaluation of pelvic masses. *Obstetrics and Gynecology.* **71**:751–6.

27 Jacobs I and Bast R (1989) The CA-125 tumour associated antigen: a review of the literature. *Human Reproduction.* **4**:1.

28 Gadducci A et al. (1992) The concomitant determination of different tumor markers in patients with epithelial ovarian cancer and benign ovarian masses: relevance for differential diagnosis. *Gynecologic Oncology.* **44**:147–54.

29 Inoue M et al. (1992) Sialyl-Tn, Sialyl-Lewis Xi, CA19-9, Ca125, carcinoembrionic antigen, and tissue polypeptide antigen in differentiating ovarian cancers from benign tumors. *Obstetrics and Gynecology.* **79**:434–40.

30 Finkler N et al. (1988) Comparison of serum CA-125, clinical impression, and ultrasound in the preoperative evaluation of ovarian masses. *Obstetrics and Gynecology.* **72**:659.

31 Jacobs I et al. (1988) Multimodal approach to screening for ovarian cancer. *Lancet.* **1**:268.

32 Semm K (1987) *Operative manual for endoscopic abdominal surgery.* Year Book Medical Publishers, Chicago.

33 Wiskind Z et al. (1990) Adhesion formation after ovarian wound repair in New Zealand white rabbits: a comparison of ovarian microsurgical closure with ovarian nonclosure. *American Journal of Obstetrics and Gynecology.* **163**:1674.

12

Laparoscopic Approach to Hysterectomy

JACOB L. GLOCK and JOHN R. BRUMSTED

Introduction

Approximately 70% of the 600 000 hysterectomies performed in the USA each year are completed abdominally[1]. While the vaginal approach is usually preferred, because of the shorter hospitalization and postoperative recuperation, this approach is often prevented by the presence of adhesions, endometriosis, lack of uterine descent or the need to explore the abdominal cavity. If these conditions are resolved initially by laparoscopy, a laparotomy can often be avoided and the hysterectomy can be completed vaginally.

Laparoscopic hysterectomy (LH) and laparoscopic assisted vaginal hysterectomy (LAVH) are designed to convert the traditional abdominal hysterectomy into laparoscopic procedures combined with vaginal removal of the uterus. Variations of the LAVH procedure include the classic abdominal Semm hysterectomy (CASH), laparoscopic supracervical hysterectomy (LSH) and Dorderlein laparoscopic hysterectomy. Regardless of which technique is used, it is imperative to understand that the laparoscopic approach to hysterectomy is a substitute not for vaginal hysterectomy but for abdominal hysterectomy in specific clinical settings. Keeping this in perspective at all times should optimize patient care and minimize the inappropriate use of this new technique.

Background

Reich and colleagues reported the first case of LH in 1989[2]. The total length of time spent in the operating room was 180 minutes, and the estimated blood loss was 25 ml. The patient was discharged on the fourth postoperative day and returned to full activity within three weeks. In 1990, Kovac and coworkers described 46 patients who were scheduled to have a total abdominal hysterectomy (TAH) based on a clinical impression of more serious pelvic pathology[3]. They used intraoperative laparoscopy to obtain decisive information in order to convert their surgery to a total vaginal hysterectomy. Based on their laparoscopic evaluation, 42 patients underwent vaginal hysterectomy and four underwent abdominal hysterectomy.

In 1992 Lui reported 72 cases of LH; there were no intraoperative complications, and 59 of 72 patients were discharged home within 24 hours[4]. Later he reported on 398 patients, the largest series of LAVHs performed by one surgeon[5]. The mean operating time was 102 minutes, mean hospital stay was 1.2 days and mean blood loss was 85 ml. Operative complications included five bladder injuries (0.8%) which were repaired laparoscopically, one vesicovaginal fistula and one partial small bowel obstruction. Five patients required laparotomy secondary to difficult laparoscopic dissection, but there were no transfusions and no life-threatening events. Although this report confirms the feasibility of performing this procedure, one could argue that many of these patients had preoperative indications for standard vaginal hysterectomy.

Comparison of methods

In 1992, Nezhat and colleagues compared 10 women who underwent TAH with 10 women who underwent LAVH in the only prospective randomized study of this kind to date[6]. Although the number of patients was small, this study demonstrated that LAVH was associated with fewer complications, shorter hospitalization and a more rapid recovery than with TAH. In a recent study, Summitt and colleagues randomized 56 women to undergo either an outpatient LAVH (29 patients) or a standard outpatient vaginal hysterectomy (27 patients)[7]. This approach was controversial because all of the patients were candidates for standard vaginal hysterectomy. There was no difference between the two groups with regard to age, gravity, preoperative indication or previous operations. The mean operating time was significantly longer for LAVH (120.1 vs 64.7 minutes). With respect to the postoperative course, no differences were noted between the two approaches, but the mean hospital charge for the LAVH group was significantly greater; mainly because of charges for disposable stapling devices and instruments, operating room time and anaesthesia time.

More recently, Boike and co-workers reported 82 cases of LAVH and compared them retrospectively with 50 vaginal hysterectomies and 50 abdominal hysterectomies[8]. The complication rate in the LAVH group (13.4%) was between that of the vaginal hysterectomy group (6%) and the abdominal hysterectomy group (26%), but the LAVH approach was associated with a significantly shorter hospital stay. These investigators concluded that LAVH was particularly useful when there was an adnexal indication for surgery. The costs of LAVH were noted to be high because of increased operating room time, and the expense associated with disposable instruments and stapling equipment. This study is important because it details the entire experience of a heterogeneous group of 29 physicians with varying levels of expertise in laparoscopic surgery. Other investigators have also reported their experience with LAVH (Table 12.1).

Definition

The term laparoscopic hysterectomy implies that the entire operation (including ligation of the uterine vessels, division of the cardinal-uterosacral ligament complex, vaginal incision, and vaginal suspension) is completed abdominally. However, since laparoscopic surgery is performed through small incisions, it is still necessary to remove the uterus either through the vaginal incision or by morcellation. The term laparoscopic assisted vaginal hysterectomy does not specify the extent of either the laparoscopic or the vaginal portion of the operation, but probably should only be used when some part of the hysterectomy is performed laparoscopically. Historically the two procedures were differentiated simply on the basis of whether the uterine vascular pedicles were ligated vaginally (as in LAVH) or laparoscopically (as in LH)[2]. The classic abdominal Semm hysterectomy involves the laparoscopic division of the infundibulopelvic ligaments and uterine vessels, followed by a unique transcervical morcellation of the fundus, with removal of the entire uterus through the abdominal trocar sleeves[15]. In the Dorderlein laparoscopic hysterectomy[16], the laparoscopic portion of the procedure is carried out up to (but not including) the uterine vessels. This is followed by delivery of the fundus through an anterior colpotomy incision and division of the uterine artery pedicle under direct vision. Laparoscopic supracervical hysterectomy (LSH) is very similar to the open abdominal version, except that the freed uterus is bifurcated or morcellated using sharp dissection and removed through the subumbilical trocar incision[17]. Regardless of the definition, parts of all procedures may be performed either laparoscopically or vaginally, and these should be viewed as a continuum of the same operation, with variations according to the patient's clinical situation and the surgeon's abilities. Fortunately, a classification system has recently been proposed to facilitate training, credentialling and outcome evaluation[18] (Table 12.2).

Indications

Although the indications for LH/LAVH are not absolute, possible specific indications include:

- adhesions
- endometriosis
- adnexal mass
- uterine size not more than 14 weeks
- nulliparity with lack of uterine descent.

Currently the only absolute contraindication for the procedure is invasive cancer of the uterus.

Indication	Number of cases	Method of dividing uterine vessels	Instrumentation	Operating room time (minutes) Mean (Range)	Days in hospital Mean (Range)	Morbidity
Reich et al.[2]	Previous pelvic surgery	1	Laparoscopically	Bipolar electrocautery	180	4	0/1
Kovac et al.[3]	Endometriosis	46	Vaginally	Not specified	Not specified	3.8	2/46
Minelli et al.[9]	Leiomyoma	7	Laparoscopically and vaginally	Bipolar electrocautery	90–180	4	0/7
Nezhat et al.[6]	Leiomyoma	10	Laparoscopically and vaginally	Bipolar electrocautery	160(130–230)	2.4(2–3)	1/10
Maher et al.[10]	Abnormal uterine bleeding	17	Laparoscopically	Bipolar electrocautery	160(90–220)	3.1(2–5)	1/17
Liu[4]	Previous pelvic surgery	72	Laparoscopically	Bipolar electrocautery	120(80–195)	1.18	2/72
Pruitt and Stafford[11]	Leiomyoma	60	Vaginally	Bipolar electrocautery and endoscopic stapler	80(60–170)	2.1(1–3)	14/60
Summitt et al.[7]	Leiomyoma	29	Not specified	Endoscopic stapler	120.1(50–245)	0.5	2/29
Padial et al.[12]	Not specified	75	Vaginally	Bipolar electrocautery and endoscopic stapler	121	2.37(1–5)	8/75
Boike et al.[8]	Leiomyoma	82	Laparoscopically and vaginally	Bipolar electrocautery and endoscopic stapler	Not specified	2.5(1–9)	12/82
Canis et al.[13]	Abnormal uterine bleeding	33	Laparoscopically	Bipolar electrocautery and endoclips	149(55–190)	4.8	2/33
Phipps et al.[14]	Abnormal uterine bleeding	114	Laparoscopically and vaginally	Endoscopic stapler	LH:82(60–120) LAVH:65(55–100)	2(1.5–8)	5/114

Table 12.1: Laparoscopic hysterectomy and laparoscopic assisted vaginal hysterectomy: review of the literature.

Type 0	Laparoscopically directed preparation for vaginal hysterectomy	
*Type I**	Dissection up to but not including uterine arteries	
	• Type IA	Ovarian artery pedicle(s) only
	• Type IB¶	A + anterior structures
	• Type IC	A + posterior culdotomy
	• Type ID¶	A + anterior structures and posterior culdotomy
*Type II**	Type I + uterine artery and vein occlusion, unilateral or bilateral	
	• Type IIA	Ovarian artery pedicle(s) plus unilateral or bilateral uterine artery and vein occlusion only
	• Type IIB¶	A + anterior structures
	• Type IIC	A + posterior culdotomy
	• Type IID¶	A + anterior structures and posterior culdotomy
*Type III**	Type II + portion of cardinal-uterosacral ligament complex; unilateral or bilateral, plus:	
	• Type IIIA	Uterine and ovarian artery pedicles with unilateral or bilateral portion of the cardinal-uterosacral complex only
	• Type IIIB¶	A + anterior structures
	• Type IIIC	A + posterior culdotomy
	• Type IIID¶	A + anterior structures and posterior culdotomy
*Type IV**	Type II + total cardinal-uterosacral ligament complex; unilateral or bilateral, plus:	
	• Type IVA	Uterine and ovarian artery pedicles with unilateral or bilateral detachment of the total cardinal-uterosacral ligament complex only
	• Type IVB¶	A + anterior structures
	• Type IVC	A + posterior culdotomy
	• Type IVD¶	A + anterior structures and posterior culdotomy
	• Type IVE	Laparoscopically directed removal of entire uterus

Table 12.2: Classification system for laparoscopically directed and assisted total hysterectomy. The system describes the portion of the procedure completed laparoscopically.
* Suffix 'o' may be added if unilateral or bilateral oophorectomy is performed concomitantly (eg type IoA).
¶ B and D subgroups may be further subclassified according to the degree of dissection involving the bladder and whether anterior culdotomy is created: (1) incision of vesico-uterine peritoneum only, (2) dissection of any portion of the bladder from cervix, and (3) creation of an anterior culdotomy.

Preoperative assessment and preparation

Patient selection

LAVH should be reserved for those patients who would otherwise have undergone abdominal hysterectomy. Although some patients may have more than one indication, each patient needs a full evaluation for pathology before surgery. This should include sampling of the endometrium in cases of dysfunctional uterine bleeding and an ultrasound evaluation of the enlarged uterus or adnexal mass. Furthermore, an appropriate course of medical therapy should be attempted before proceeding to surgery in those patients with pelvic pain or dysfunctional uterine bleeding.

Patient counselling

During the preoperative period, the patient should be allowed to discuss the details of the procedure, and be informed that it may not be possible to complete the procedure vaginally. In general, the risks and complications of LH and LAVH are similar to those of a traditional vaginal hysterectomy: eg possible injury to the bowel, bladder, ureter or blood vessels, which could result in the need for a blood transfusion and prolonged hospital stay. Energy injuries from bipolar cauterization, and injuries from trocars and misapplied staples, are specific to the laparoscopic technique. Overall, the complication rate for the laparoscopic approach to hysterectomy is 10%.

Patient preparation

The patient should be placed on a clear liquid diet for 24 hours preoperatively. In addition, cathartics can be given on the day before surgery to prepare the intestine. An adequate preoperative bowel preparation will reduce distention and allow for primary closure of injuries sustained during surgical dissection. The patient must be made aware of the need for adequate fluid intake if potential anaesthetic complications are to be avoided. Patients should receive antibiotics intravenously 30 minutes preoperatively for prophylaxis; 2 g cephalozin is commonly used. Finally, autologous blood donation should be considered in women with significant distortion of pelvic anatomy.

Technique

The operation is performed under general endotracheal anaesthesia with the patient in the dorsal lithotomy position. Careful positioning is crucial to optimize exposure while avoiding the risk of complication. For the laparoscopic portion of the procedure, the legs should be low and supported by Allen-type stirrups. When the vaginal portion of the procedure is approached, the hips must be flexed. Once the procedure has been completed from above, a single adjustment is made to abduct the lower extremities and thus gain better access for completing the vaginal portion of the procedure.

With the patient in the appropriate position, a Foley catheter is put in place. An alternative is to empty the bladder and place 15 ml of indigo carmine into the bladder as a precautionary measure[6]. This allows the early recognition of an inadvertent bladder injury which may occur during dissection of the bladder from the lower uterine segment. It is extremely important to be able to manipulate the uterus during the operative procedure. A uterine sound taped to a single tooth tenaculum already applied to the cervix is effective for maximum uterine elevation. This provides easy access to the posterior and lateral pelvic walls, and relieves the surgeon of the burden of using an abdominal instrument to manipulate the uterus.

Trocar placement

The procedure may begin with either a laparoscopic or a vaginal approach. When starting laparoscopically, the abdomen is insufflated and three trocar sites are chosen. A 10 mm trocar is placed infra-umbilically for the viewing laparoscope, and two trocars are placed suprapubically just above the pubic hair line and lateral to the inferior epigastric vessels. Laparoscopic visualization of the inferior epigastric vessels is imperative before and during trocar placement. A trocar injury to these vessels can be a challenging complication and may even lead to the need to perform a laparotomy. There is no set rule as to the sites of the two suprapubic punctures, and placement will vary in accordance with the size of the uterus and the pathology noted in the pelvis. Sometimes an additional trocar (10–12 mm) may be placed in the midline suprapubically. This will enable the surgeon to pass curved needles and suture material into the abdominal cavity. When using electrosurgical techniques (eg bipolar electrocautery) with laparoscopic scissors for division of the vascular pedicles, 5 mm accessory trocars are used. However, when using the endoscopic stapling device for division of pedicles, two 12 mm trocar sites are placed in the lower abdomen, halfway between the iliac crest and umbilicus and lateral to the inferior epigastric vessels. The use of bipolar electrocautery with laparoscopic scissors avoids the high cost of the disposable staplers and does away with the need for the high abdominal puncture sites required for most stapling devices.

Incisions

When the procedure begins vaginally, a tenaculum is attached to the cervix and traction is applied to expose the junction of the cervix and vagina anteriorly. A scalpel is used to make a 180° incision across the anterior aspect of the cervix. A sponge-covered finger is then used to dissect the bladder bluntly off the lower uterine segment. A moistened 4 × 4 inch sponge is packed into this space and left in place. The sponge may be moistened with a dilute pitressen solution to improve haemostasis. This technique elevates the bladder from the cervix and produces a tense distension of the vesico-uterine peritoneum which can be easily visualized during laparoscopy. The anterior colpotomy incision can then be safely and quickly executed at laparoscopy.

Visualization

With the patient in the Trendelenburg position, the pelvis and abdomen are inspected for any visible pathology. If adhesions, endometriosis or an adnexal mass are present, adhesiolysis is carried out until the uterus and adnexa are mobile. The goal is to restore the pelvic anatomy to normal, before extirpation of the pelvic viscera. This minimizes the potential for injury to vital structures, particularly the pelvic ureters. Usually the surgeon can visualize the right ureter passing into the pelvis at the bifurcation of the common iliac vessels, and coursing along the pelvic side wall before diving beneath the uterine artery. The sigmoid colon, which often covers the bifurcation of the common iliac artery and vein on the left pelvic side wall, may need to be reflected to visualize the left ureter. Its course can be made obvious by gentle stroking to elicit peristalsis. In rare cases, preoperative ureteral stent placement will facilitate identification of the ureter.

Ovaries

If oophorectomy is to be performed, isolation of the infundibulopelvic ligament (IP) is required. This is best accomplished by grasping and elevating the ovary and tube through the contralateral trocar. This allows adequate exposure of, and traction on, the IP. The bipolar cautery is then placed over the IP well away from the ureter. By applying brief and intermittent bipolar cautery, thermal damage to adjacent tissue is limited while complete desiccation of the IP is assured. If the ovaries are to be conserved, the utero-ovarian ligaments and round ligaments are desiccated, often with one application, via bipolar cautery. The laparoscopic scissors are then used to cut the desiccated portion.

Bladder dissection

The bladder must be dissected off the lower uterine segment and cervix. A grasper is used to elevate the vesico-uterine peritoneum in the midline, which is then opened using the laparoscopic scissors. With the moistened sponge in place vaginally, it will protrude through the anterior colpotomy while preventing loss of pneumoperitoneum. If no sponge was placed vaginally, both sharp and blunt dissection are used to separate the bladder from the uterus. It is important to keep the scissor points as well as blunt instruments closely applied to the cervix to avoid injury to the bladder. Bipolar cautery may be required as one dissects laterally along the lower uterine segment, because this area is typically more vascular. Laparoscopic scissors, equipped both as a cutting instrument and as a unipolar electrode, are ideal for this dissection. The dissection continues laterally to the bladder pillars which are coagulated to ensure haemostasis, then cut using the laparoscopic scissors. An alternative technique involves opening the anterior leaf of the broad ligament following the division of the round ligament. The suction irrigation tip is then placed beneath the peritoneum, between the anterior and posterior leaves of the broad ligament, to separate the peritoneum from the underlying bladder. With a combination of blunt dissection, sharp dissection and hydrodissection, the bladder is freed from the lower uterus and cervix.

Uterus

Once the bladder is adequately displaced, attention is returned to the uterine vessel pedicles. Because of the close proximity of the uterine vessels and the ureter, exposure of the uterine artery is achieved by incising the posterior leaf of the broad ligament all the way to the uterine artery. Then the uterus is elevated and maximally displaced toward the opposite side. This allows for access of the uterine vessels away from the ureter. The bipolar cautery forceps are placed across and at a right angle to the vessels. Energy is then applied until complete desiccation occurs. Both uterine arteries are desiccated prior to division to avoid troublesome back bleeding. Care must be taken during this portion of the procedure to remain well away from the ureter. If there is any uncertainty, the ureter must be dissected and visualized before applying the bipolar forceps. When the procedure is to be completed laparoscopically, the bipolar cautery is carried across the cardinal and uterosacral ligaments and both are transsected with the laparoscopic scissors. Alternatively, the uterine vessels, cardinal ligaments and uterosacral ligaments can be transsected using an endoscopic stapling device when adequate lateral displacement of the ureter allows safe application of this instrument.

In most instances, transsection of the uterine arteries, cardinal and uterosacral ligaments, and the posterior colpotomy can all be accomplished vaginally. Although both electrosurgical and stapling instrumentation are effective in achieving large vessel haemostasis, ultimate safety with either technique is dependent on the surgeon's knowledge of the pelvic anatomy and identification of the ureters. If one wishes to complete the hysterectomy laparoscopically, a sponge stick may be placed in the vagina from below to elevate and distend the posterior vaginal fornix. If the location of the rectum is uncertain, a digital exam can be performed or a probe can be placed in the rectum. An incision over the sponge stick is then made using the CO_2 laser, unipolar cautery or laparoscopic scissors, thereby creating the posterior colpotomy. Once the sponge is seen through the incision, any remaining portion of the uterosacral ligaments is transsected using bipolar cautery and sharp dissection. Finally, the vaginal cuff is closed and supported to the cardinal ligament at each angle using 0-vicryl extracorporeal suturing. The uterine vascular pedicles and the vaginal vault are then reinspected through the laparoscope. Any residual blood is aspirated from the peritoneal cavity.

Many gynaecologic surgeons have combined various aspects of different techniques for the satisfactory performance of LAVH. However, at the point where the surgeon is about to embark on dividing the uterine vessels, the relationship of the ureter to uterine vessels must be apparent; if not, it should be considered dangerous to try and secure the uterine arteries from above. The laparoscopic phase of LAVH proceeds only up to the point where a vaginal hysterectomy can be more safely and easily accomplished. This would include lysis of adhesions that might interfere with the vaginal hysterectomy, transsection of the infundibulopelvic ligament to guarantee removal of the adnexa or division of the round ligaments with detachment of the adnexa, if the adnexa are to be conserved. Additionally, in nulliparous women with minimal uterine descent, laparoscopic transsection of the uterosacral ligaments may make a vaginal hysterectomy less difficult. When the procedure is to be completed vaginally, it is important to avoid completely dissecting the uterine arteries free from surrounding tissue as traction applied to the uterus may lead to inadvertent avulsion of the vessels. Developing the vesico-uterine space, dividing the uterine arteries and endosuturing the vaginal cuff, may be technically feasible but should not be necessary for the experienced vaginal surgeon.

Variations on the LAVH

Classic abdominal Semm hysterectomy

The round ligaments, and either the infundibulopelvic or the utero-ovarian ligaments, are ligated as described above. Next, the body of the uterus is centralized by introducing the rod of the calibrated uterine resection tool (CURT) through the cervix, perforating the uterine fundus in the midline. The anterior and posterior leaves of the broad ligament are opened with laparoscopic scissors to expose the uterine vessels. The bladder is partially dissected free from the lower uterine segment. A Roeder loop or endoligature is placed over the uterus encircling the lower uterine segment. The CURT is then placed over the rod and the cervix is cored out, removing a cylinder of tissue from the exocervix to the fundus. The CURT is retracted and the Roeder loop closed over the uterine cervix at the level of the uterosacral ligaments. Securing the uterine vasculature in this manner is possible because the cervix has been debunked centrally by the CURT. Two additional loops are placed to ensure that the uterine vessels are securely tied. The uterus is then amputated above the ligatures. The stumps of the round ligament and utero-ovarian ligament are sutured to the cervical stump. The specimen is then morcellated and removed through a 15 or 20 mm trocar sheath. The benefits of the CASH procedure include not having to cut into the vagina and preserving the cardinal and uterosacral support to the pelvic floor.

Dorderlein laparoscopic hysterectomy

The laparoscopic portion of the procedure stops when it is time to secure the uterine vessels. After this has been done, an anterior colpotomy incision is made through which the uterine fundus is delivered into the vagina. Haney clamps are next applied to the uterine artery pedicles, which are cut and suture-ligated, under direct vision, vaginally. The cardinal and uterosacral ligament pedicles are also clamped, cut and sutureligated to complete the procedure. This approach is designed to avoid ureteral injury.

Laparoscopic supracervical hysterectomy

The infundibulopelvic ligaments, round ligaments and uterine arteries are desiccated and divided laparoscopically. Next, with a uterine manipulator in place, the uterine fundus is amputated at the level of the internal os by cutting down onto the uterine manipulator. The uterus is then bifurcated or morcellated using sharp dissection and removed through the subumbilical incision. Any bleeding on the cervical cuff is coagulated. The endocervical epithelium can be destroyed by applying laser or electrosurgical energy after removal of the fundus. The anterior and posterior folds of peritoneum are then placated over the cervical stump, with sutures placed laparoscopically. By not removing the cervix, the potential for damage to the ureters, bladder and bowel is reduced, while still enabling the removal of the uterine fundus. Other proposed advantages include improved sexual performance and decreased postoperative pain[19]. Possible disadvantages include the development of cervical cancer, menstrual bleeding from incomplete removal of the lower uterine segment, and technical difficulties in removing the uterus after detachment from the cervix.

Postoperative care

Postoperative care after LAVH or LH is similar to that following a vaginal hysterectomy. The Foley catheter is removed after 12 hours. A liquid diet is allowed on the day of surgery, with advancement to a regular diet as tolerated. The majority of patients are discharged on the first postoperative day. Physical activity is limited for one week, after which there should be a gradual increase in activity level. After a routine postoperative visit at four weeks, normal activity can resume.

Conclusion

The route selected for removal of the uterus in specific clinical settings needs to be evaluated critically as the techniques continue to evolve. Although LAVH can be beneficial to the patient who would otherwise have undergone an abdominal hysterectomy, one could argue that a skilled vaginal surgeon can provide this same benefit. Clearly, the best patient care is provided by the surgeon who is accomplished at both operative endoscopy and vaginal surgery.

Although there has been an exponential growth in the application of LAVH, well designed clinical trials to determine efficacy and safety are still lacking. A classification system has been devised to compare outcome data, standardize terminology and simplify credentialling in an effort to improve overall safety[18]. Although this is a commendable approach for the training of residents and practising physicians, the overall goal of any surgeon should still be to provide the best care to the patient and with the least amount of morbidity.

References

1   Dicker RC *et al.* (1982) Complications of abdominal and vaginal hysterectomy among women of reproductive age in the United States. *American Journal of Obstetrics and Gynecology.* **144**:841–8.

2   Reich H *et al.* (1989) Laparoscopic hysterectomy. *Journal of Gynecologic Surgery.* **5**:213–16.

3   Kovac SR *et al.* (1990) Laparoscopically-assisted vaginal hysterectomy. *Journal of Gynecologic Surgery.* **6**:185–93.

4   Liu CY (1992) Laparoscopic hysterectomy: a review of 72 cases. *Journal of Reproductive Medicine.* **37**:351–4.

5   Liu CY (1992) *Laparoscopic hysterectomy. (Abstract.)* American Association of Gynecologic Laparoscopists, Chicago.

6   Nezhat F *et al.* (1992) Laparoscopic versus abdominal hysterectomy. *Journal of Reproductive Medicine.* **37**:247–50.

7   Summitt RL *et al.* (1992) Randomized comparison of laparoscopy-assisted vaginal hysterectomy with standard vaginal hysterectomy in an outpatient setting. *Obstetrics and Gynecology.* **80**:895–901.

8   Boike GM *et al.* (1993) Laparoscopically assisted vaginal hysterectomy in a university hospital: report of 82 cases and comparison with abdominal and vaginal hysterectomy. *American Journal of Obstetrics and Gynecology.* **168**:1690–701.

9   Minelli L *et al.* (1991) Laparoscopically-assisted vaginal hysterectomy. *Endoscopy.* **23**:64–6.

10   Maher PJ *et al.* (1992) Laparoscopically assisted hysterectomy. *Medical Journal of Australia.* **156**:316–18.

11   Pruitt AB and Stafford RH (1992) Laparoscopic-assisted vaginal hysterectomy: a continuing evolution of surgical technique. *Journal of South Carolina Medical Association.* **8**:433–6.

12 Padial JG *et al.* (1992) Laparoscopic-assisted vaginal hysterectomy: report of seventy-five consecutive cases. *Journal of Gynecologic Surgery*. 8:81–5.

13 Canis M *et al.* (1993) Laparoscopic hysterectomy: a preliminary study. *Surgical Endoscopy*. 7:42–5.

14 Phipps JH *et al.* (1993) Laparoscopic and laparoscopically assisted vaginal hysterectomy: a series of 114 cases. *Gynaecological Endoscopy*. 2:7–12.

15 Semm K (1991) Hysterectomy via laparotomy or pelviscopy. A new CASH method without colpotomy. *Geburtshilfe und Frauenheilkunde*. 51:996–1003.

16 Saye W *et al.* (1993) Laparoscopic Dorderlein hysterectomy: a rational alternative to traditional abdominal hysterectomy. *Surgical and Laparoscopic Endoscopy*. 3:88.

17 Lyons T (1993) Laparoscopic supracervical hysterectomy: a comparison of morbidity and mortality results with laparoscopically assisted vaginal hysterectomy. *Journal of Reproductive Medicine*. 38:763–7.

18 Munro MG and Parker WH (1993) A classification system for laparoscopic hysterectomy. *Obstetrics and Gynecology*. 82:624–9.

19 Kiilku P *et al.* (1985) Supravaginal uterine amputation with preoperative electrocoagulation of endocervical mucosa: description of method. *Acta Obstetrica et Gynecologica Scandinavica*. 64:175–7.

13

Laparoscopic Treatment of Urinary Stress Incontinence

THOMAS LYONS

Introduction

Most gynaecological urologists agree that a retropubic approach to urinary stress incontinence has a high likelihood of being successful.

Various authors[1,2] have described failure rates approximating 11% with the abdominal approach (MMK, Burch), compared with a 40% failure rate with needle procedures (Peyrera, Raz, Gittes)[3,4] over a one- to five-year observation period. Vaginal techniques have met with a greater failure rate in most hands[5,6]. For this reason and with the conversion of numerous other abdominal procedures to the laparoscopic approach, endoscopic or minimal access retropubic urethropexy could be an excellent alternative. This procedure may be combined with other laparoscopic procedures including hysterectomy and posterior supportive procedures to provide a complete approach to abdominal and pelvic pathology.

Several endoscopic surgeons have described alternatives to the classic retropubic culpo suspension performed via minimal access techniques. VanCaillie and Schuessler[7] reported the first series of laparoscopic Burch procedures in 1991. More recent case reports[8,9] have reported success rates comparable to those of classic Burch procedures. Davis and Lobel[10] described a modification of this using a combination of needle techniques with Burch suture placement. Lyons[9] presented a suture stapling technique with comparable follow-up and equivalent results. Ou et al[11] have performed the Burch using surgical mesh and endoscopic stapling devices. Other modifications will most assuredly follow. The need for a simple but effective minimal access approach in appropriately selected patients is obvious, and each of these techniques must be evaluated for reliability and long-term patient outcome.

Patient selection

Success with this new technique depends on the accurate selection of patients. Each patient selected for culpo suspension should be carefully evaluated and be noted to have genuine stress incontinence with or without associated detrusor symptoms. The urethral sphincter mechanism must be intact, and urethral support (anterior vaginal wall mobility) should be poor. The surgeon must have a detailed knowledge of the patient's other gynaecological problems, voiding habits, neurological symptoms and current medication history. The *symptoms* of stress incontinence must be expressed by the patient as the incorrect or misdiagnosis of urinary stress incontinence will usually lead to surgical failure. The pelvic examination should concentrate on other pelvic pathology, neurological assessment of S2–S4, urinalysis and urine culture, demonstration of the *signs* of stress incontinence, and a Q-tip or Marshall's test. A timed void can be used to rule out decreased bladder capacity and voiding disorders. If a confusing clinical picture is presented, multichannel urodynamics and/or voiding cystometrics may be indicated. Patients with medical conditions which would preclude surgery, those who have not previously tried medical approaches and those with voiding disorders (including a shortened or scarred anterior vaginal wall) should be excluded as candidates for this procedure. Detrusor instability and prior surgery are not absolute contraindications for the procedure, but preoperative evaluation should be more extensive in these patients. Patients with type 1–2 urinary stress incontinence will benefit most from this new technique. Type 3 incontinence is best managed by other methods.

Procedure

Consent must be obtained for retropubic suspension, after a full discussion of laparotomy as for all laparoscopic procedures. Prophylactic antibiotics are given. A 30 cc Foley inflated to 20 cc is used to aid in identification of the U/V junction. Foley catheter manipulation allows definition of the bladder, urethral vesical angle and the endo pelvic fascia. Irrigation of the bladder at the termination of the procedure will identify bladder perforations. The patient should be placed in the modified lithotomy position to allow access to the vagina. Either of the two approaches may be used to enter the space of Retzius. In the preperitoneal approach, an open (Hasson) trocar is inserted at the umbilicus below the anterior leaf of the rectus fascia and the pneumoperitoneum is created in the preperitoneal space. The space is dissected via blunt dissection through the operating channel of the laparoscope. Once the space has been opened, a second 10/12 mm trocar is placed in the midline, one or two finger breadths above the symphysis under direct visualization. A 5 mm trocar is then placed lateral to the rectus avoiding the epigastric vasculature (Figure 13.1).

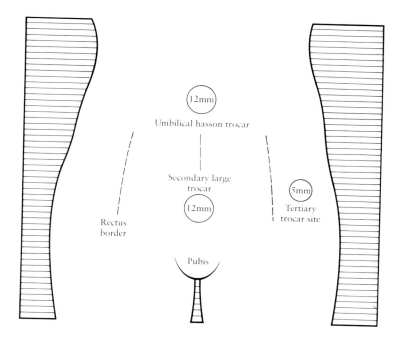

Figure 13.1: Trocar placement for preperitoneal approach – a technically demanding procedure which at times limits exposure.

In the transperitoneal approach, the trocar placement uses the traditional four-puncture technique, with one 10/12 mm trocar at the subumbilical site, another at the midline superpubic site, and a 5 mm trocar lateral to the rectus muscles bilaterally (Figure 13.2). The entry to the retroperitoneal space is made by incising the peritoneum approximately 2.5 cm above the symphysis pubis in a transverse cut extending to the obliterated umbilical ligaments.

Blunt dissection is then carried out using an endoscopic Kittner over the operator's fingers, which are placed in the vaginal vault to identify the fascia lateral to the U/V junction. Cooper's ligaments are also readily identified bilaterally. These structures are cleaned of excessive fat and areolar tissue. 0-Vicryl or 0-Ethibond suture on a CT-3 needle is then placed 1–2 cm lateral to the U/V junction bilaterally in a figure-of-eight technique. This suture is placed with the operator's fingers in the vagina, palpating the U/V junction. One of two techniques is then employed: an endknot loop can be created and the loop stapled into Cooper's ligament with the endoscopic stapler. As the loop is shortened, the U/V angle is increased with elevation. Alternatively the figure-of-eight suture can be placed at the U/V angle, and then one arm of the suture is stapled to the Cooper's ligament with the endoscopic stapler and tied in an extracorporeal technique (Nolan–Lyons modification — see Figure

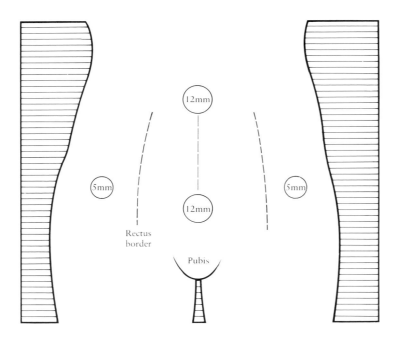

Figure 13.2: Trocar placement in triangular shape. Diamond and horseshoe shapes are also used, depending on surgeon's preference.

13.3). These sutures can also be passed in the classic Burch fashion through Cooper's ligament with a curved needle; however this manoeuvre is extremely difficult, and hence has led to the development of the Nolan–Lyons technique. The secondary sutures can then be placed to further lengthen the urethra and adequately elevate the U/V angle if necessary. With haemostasis assured, the laparoscope and trocars are removed and the incisional sites closed. In the transperitoneal approach, the peritoneum is closed with a pursestring suture. A posterior culdoplasty (Moschowitz or Halban) is also performed to prevent enterocele formation in appropriate patients. A drain may be left in the space of Retzius for a period of 24–48 hours.

The Foley catheter is removed postoperatively and the patient is allowed to void. If difficulty in voiding is noted, a leg bag is fitted with a Foley in place and the patient is sent home. The catheter can be removed 24–48 hours later. Postoperative instructions limit vigorous activity or straining for at least two weeks. The patient is allowed to resume other normal activities immediately.

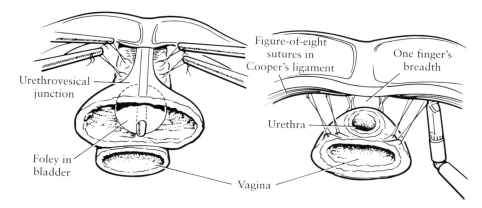

Figure 13.3: Nolan–Lyons modification. Sutures in Cooper's ligament are tied extracorporeally.

Discussion

Urinary stress incontinence is an endemic problem which impacts significantly on the patients' lifestyles and long-term psychological and physical health. Medical therapy is and should remain the mainstay of therapy, as these modes are successful in up to 70% of patients with urinary stress incontinence. With severe stress incontinence, however, surgery may be mandated or best considered because of other associated gynaecological pathology. In the past, needle procedures (eg Raz, Perrer, Stamey, Gittes) and anterior culporraphy offered the lowest morbidity procedures but were associated with the highest failure rates (40–50% in most studies). Retropubic approaches (MMK, Burch) have become the gold standard, with long-term success rates approaching 80–90%. Unfortunately these highly effective procedures have produced the highest morbidity of all procedures designed to correct urinary stress incontinence, with complications secondary to the large abdominal incisions necessary to accomplish them. Therefore these procedures have usually been reserved for patients in whom vaginal approaches have failed, or who are having other indicated abdominal surgery.

Since 1989, when the first laparoscopic retropubic culpopexy was performed, there has been much interest in the minimal access approach to the space of Retzius. Case reports of laparoscopic Burch procedures have demonstrated success rates comparable to those of open procedures[7,8]. Unfortunately, no authenticated comparisons have so far been made of clinical outcomes, although initial results suggest there may be considerably decreased morbidity when laparoscopic cases are compared with open procedures. Morbidity from the Burch procedure is usually isolated around hospital recovery time, length of catheterization, and other surgical parameters. Significant changes in these areas are conclusively demonstrated when laparoscopic procedures are compared with open procedures, and no differences have been noted between the prospectively studied Nolan–Lyons modification and the more traditional laparoscopic suture technique[9]. The Nolan–Lyons technique alleviates the need to place the most difficult Cooper's ligament suture pass by utilizing existing endoscopic equipment. It is not surprising that these patients have performed as well in traditional open Burch procedures, since the procedure is performed in the same fashion but with the superior visualization afforded by laparoscopy; nor is it unexpected that the surgical morbidity is reduced. Of particular interest is the decreased need for lengthy catheterization and the decreased incidence of long-term (> 2 weeks) detrusor symptomatology. In fact, when comparing preoperative detrusor symptoms with postoperative ones, the rate actually declined. The significant economic benefits of these procedures stem from the decreased hospital stay and the earlier return to work.

All patients with urinary stress incontinence must be evaluated thoroughly to rule out non-mechanical causes for urinary tract irregularities[12–14]. However, when an appropriate patient has been selected for a retropubic repair, the laparoscopic approach should be considered. The advantages of this procedure include results that are identical to those with laparotomy, with a significantly decreased morbidity associated with the minimal access approach. The operator's visualization is excellent, leading to superior surgical precision. However, the procedure is technically demanding because of the suturing manoeuvre of the suspension. Furthermore, the laparoscope allows the operator to select the same combined procedures anticipated at laparotomy including procedures to prevent enterocele or rectocele, the incidence of which may be increased after an anterior suspension surgery.

Only long-term follow-up will determine the efficacy of these procedures, but there is no reason why the results should be different from those with the traditional Burch suspension. The suture material and placement are the same as with the procedure performed at laparotomy. In several reported case reviews, one-year follow-up appears to show at least 90% success rates[7–9,15]. Surgical morbidity is certainly reduced even in the limited number of cases available for review, despite technical demands which are evident when the procedure is performed laparoscopically.

The technical abilities of laparoscopic surgeons continue to improve in procedures which were formerly the only available form of laparotomy. Technical advances in equipment will heighten the surgical expertise in this type of surgery. Several products are currently being developed that will allow knotless bladder suspensions. Suture anchors and clips are a reality and will eventually eliminate laparoscopic knot tying. Evaluations of Lapa-Ty (Ethicon, Inc) already allow a knotless suture. Nonabsorbable materials are in development for use with bladder neck suspensions. However, education and training remain important. Despite some obstacles, procedures continue to be developed because they are *better for patients*, the true test of any medical advance. With this promise as background, continued improvements like Minimally Invasive Retropubic Urethopexy will slowly replace traditional procedures as standard care.

References

1   Marshall VF, Marchetti AA and Krantz KE (1949) The correction of stress incontinence by simple vesicourethral suspension. *Surgery, Gynecology and Obstetrics*. **88**:590.

2   Burch JC (1961) Urethrovaginal fixation to Cooper's ligament for correction of stress incontinence, cystocele and prolapse. *American Journal of Obstetrics and Gynecology*. **81**:281.

3   Karram MM and Bhatia NN (1989) Transvaginal needle bladder neck suspension procedures for stress urinary incontinence: a comprehensive review. *Obstetrics and Gynecology*. **73**:906–14.

4   Gittes RF and Loughlin KR (1987) No incision pubovaginal suspension for stress incontinence. *Journal of Urology*. **138**:568.

5   Bergman A, Ballard C, Koonings P (1989) Primary stress urinary incontinence and pelvic relaxation: prospective randomized comparison of three different operations. *American Journal of Obstetrics and Gynecology*. **161**:97–101.

6   Bergman A, Ballard C, Koonings P (1989) Comparison of three different surgical procedures for genuine stress incontinence: prospective randomized study. *American Journal of Obstetrics and Gynecology*. **160**:1102–6.

7   VanCaillie TG and Schuessler W (1991) Laparoscopic bladder neck suspension. *Journal of Endolaparoscopy*. **1**.

8   Liu CY (1993) Laparoscopic retropubic colposuspension (Burch procedure). *Gynecolgic Endoscopy*. **2**.

9   Lyons TL (1993) Minimally invasive retropubic urethropexy. The Nolan/Lyons modification of the Burch procedure. Paper presented at the World Congress of Gynecologic Endoscopy, 22nd Annual Meeting.

10 Davis GD and Lobel RW (1993) Laparoscopic retropubic colposuspension: the evolution of a new needle procedure. Paper presented at the World Congress of Gynecologic Endoscopy, 22nd Annual Meeting.

11 Ou CS, Presthus J, Beadle E (1993). Laparoscopic bladder neck suspension using hernia mesh. Paper presented at the World Congress of Gynecologic Endoscopy, 22nd Annual Meeting.

12 Walters M and Shields L (1988) The diagnostic value of history, physical examination and the Q-tip cotton swab test in women with urinary incontinence. *American Journal of Obstetrics and Gynecology*. **159**:145–9.

13 Norton PA (1992) Nonsurgical management of stress urinary incontinence. *Contemporary Obstetrics and Gynecology*. **37**. (special issue: Urogynecology).

14 Walter MD and Realini JP (1992) The evaluation and treatment of urinary incontinence in women: a primary care approach. *Journal of American Board of Family Practitioners*. 5.

15 Horbach NS and Genuine SUI (1992) Best surgical approach. *Contemporary Obstetrics and Gynecology*. 37. (special issue: Urogynecology).

14

Operative Endoscopy in the Treatment of Infertility
STEPHEN COHEN

Introduction

In the USA, almost one couple in five have a problem with infertility. In the older age group, that proportion is even higher. Forty per cent of these couples will be found to have pathology at the time of laparoscopy/hysteroscopy. Thus, endoscopic assessment of the infertile couple is an essential part of the infertility investigation.

In addition to infertile couples, one encounters many couples who are able to produce a pregnancy, but have repeated early or mid-pregnancy losses (so-called 'habitual abortion' or 'second-trimester loss' patients). The spontaneous abortion group is more likely to have a medical or genetic problem, whereas the second-trimester loss group is often found to have a structural uterine or cervical abnormality. Since the investigations for infertility and for pregnancy loss are intimately related, both will be described in this chapter.

Preoperative investigations

When a couple present with infertility, a complete history is obtained from both husband and wife. Significant findings at the time of laparoscopy and hysteroscopy can often be predicted from the history alone. A positive history of salpingitis, ruptured appendix, ovarian cystectomy, myomectomy, abdominal surgery, diverticulitis, termination of pregnancy or IUD use may lead one to anticipate finding pelvic adhesions. A history of cyclic pelvic pain, dyspareunia, painful bowel movements, dysuria or changing menstrual pattern might raise one's expectations of finding endometriosis. Tubal obstruction is certainly more likely when the patient reports one or more episodes of salpingitis. Tubal obstruction, however, — especially proximal block — often occurs without any previous symptoms.

The provider should conduct a standard infertility investigation on each couple. It is usually most expedient to complete the diagnostic part of the investigation prior to proceeding with treatment, although there are exceptions, such as with the anovulatory female or the azoospermic male. The standard infertility investigation can be accomplished in two months. The first month is devoted to office studies, when tests should include semen analysis, sperm antibodies, sperm penetration assay, post-coital test, endometrial biopsy, serial ultrasounds of follicular development, and mycoplasma cultures. During the second month, a laparoscopy and hysteroscopy are performed. Some practitioners perform a hysterosalpingo-gram prior to the laparoscopy and hysteroscopy. The advantage of a preoperative hysterosalpingogram is that the operator will have more information on the anatomy of the endometrial cavity and tubes, which might allow him to predict the length and type of the surgical procedure more accurately. Disadvantages, however, include the potential for postoperative endometritis/salpingitis and subsequent tubal obstruction, the possibility of perforation of the uterus, patient discomfort and the additional cost.

The physical exam is a vital part of the preoperative investigation of the infertile couple. During the examination of the female patient, one should pay particular attention to the overall build of the patient, hair distribution, thyroid, breast development and pelvic anatomy.

The pelvic examination is a critical part of the evaluation. It is a mistake to believe that this examination can be less than intensive, just because one is planning a laparoscopy. These two examinations are complementary. A large rock-hard mass in the rectovaginal septum may be missed entirely, or its extent underestimated at laparoscopy, if one has not done an adequate pelvic exam. Thickened uterosacral ligaments, vaginal endometriosis, or a rectal lesion may all be missed entirely if the preoperative exam is less than thorough.

The family history may also add some clues about the patient's problem. Congenital birth defects, chromosomal problems, endometriosis and endo-crine problems in the family may suggest that further investigations in these areas should be performed; and of course a sexual history must be asked for and reviewed.

Preoperative preparation

The patient and provider need to discuss endoscopic surgery in depth prior to scheduling. There needs to be a complete understanding as to why the surgery is being performed. The patient needs to know whether this is purely a diagnostic procedure, or whether a treatment will be provided if pathology is noted. If treatment is to be provided, the patient will need to know how extensive that therapy will be. Will only minimal disease (stage I/II endometriosis, filmy adhesions, etc) be treated? Will laparoscopic distal salpingostomies, cornual catheterizations or removal of extensive adhesions be performed during this procedure, or will additional surgery be scheduled if necessary? Will a laparotomy be performed electively if necessary, or will it be scheduled at another time? Does the patient want a laparotomy or does she want only to have minimal access surgery?

Informed consent from the patient must include knowledge of the inherent risks. These risks should not be underplayed, as this is an elective procedure. Associated anaesthetic risks, bleeding and infections, complications of insufflation and trocar placement, and injuries that can occur to abdominal organs (bowel, bladder, uterus, and vessels) must be described to the patient. Any circumstances that may increase risk, such as known pelvic adhesions, should be discussed. Reasons for deciding on a particular approach — ie open vs closed laparoscopy — should be documented prior to surgery.

Operative procedures

The most common pathological conditions found during endoscopy for infertility include endometriomas, endometriosis, pelvic adhesions, tubal obstruction (distal or proximal) or a combination of these. In this chapter, the operative treatment of pelvic adhesions and tubal obstruction will be described. The treatment of endometriosis and ovarian cysts is described in other chapters.

Pelvic adhesions

The operative endoscopic treatment of pelvic adhesions can be the simplest or the most difficult operation that the gynaecological surgeon is called upon to perform. One may find a few transparent adhesions covering the ovaries, which can be removed safely, quickly and easily; on the other hand, one may encounter a pelvis so encompassed with dense adhesions that no pelvic structure is even recognizable.

Trocar placement

Entry and trocar placement are dictated by previous knowledge of the pathology. Some operators prefer to use open laparoscopy when the patient is known to have or is suspected of having extensive pelvic adhesions. However, others will use closed trocar placement even with known adhesions, as published reports do not show any lower incidence of bowel perforation using the open technique. If the patient has known periumbilical adhesions, initial trocar placement should occur higher in the abdomen, usually in the left upper quadrant approximately two finger-breadths below the costal margin. Additional trocar placements are dictated by the pathology. One should try to keep trocars as far apart as possible, and of course the inferior epigastric vessels must be avoided.

Instrumentation

The equipment necessary to remove adhesions is not extensive or complex. Most importantly one must have good graspers: atraumatic graspers (fallopian tube) and graspers for thick tissue (omentum), thin tissue (filmy adhesions) and bowel. It is crucial to be able to put adhesions on constant stretch during division and removal, regardless of the energy source used to divide these bands. There are many ways to separate adhesions, including scissors (unipolar or bipolar), unipolar electrosurgery, harmonic scalpel and lasers (CO_2, Nd:YAG, Argon and KTP). Each of these modalities has specific advantages and disadvantages as described elsewhere in this book.

Procedure

The surgeon should begin the operation with a careful and in-depth study of the anatomy. One should make sure that vital structures (such as great vessels, ureters, bowel and rectum) are located as far as the pathology will allow. The operator must then decide what operation should be performed. For example, in a pain-free patient with infertility, removal of pericaecal adhesions above the pelvic brim is usually not indicated, and in fact may lead to increased postoperative adhesions. If extensive bowel adhesions are encountered, one should take down those adhesions which can be removed safely. A second procedure may be necessary, following a bowel prep and general surgery standby, and after telling the patient about the increased likelihood of bowel perforation and obtaining informed consent.

One should begin taking down adhesions in the areas that are best visualized and most accessible. One should constantly be asking whether any bleeding that occurs will be able to be controlled and stopped. Cutting in a deep hole can be dangerous. Always try to remove adhesions evenly, so that access is improved. Periodically back away from the restricted field to get an overview. It is possible to be concentrating so intently within a limited field that one loses the overall perspective. One cannot reassess too often.

When using an energy source, one must be constantly thinking about the path of the energy after it hits the intended adhesion target. With the CO_2 laser, tissue behind the adhesions must be protected with rods or fluid. With fibre lasers, adjacent organs must be kept away from the fibre. With unipolar electrosurgery, one must protect against deep thermal spread and electron flow through the path of least resistance to vital organs or vessels.

After the removal of the adhesions is completed, it is often useful to place an adhesion barrier to prevent readhesion formation. It has been reported that 15–25% of patients will develop postoperative adhesions following laparoscopic surgery. Interceed, Gore-Tex and lactated Ringer's solution are currently the most commonly used agents for adhesion prevention[1].

Interceed can be pushed down through an open trocar and positioned by picking up a corner with a grasper. Recently, an Interceed applicator has been released. Gore-Tex can be positioned in the same fashion, but needs to be sutured or stapled in place. If lactated Ringer's solution is used, 1–2 l should be placed with the irrigator prior to closure. Lactated Ringer's cannot be used with Interceed as this will cause the Interceed to float off the serosal surface.

In the operative report it is important to document the condition of the pelvis both preoperatively and postoperatively. A detailed operative report, including the American Fertility Society adhesion scoring sheet, should be completed. Still pictures, videos, and slides are also helpful in certain circumstances.

Distal tubal obstruction

Distal tubal obstruction (clubbed tubes) is a common condition in the infertile female. Distal obstruction is usually caused by salpingitis, or occasionally by other intra-abdominal sources of infection such as appendicitis or diverticulitis. Although the prognosis for intra-uterine pregnancy is poor, (with a pregnancy rate of approximately 30%), these tubes can usually be repaired during laparoscopic surgery.

If adhesions to the adnexa are found, they should be removed prior to opening the tubes. The tubes should then be distended by insufflating through an intra-uterine catheter (HUI, Foley etc). Then one must carefully examine the tube to determine the most distal end. Often the tube is knuckled on itself, and the apparent distal end is not the true distal tube.

As one separates the tube from the ovarian capsule, the true distal end will often become apparent. Keeping the tubal wall on stretch, a linear incision is made, using any of the previously mentioned energy sources. One should use the highest energy that can be safely controlled, to minimize thermal damage. Once the mucosa is visible, the walls of the incision are grasped with atraumatic forceps. After exploring the inside of the tube, additional incisions are placed through areas of scar, so that the distal end is completely relaxed and easily rolled open.

To fix the distal tubal cuffs in the open position, one may use a low-power energy source on the distal tubal serosa, to accomplish the Bruhat technique of eversion; alternatively one may suture the cuff in place using the intracorporeal suturing technique.

Following the salpingostomy the pelvis should be lavishly irrigated, and an adhesion barrier or hydroflotation should be considered. The use of prophylactic antibiotics and early second-look laparoscopy are controversial.

Proximal tubal obstruction

Obstructed fallopian tubes are a common cause of infertility. Salpingitis is the leading cause of both proximal and distal obstruction. Salpingitis isthmica nodosa, a cause of proximal obstruction whose aetiology still eludes us, is a much less likely cause of proximal block.

The treatment of proximal block has continued to evolve over the last three decades. In the 1970s, proximal block was treated with exploratory laparotomy and tubal implantation. The site of the implant was either the back wall or the cornual area of the uterus. In the 1980s, microsurgical cornual-isthmic anastomosis succeeded implants as the surgical method of choice. Pregnancy rates improved, but laparotomy was still required. In the 1990s, tubal catheterization via hysteroscopy has become the preferred method of treating proximal obstruction. The surgery requires minimal access and gives comparable results to the more invasive procedures of the previous decades. Patency rates of 70–90% and pregnancy rates of 50–60% have been reported[2–5].

Hysteroscopic tubal catheterization

Hysteroscopic tubal catheterization is one of the easier operative endoscopic procedures to perform. It is advisable always to perform a laparoscopy with the hysteroscopic procedure, so that the patient's fertility status can be assessed fully. Pelvic adhesions and endometriosis can be treated at the same time. More importantly, one can observe the tube as the catheter is passing into it. The operator can avoid perforations by moving the tube with a grasper so that it lines up with the advancing catheter. This makes the procedure easier and safer, and increases the chances of success.

Once the laparoscope is in the abdomen, the cervix is dilated and a continuous flow operative hysteroscope is placed in the endometrial cavity. Any liquid distending medium is acceptable for this procedure, since no energy source will be used. The entire endometrial cavity should be assessed and the cornual openings identified. A Novy catheter system (Cook) is then placed through the operative channel of the hysteroscope. The outer rigid catheter (5.5 F) is placed within a few millimetres of the cornual opening. Once the outer catheter is in place, the inner catheter (3 F) and guide wire (0.46 mm) are advanced into the tube. Gentle manipulation of the wire and catheter will usually allow one to slide through the obstruction. Once the inner catheter is well beyond the obstruction, indigo carmine dye is injected through it to confirm distal patency. The catheter is then removed from the tube and uterus. The hysteroscope is then removed and replaced with a HUMI catheter and indigo carmine is insufflated into the uterus to document patency.

Postoperative procedure

If conception has not occurred within six months, the patient should have a hysterosalpingogram performed. Patients who conceive after the hysteroscopic tubal catheterization must be carefully followed early in pregnancy to exclude ectopic pregnancy.

Hysteroscopic metroplasty

There are many causes of second-trimester loss, including incompetent cervix, premature rupture of the membranes, congenital foetal abnormality and congenital uterine deformity. The uterine deformities which are responsible for most of these losses are the septate and bicornuate uterus.

Habitual abortion patients also have been found to have varied aetiologies, including chromosome abnormalities, infections, connective tissue disorders, antibody problems, embryo toxic factors and luteal phase defects. The septate and bicornuate uterus also seem to increase the rate of habitual abortion.

Until recently, the treatment of choice for septate uterus was exploratory laparotomy and Tompkins or Jones metroplasty. With the advent of hysteroscopic metroplasty, the procedure can be performed in less than an hour with minimal access. Vaginal delivery can be allowed when these patients become pregnant, as no myometrial incision has been made.

Laparoscopy

To begin the procedure, a laparoscopy must be performed to assess the uterine shape. One must know that the uterus is not bicornuate. Other surgeon's operative reports can be misleading, as some surgeons use the words septate and bicornuate interchangeably. When any doubt exists, perform a laparoscopy. Some operators always perform laparoscopy when doing a hysteroscopic metroplasty, but others do not. If the uterine configuration is known for certain, laparoscopy is optional.

Placement of instruments

The cervix should then be mechanically dilated if laminaria has not already been put in place. The septum can be removed using scissors, laser or electrosurgery. If scissors or fibre laser are used, an operative hysteroscope is placed in the endometrial cavity, while infusing any of the liquid distending media. If electrosurgery is to be used, a continuous flow resectoscope is placed into the uterus. Distending media that contain electrolytes (lactated Ringer's or saline) must not be used, as they will diffuse the current. Sorbitol and Glycine are the most commonly used media for resectoscopic surgery. The cavity must be carefully and thoroughly explored. No resection should begin until the anatomy is surely known and the view is clear. Both cornual openings must be identified before beginning.

Resection

Regardless of the method chosen, the resection should begin at the end of the septum closest to the cervix and progress up toward the fundus. With scissors or laser, this involves whittling away from bottom to top. When using the resectoscope, either a loop or Collin's blade may be used. The element should be turned at 90° to the septum. If using the loop, sections of the septum are removed as the loop is brought toward the operator. If using the Collin's blade, this is placed up against the base of the septum and advanced down the midline as the current is turned on. The generator should be set at 125 W, (cutting) blend 1 (15% coagulation). One should constantly reassess the anatomy so that the incision line remains in the midline. A common mistake is to let the resection line drift toward the posterior wall of the uterus. One must also repeatedly check the location of the cornual openings in relation to the base of the septum, so that the ostia are not damaged. Knowing when to stop the resection takes experience. The texture of the tissue will change as one begins to progress into the myometrium. The area also becomes less scar-like and has more characteristics of muscle, and more vascularity is encountered. One should not try to level the top of the endometrial cavity with the ostia, as this is too deep and perforation is likely to occur. Sinografin can be instilled through the hysteroscope and the uterus can be imaged with fluoroscopy intraoperatively, although this is rarely necessary.

Postoperative procedure

Postoperatively, patients should be placed on oestrogen replacement to encourage endometrial regrowth over the scar. This is especially important if the patient has been on oestrogen suppression with drugs such as danazol or a GnRH agonist. Term pregnancy rates following metroplasty have been excellent: successful pregnancies occur in over 90% of patients[6].

Conclusions

Infertile couples have greatly benefited from minimal access surgery. Success rates are higher, and procedures are safer, easier and more comfortable, than ever before. Minimal access procedures will continue to evolve as we head into the 21st century. Already experimental work with tuboscopes and hysteroscopic GIFT is being reported. The area of infertility is certainly a fertile ground for minimal access surgery.

References

1   Giannacodimas G, Douligeris N and Lappas K (1992) *Prevention of post surgical adhesions by Interceed (TC7) in polycystic ovary syndrome treated by CO_2 laser vaporization laparoscopy.* Abstract, 8th Annual Meeting of the European Society of Human Reproduction and Embryology, July 5–8, p.39.

2   Sulak PJ, Letterie GS, Hayslip CC, Coddington CC and Klein TA (1987) Hysteroscopic cannulation and lavage in the treatment of proximal tubal occlusion. *Fertility and Sterility.* **48**:437.

3   Deaton JL, Gibson M and Riddick DH *et al.* (1988) *Diagnosis and treatment of cornual obstruction using a flexible tip guide wire.* Abstract AFS, p.35.

4   Thurmond AS (1991) Selective salpingography and Fallopian tube recanalization. *American Journal of Roentgenology.* **156**:33.

5   Rosch J, Thurmond AS, Uchida BT and Sovak M (1988) Selective transcervical Fallopian tube catheterization: technique update. *Radiology.* **168**:1.

6   Buttram VC and Reiter RC (1985) *Surgical treatment of the infertile female.* Williams and Wilkins, Baltimore. p.185.

15

Minimally Invasive Treatment of Endometriosis

CHRIS SUTTON

Introduction

Endometriosis remains one of the most perplexing diseases encountered by the gynaecologist. In spite of intense research into its aetiology and pathogenesis, we are not a great deal further forward than when Sampson, in 1927, suggested that it was due to menstrual dissemination of endometrial tissue into the peritoneal cavity[1]. For this reason the disease presents with particular severity in patients with cervical stenosis, müllerian abnormalities and retroverted uterus, and the transplantation theory is supported by large epidemiological studies[2,3] which have shown that the greater the exposure to regular spontaneous menstruation, the greater the likelihood of developing endometriosis. This is further supported by observational studies[4] which have shown that endometriosis is more commonly found in sites where endometrial cells from retrograde menstruation may settle undisturbed, such as the ovaries, posterior cul-de-sac and the back of the broad ligament, whereas it is relatively uncommon on mobile structures such as the small intestine or fallopian tube.

Obviously other mechanisms of spread must account for endometriosis at distant sites but work in the experimental animal[5] has shown that, if an endometrial implant is sutured into the abdominal cavity, deep infiltration occurs and three weeks later the glandular structure is covered by an intact serosal surface with neovascularity. The development of ovarian endometriomas within the substance of the ovary can be explained by the finding of endometrial fragments in the plentiful lymphatic and vascular connections between the uterus and ovary[6]. Other types of ovarian endometrioma — where the ovary is densely stuck to the back of the broad ligament and is liable to burst with the release of old blood and haemosiderin when attempts are made to mobilize it — are possibly due to invagination of the external surface with an adhesion sealing off the cavity and thus binding the ovary to the peritoneum of the ovarian fossa. This concept is supported by the observation that the ovarian cortex can be clearly identified around the outer edge of the endometrioma cavity by the presence of primordial follicles (Figure 15.1)[7]. Brosens has also suggested that there is another type of 'chocolate cyst', in which late secretory changes and menstrual bleeding are absent and the bleeding comes from congested vessels at the hilus of the ovary[8].

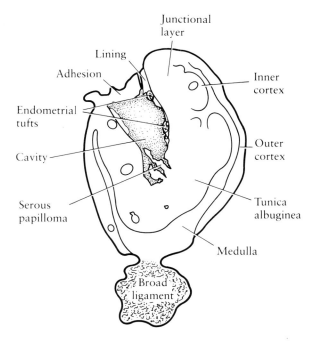

Figure 15.1: Ovarian endometrioma.

Medical vs surgical treatment

In addition to these problems with the pathogenesis, the clinical presentation bears little relationship to the severity of the disease, the natural history is unpredictable and attempts to provide rational treatment are often based on anecdotal experience rather than on scientific logic[9]. It is therefore not surprising that there are many different approaches to treatment, often straying beyond the confines of orthodox medicine and, to add to the confusion, most of the treatments are based on studies that have been largely uncontrolled and retrospective[10]. Against this background, both patients and doctors often find themselves confused and frustrated, as approaches to treatment tend to flow with fashion. Although medical treatment reigned supreme in the 1980s there has recently been a discernible trend away from traditional medical therapy for endometriosis, particularly in North America, to a more conservative surgical approach, preferably with minimally invasive endoscopic techniques[11].

There has been widespread disappointment with drug therapy, particularly since an elegant prospective study showed that if the second-look laparoscopy is performed two months after cessation of anti-endometriosis drug treatment there is already a significant recurrence[12]. The effects of these drugs appear to be only temporary, and the real role of drug therapy is probably the long-term suppression of the disease after removal of all visible deposits by surgical ablation[13].

The surgical treatment of endometriosis

It is intellectually dishonest to sustain the hypothesis that removal of ectopic endometrial implants is likely to cure this strange disease. Any gynaecologist embarking on the surgical treatment of endometriosis must be aware of the limitations of conservative surgery. It is a relatively crude approach (as imprecise at a cellular level as surgery for malignant disease) and can only realistically be expected to provide temporary relief of symptoms or to remove physical barriers, usually adhesions, that are preventing conception. Nevertheless, several retrospective studies have reported good pain relief[14–18] and impressive pregnancy rates[18–21].

The best way to vaporize ectopic endometrial tissue on the surface of the peritoneum is to use a CO_2 laser transmitted down the central channel of the laparoscope or, to provide greater safety and optimal visualization, through a second portal placed in the right or left iliac fossa (Figure 15.2). The CO_2 laser is still the most precise laser in routine clinical use, and in skilled hands,

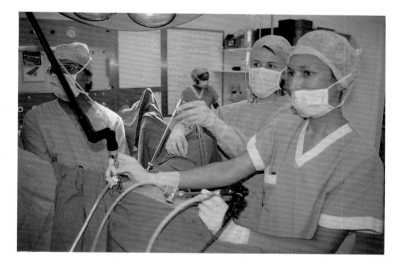

Figure 15.2: CO_2 laser laparoscopy viewed via a TV monitor. The laser energy is transmitted via rigid tubes and mirrors.

it is able to remove endometriotic implants to an accuracy of 100 μm even when they are sited on the bowel (Figures 15.3 and 15.4), bladder or ureter (Figure 15.5). With the new ultrapulse lasers (Coherent, Palo Alto, California, USA; Coherent, Cambridge, UK), whereby the laser beam is delivered as very high-pulse energy bursts of up to 250 mJ and average powers of 950 mW, it is possible to achieve precise char-free cutting with the lateral thermal damage of only 50 μm.

Laser tissue reactions with the carbon dioxide laser

The CO_2 laser beam, providing energy at a wavelength of 10 600 nm, is maximally absorbed by water. Since the majority of biological tissue volume is water, the penetration of the CO_2 laser is very superficial; 99.9% of the incident power is absorbed in the first 0.1 mm of soft tissue. The superficial cells are vaporized by energy which is converted to heat. Carbonization then occurs due to the ignition of the debris coming out of the laser crater, resulting in a plume of smoke which has to be evacuated by a special smoke removal system.

The power output can be varied from 4–100 W and spot sizes selected from 2–10 mm. Average power densities can therefore be varied from 10–1 500 000 W cm^{-2}. Greater average power densities improve surgical precision and speed, but at the expense of reduced haemostasis; because all the tissue debris is removed as smoke in the laser plume the wound heals with virtually no fibrosis, scarring or contracture, and because there is very little oedema healing tends to be virtually painless. It is very impressive at second-look laparoscopy to observe this beautiful healing, usually without adhesion formation. It is important, however, particularly with endometriosis, to note that the carbon debris is covered by the peritoneum but is not removed by the macrophages in the way that it is when laser surgery is performed on the cervix. It is therefore important not to confuse the subperitoneal carbon fragments with recurrent endometriosis which visually looks very different, although the unwary observer might not realize this.

Disadvantages of the carbon dioxide laser at laparoscopy

Due to the long wavelength, the CO_2 laser cannot yet be passed down a standard flexible fibre and the various devices that bend it between 10° and 15° usually result in considerable loss of power. It is therefore transmitted from the laser generator by a series of articulated arms and mirrors which make it a little cumbersome to use, and which also means that the equipment cannot be moved easily from one operating room to another (although some of the new sealed tube systems have gone a long way to solving these problems).

Although haemostasis can be achieved by defocusing the beam and sealing small vessels, it is very difficult to stop large vessel haemorrhage and the

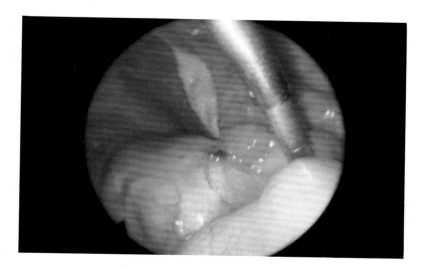

Figure 15.3: Deposit of endometriosis on sigmoid colon.

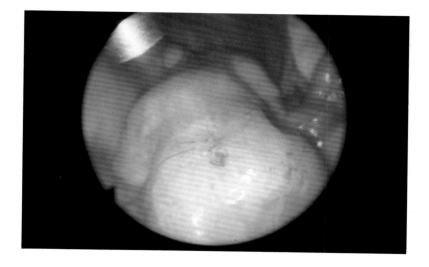

Figure 15.4: Same deposit precisely vaporized with ultra-pulse CO_2 laser.

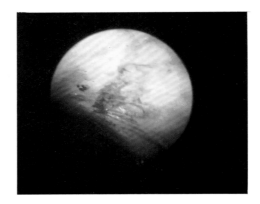

Figure 15.5: Endometrial implant precisely vaporized by the CO_2 laser down to the serosa of the ureter.

operator must have instant access to haemostatic clips, bipolardiathermy or endocoagulation to stem the blood flow if anything larger than a capillary vessel is accidentally severed. This, combined with greater char and smoke generation, necessitating pressurized irrigation systems and smoke evacuation equipment, makes it a difficult laser to use and requires a larger amount of teamwork from the operating room personnel. The other disadvantage of the long focal length means that the beam retains effective power and can easily damage tissue distal to the target. This is not a great problem if the beam hits a safe area on the pelvic side wall or if the adhesion can be pulled over the fluid-filled cul-de-sac, since the laser energy will be absorbed. However, when performing a complicated adhesiolysis procedure (particularly one involving loops of bowel), this is not always possible; then it is necessary to employ a backstop on the end of the probe or to use another nonreflective instrument to absorb the energy.

The Nd:YAG laser

This laser was the first of the flexible fibre lasers to be introduced into gynaecology (Figure 15.6) and it has a wavelength of 1064 nm which is approximately one tenth the wavelength of the CO_2 laser. It also lies within the invisible part of the spectrum, however, and like the CO_2 laser it requires the incorporation of a helium neon laser to provide an aiming beam. The laser medium is a YAG crystal contaminated with a solution of neodymium ions. The effect is to produce a powerful laser beam which can be delivered easily through a flexible optical fibre, with extensive tissue penetration and scatter. This makes it an excellent coagulating laser. It is ideal for procedures such as endometrial ablation, but the standard bare fibre is unsafe for use laparoscopically in the pelvis. This has led to the introduction of synthetic sapphire probes (Surgical Laser Technologies) which concentrate the beam as it leaves the fibre, resulting in 'laser scalpels' and thus restoring a tactile sense

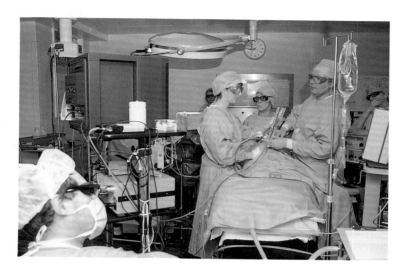

Figure 15.6: Nd:YAG laser laparoscopy.

to what was previously 'no touch' surgery. Scatter of the laser beam has not only been greatly reduced but the energy can be focused and the depth of tissue damage lessened by selection of different probe profiles. For precision cutting a scalpel tip is selected which produces a lateral laser scatter, but if coagulative properties are needed to deal with a large bleeding vessel a frosted or rounded probe may be selected.

Disadvantages with the Nd:YAG laser

Less power is required to produce the desired tissue effect due to concentration of the beam, and there is certainly less smoke production than with the CO_2 laser. Adhesions can be cut effectively only if they are put on stretch, however, and the active cutting is more clumsy than the neat trench achieved by the precise tissue vaporization of the CO_2 laser, particularly when delivered in superpulse or ultrapulse bursts of energy. In addition it has been shown experimentally that these devices do not work until they are contaminated with tissue debris which ignites, causing a great increase in their temperature. Following this, cutting is achieved by a purely thermal effect, which could easily be performed with an electrodiathermy needle[22].

Artificial sapphire tips are expensive and very fragile, with a limited life-span and an unfortunate tendency to fracture in use within the abdominal cavity from where retrieval can sometimes be very difficult. In order to get around some of these problems, other manufacturers have produced sculpted quartz fibres (SharPlan Laser Industries, Tel Aviv, Israel) in which the bare fibre is moulded in such a way as to produce convergence of the laser energy. Although these are considerably cheaper than the sapphire tips, their life-span is even shorter: and when the fibre tip eventually undergoes a significant degree of melting, the whole fibre must be replaced.

Fibretom

The latest refinement in Nd:YAG laser technology has been the introduction of the fibretom (Medilas, MBB, Munich, Germany). The laser manufacturers have realized that they have produced a sophisticated 'hot needle', and have cunningly incorporated an opto-electronic servo-mechanism to regulate the heat production. A sensor in the laser measures the temperature with a fibre tip during cutting and the laser power is automatically controlled to keep the temperature at the tip at an effective and safe level below the meltdown threshold.

KTP laser

This is basically an Nd:YAG laser in which the energy is passed through a crystal of potassium titanyl phosphate (KTP) which results in halving the wavelength to 532 nm, in the visible part of the spectrum (Figure 15.7). The emerald green light avoids the need for an aiming beam and has the advantage at this wavelength of being selectively absorbed by pigmented tissue, such as that found in typical endometrial implants. This laser penetrates soft tissue to a depth which is between those penetrated by the CO_2 and the Nd:YAG lasers. It can be passed through optical fibres and transmitted through clear fluids and, since lateral scatter occurs only in moderate amounts, it is relatively safe to use the bare fibre within the abdominal cavity[23].

The major advantages of this laser are that it is not necessary for all operating room personnel to wear protective goggles since it is a visible light laser and the protective blink reflex can be utilized. It is also unnecessary to use specially designed probes since the fibre can be repeatedly recleaved and thus one is able to use a single fibre 20 or 30 times. Tissue is effectively incised, again by the hot needle effect, by dragging the fibre across stretched tissue, and cutting is more effective if the small 300 µm fibre is used. If the end of the fibre is moved away from the surface and the tissue effect changes from vaporization to coagulation, it will seal bleeding vessels, especially if the blood is removed by an irrigating stream of fluid and the laser beam is activated through the jet of fluid.

Although this laser is expensive and requires considerable initial capital outlay, it is very cheap to run and there is little need for disposable fibres or tips and ongoing maintenance costs are extremely low. Most newer models have the added advantage that, at a switch of a mirror, the Nd:YAG beam bypasses the KTP crystal and pure YAG energy emerges from the laser

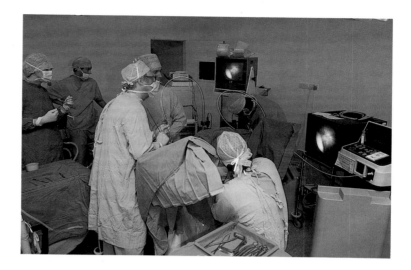

Figure 15.7: KTP/532 visible light laser being used for endo-ovarian surgery.

generator, so one is effectively getting two lasers with widely differing tissue actions for the price of one.

Holmium:YAG laser

When the YAG crystal of the lasing medium is impregnated with holium particles, laser energy is generated with a wavelength of 2100 nm which is approximately twice the wavelength of the Nd:YAG laser. The beam can be directed through a flexible fibre and, as scatter is minimal, the bare fibre can be used laparoscopically with relative safety. Energy at this wavelength is highly absorbed by fluids, and thermal necrosis to surrounding tissue is slight. This laser also incorporates a superpulse facility and it handles in a way that is similar to the KTP–532 laser, with a slightly greater degree of coagulation but significantly more smoke. As with the CO_2 laser, it is unnecessary to wear special tinted safety glasses or automatic shutters in the endoscopes, and although it can be used for laparoscopic surgery, its ineffectiveness within the fluid-filled uterine cavity makes it unsuitable for hysteroscopic surgery.

Argon laser

The argon laser produces a mixture of several different wavelengths between 488 and 514 nm, producing a blue light in the visible part of the

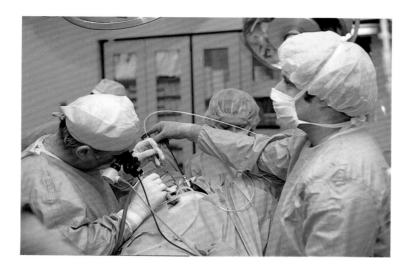

Figure 15.8: Argon laser laparoscopy.

spectrum (Figure 15.8). These wavelengths are similar to those of the KTP laser, and the physical properties are also very similar, but it does not appear to cut as effectively. It is mainly a coagulating laser and the energy at these wavelengths is strongly absorbed by blood and pigmented tissue.

When used in contact mode with 300 and 600 μm fibres, the cutting efficiency with the argon laser depends only on the power transmitted through the fibre (1 mm cutting depth at 8 W and 0.35 mm coagulation zone). This means that both the argon and KTP lasers cut more efficiently than the Nd:YAG laser, by a factor of 1.5. There is a problem with the argon laser, however, in that the end of the fibre burns off during the cutting procedure. Continuous measurements of the loss of laser power at the fibre tip during cutting shows a nearly exponential decrease of power output with length of cut. After 50 cm only 10% of the laser power exits from the fibre tip. Correspondingly, the cutting efficiency is reduced to 30% but without any influence on the coagulation zone[24].

Laser laparoscopy for the treatment of endometriosis

A decade of experience has now been gained with the use of these lasers. With skill and experience of laser-tissue interactions, the surgeon can remove endometriotic implants precisely and with minimal damage to surrounding tissue. Since all tissue debris is removed as smoke in the laser plume, and residual carbon is removed from the laser crater by a jet of irrigating fluid, healing occurs with minimal fibrosis and tissue contracture.

Laparoscopy is mandatory for the diagnosis of endometriosis, and therefore it would appear logical to try to remove as many of the ectopic endometrial implants and to divide as many of the adhesions as possible at the same time. However, it is important to be aware of the aims and limitations of the conservative endoscopic surgical approach. Surgery cannot realistically be expected to cure this disease, and the aims of the treatment are cyto-reduction of ectopic endometrium, restoration of normal tubo-ovarian anatomy to restore fertility prospects, division of afferent-sensory pain fibres in patients with dysmenorrhoea and dyspareunia, and finally the removal of ovarian endometriomas which are notoriously resistant to drug therapy.

Cyto-reduction of endometriosis and infertility

There is considerable controversy about the relationship of the milder forms of endometriosis to infertility. Nevertheless, many retrospective studies have shown that laser laparoscopy results in excellent fecundity rates, as high as 5.79%, even in patients with severe stage 4 disease — much more impressive than that achieved by the use of anti-endometriosis drugs. Our original five-year follow-up of 228 patients with a pregnancy rate of 80% has recently been extended to seven years involving 310 patients, of whom 85 presented with infertility. Of the patients with endometriosis alone, 75% became pregnant resulting in a successful outcome (excluding TOPs) in 74%. Several series in the literature give results ranging between 50 and 81% (Table 15.1), compared to the average pregnancy rate following danazol therapy of 37% and a fecundity rate 0.068%. All the laser laparoscopy series suffer from the disadvantage that they are retrospective. At the moment we are involved in a prospective randomized doubleblind controlled study comparing laser laparoscopy with expectant management alone — removal of peritoneal fluid and dye-hydrotubation — which can be expected to give a background pregnancy rate of about 50% in minimal and mild disease, and this background rate has to be taken into account when interpreting results. Until such a study has been successfully completed, the true role of laser laparoscopy in endometriosis-related infertility and pelvic pain remains unknown.

Laparoscopic uterine nerve ablation (LUNA) (and presacral neurectomy)

Although many patients with endometriosis experience pain throughout the month, the most crippling symptom is often severe dysmenorrhoea, both congestive and spasmodic, and deep dyspareunia which causes profound sexual problems often resulting in marital disharmony and certainly contributing

	Patients N	Pregnancies N	%	Viability %
Daniell (1984)[14]	75	48	62	–
Feste (1985)[15]	29	21	72	–
Davis (1986)[25]	65	37	–	57
Nezhat (1986)[26]	102	62	61	51
Martin and Olive (1986)[27]	80	33	41	–
Donnez (1987)[20]	70	40	–	57
* Sutton (1990)[9]	56	45	80	69
Feste (1989)[28]	178	93	73	–
* Feste (1989)[28]	64	52	81	–
Nezhat (1989)[29]	243	168	69	–

Table 15.1: Results of laser laparoscopy for endometriosis.
    *   Endometriosis only, no other infertility factors.

to infertility. The symptoms are likely to be particularly pronounced when endometriosis is present in the utero-sacral ligaments which transmit the afferent-sensory nerve fibres to the lower uterine segment and also supply some of the fundus. These ligaments can easily be vaporized by the laser at laparoscopy (Figure 15.9), and all endometriotic deposits and nodules should also be removed since they can penetrate as deeply as 11 mm into the utero-sacral ligaments. It is not surprising, therefore, that cyclical bleeding around the sensory nerves and ganglia of the Lee-Frankenhauser plexus results in such severe discomfort and disabling dysmenorrhoea. Great care must be taken to avoid the ureter, which runs parallel to the utero-sacral ligament at this point; it should be palpated carefully with a blunt probe and recognized by the characteristic peristaltic movements. Care must also be taken to avoid injuring the thin-walled veins which run just lateral to the utero-sacral

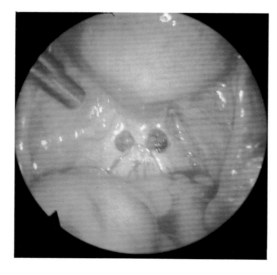

Figure 15.9: Laparoscopic uterine nerve ablation (LUNA) by vaporizing the uterosacral ligaments with the CO_2 laser.

ligaments because these can bleed profusely. Vaporization continues until the fibres and nerve bundles in the utero-sacral ligament stop splitting, but if the surgeon goes too deep there are some large arteries at the base of the utero-sacral ligament which can cause troublesome bleeding. It is therefore mandatory to have appropriate haemostatic equipment (such as an endocoagulator, bipolar diathermy or haemostatic clips) on immediate standby should heavy bleeding be encountered.

This simple operation, easily performed at the time of diagnostic laparoscopy with the CO_2 or KTP laser, provides spectacular relief of severe dysmenorrhoea and deep dyspareunia, and is particularly effective when the utero-sacral ligaments are infiltrated with endometriosis. It is also one of the few procedures in the entire literature produced by endoscopic surgery that has been subjected to a randomized prospective double-blind trial[30].

Another prospective study has shown that presacral neurectomy performed by laparotomy is effective in relieving mid-line dysmenorrhoea in patients with advanced endometriosis[31]. A similar procedure can be performed laparoscopically using lasers and aquadissection to expose the presacral nerve bundle which is then transsected. This very advanced laparoscopic surgery is technically difficult, but in skilled hands it gives excellent results. The retroperineal space in front of the sacral promontory is extremely vascular, and this operation is facilitated by the argon beam coagulator in which a unipolar diathermy current passes down a jet of argon gas which blasts tissue debris and blood out of the surgical field, thus allowing extremely effective haemostasis directly applied to the exposed bleeding vessel. Of more recent note, ultrasonic vibration delivered laparoscopically has shown promising results as an adjunctive tool for this procedure.

Laparoscopic surgery for ovarian endometriomas

KTP laser

In patients with severe and extensive disease and in those with endometriomas of the ovary (chocolate cysts) with gross distortion of pelvic anatomy, a potassium titanyl phosphate (KTP–532) visible light laser is more suitable (Laserscope, San Jose, California). This visible light laser produces a pure emerald-green laser at a wavelength of 532 nm which is close to the absorption band for haemoglobin and is therefore selectively taken up by pigmented endometrial tissue. This wavelength is close to the absorption band for argon laser light. The argon laser itself produces a mixture of blue wavelengths but is more of a photocoagulating laser and does not cut as effectively as the KTP laser. Both these lasers can be transmitted by flexible silicon quartz fibres to allow access to inaccessible sites and both have the advantage of being able to work in the presence of blood and haemosederin, whereas the CO_2 energy — being almost totally absorbed by water — will not work in the presence of blood and fluids.

The KTP laser is particularly suitable for laparoscopic treatment of ovarian endometriomas. The cyst is fenestrated at the thinnest point of the capsule and the thick chocolate fluid is aspirated and irrigated until clear. The edges of the cyst wall are steadied by two pairs of grasping forceps, and the flexible laser fibre is introduced into the cavity of the endometrioma. After close inspection and biopsy of the cyst wall, the entire lining is photocoagulated at a power of 12 W. This endoscopic surgery is very difficult and time-consuming, but appears to be associated with a low recurrence rate. Daniell[23] has recently reported a series of 47 patients with endometriomas varying in size from 3–12 cm. Pain relief was reported in nearly 80% of the patients and, of the 32 trying for pregnancy, 12 had conceived. This resulted in a 37.5% pregnancy rate, which is very reasonable bearing in mind the severity of the disease process when large endometriomas are present.

Nd:YAG laser

Although the Nd:YAG laser has been used by some surgeons, this laser produces an unacceptably large zone of tissue necrosis beneath the surface, making it less suitable for delicate fertility surgery and particularly intra-ovarian surgery. Attempts to minimize this laser tissue effect by the use of artificial sapphire tips or sculpted quartz fibres rely on a purely thermal effect which can be achieved much more cheaply by electrodiathermy. However, several investigators report satisfactory results using the Nd:YAG laser.

Argon laser

Brosens (1989) described an interesting technique of endo–ovarian surgery using a flexible argon laser inserted through an ovarioscope[8]. In these cases, complete excision of the endometrioma is achieved. If flexible fibre lasers are not available, the capsule can be removed by conventional operative laparoscopy by grasping the capsule with ovarian biopsy forceps and applying countertraction with another pair of grasping forceps applied to the healthy ovarian tissue[32]. This technique has the advantage of providing a complete specimen for histological examination and any bleeding can usually be stopped by electrocautery or the argon beam coagulator.

Closing the ovarian defect

At the end of the procedure some surgeons close the ovarian defect with sutures, but this is illogical since the primary stimulus to postoperative adhesion formation is tissue ischaemia produced by surgical knots[33]. An alternative technique is to use fibrin glue. We have found that the wounds heal well if left alone. We always finish our procedures by leaving heparinized Hartmann's solution (0.5 l) in the hope of preventing initial fibrinous adhesion formation which usually occurs in the first four hours following surgery. In North America, a cellulose barrier 'Interceed', has been utilized to prevent postoperative adhesions of the ovary after cystectomy. This material is manipulated over the operative site and 'laid down' over the lower surface at the completion of the laparoscopy.

Conclusion

The past decade has witnessed a revolution in the laparoscopic treatment of endometriosis due to technological developments and increasing sophistication of the instrumentation as well as an enormous increase in the surgical skill required to master the challenges of this new kind of surgery. Most attempts at laparoscopic surgery have been conservative, with a view to restoring fertility potential, but there is inevitably a significant recurrence associated with surgical ablation.

The only way to achieve a permanent cure is to remove the uterus and all ovarian tissue which up to now required a laparotomy. Operative laparoscopy is now entering a new phase to treat severe endometriosis. Some of these advanced surgical endoscopy procedures can take many hours, and the excision of dense fibrotic endometriosis that has obliterated the cul-de-sac requires ureteric dissection, mobilization of the rectum and even the sigmoid colon from the back of the uterus, and sometimes laparoscopic resection of a segment of colon that has been infiltrated by endometriosis throughout the entire thickness of the wall.

Advanced operative laparoscopy can also be used to mobilize and remove the ovaries and perform bowel adhesiolysis, thus allowing the uterus to be easily removed vaginally. It is therefore possible to convert a difficult laparotomy to a minimally invasive procedure with smaller scars and a decrease in postoperative adhesion formation. There is animal work to support this contention and even a prospective double-blind clinical study showing that there are fewer adhesions following laparoscopic surgery than with salpingostomy for ectopic pregnancy performed by laparotomy[34].

Some of these difficult procedures can take a long time in the operating theatre, requiring immense concentration and patience on the part of the surgeons and an efficient, enthusiastic and dedicated team of nurses and technicians to anticipate instrument requirements and operate the array of advanced technology equipment. The results, however, can be very gratifying, particularly for the patient who often has a short stay in hospital and convalescence, and an early return to work or family commitments.

References

1   Sampson JA (1927) Peritoneal endometriosis due to menstrual dissemination of endometrial tissue into peritoneal cavity. *American Journal of Obstetrics and Gynecology.* **14**:422.

2   Mahmood TA and Templeton A (1990) Mahmood TA and Templeton A (1991) The prevalence and genesis of endometriosis. *Human Reproduction.* **6**:544–9.

3   Candiani GB *et al.* (1991) Reproductive and menstrual factors and risk of peritoneal and ovarian endometriosis. *Fertility and Sterility.* **56**:230–4.

4   Jenkins S *et al.* (1986) Endometriosis: pathogenetic implications of the anatomic distribution. *Obstetrics and Gynaecology.* **68**:335–8.

5   Ishimaru T and Masuzaki H (1991) Peritoneal endometriosis: endometrial tissue implantation as its primary aetiologic mechanism. *American Journal of Obstetrics and Gynecology.* **165**:210–14.

6   Ueki M (1991) Histological study of endometriosis and examination of lymphatic drainage in and from the uterus. *American Journal of Obstetrics and Gynecology.* **165**:201–9.

7   Hughesdon PE (1957) The structure of endometrial cysts of the ovary. *Journal of Obstetrics and Gynaecology of the British Empire.* **64**:481–7.

8   Brosens IA (1989) Ovarian endometriosis. In: Brosens IA and Gordon A (eds). *Tubal infertility.* Gower Medical Publishing, London. pp.13–17.

9   Sutton CJG (1990) The treatment of endometriosis. In: Studd JWW (ed). *Progress in obstetrics and gynaecology, volume 8.* Churchill Livingstone, Edinburgh. pp.293–313.

10   Olive DL (1992) Endometriosis: advances in understanding and management. *Current Opinion in Obstetrics and Gynaecology.* **4**:380–7.

11   de Cherney AH and Semm K (1991) Gynaecological surgery and endoscopy. Editorial overview. *Current Science.* **3**:359–61.

12   Evers J (1987) The second look laparoscopy for the evaluation of the results of medical treatment of endometriosis should not be performed during ovarian suppression. *Fertility and Sterility.* **52**:502–4.

13   Sutton CJG (1991) Laser laparoscopy in the treatment of endometriosis. In: Thomas E and Rock J (eds). *Modern approaches to endometriosis.* Kluwer Academic Publishers, Dordrecht. pp.199–200.

14   Daniell JF (1984) Laser laparoscopy for endometriosis. *Colposcopy and Gynaecological Laser Surgery.* **3**:185–92.

15   Feste JR (1985) Laser laparoscopy. A new modality. *Journal of Reproductive Medicine.* **30**:413–18.

16   Keye WR *et al.* (1987) Argon laser therapy of endometriosis: a review of 92 consecutive patients. *Fertility and Sterility.* **47**:201–12.

17   Nezhat C *et al.* (1988) A comparison of the carbon dioxide, argon and KTP–532 lasers in the videolaseroscopic treatment of endometriosis. *Colposcopy and Gynaecology Laser Surgery.* **1**:41–7.

18 Sutton CJG and Hill D (1990) Laser laparoscopy in the treatment of endometriosis: a five year study. *British Journal of Obstetrics and Gynaecology.* **97**:901–5.

19 Nezhat C *et al.* (1989) Videolaseroscopy for the treatment of endometriosis associated with infertility. *Fertility and Sterility.* **51**:237–40.

20 Donnez J (1987) Carbon dioxide laser laparoscopy in infertile women with endometriosis and women with adnexal adhesions. *Fertility and Sterility.* **3**:390–4.

21 Feste JR (1992) Gynaecological microsurgery using the CO_2 laser. In: Sutton CJG (ed). *Lasers in gynaecology.* Chapman and Hall, London. pp.25–54.

22 Keckstein J (1989) Laparoscopic treatment of polycystic ovarian syndrome. In: Sutton CJG (ed). *Laparoscopic surgery. Baillière's clinical obstetrics and gynaecology, vol. 3, no. 3.* Baillière Tindall, London. pp.563–82.

23 Daniell JF (1989) Fibre optic laser laparoscopy. In: Sutton CJG (ed). *Laparoscopic surgery. Baillière's clinical obstetrics and gynaecology, vol. 3, no. 3.* Baillière Tindall, London. pp.545–62.

24 Keckstein J *et al.* (1988) Laser application in contact and non-contact procedures: sapphire tips in comparison to 'bare fibre' argon laser in comparison to Nd:YAG laser. *Lasers in Medicine and Surgery.* **4**:158–62.

25 Davis GD (1986) Management of endometriosis and its associated adhesions with the carbon dioxide laser laparoscope. *Obstetrics and Gynecology.* **68**:422–5.

26 Nezhat C, Growgey SR and Garrison CP (1986) Surgical treatment of endometriosis via laser laparoscopy. *Fertility and Sterility.* **45**:777–83.

27 Martin DC and Olive DL (1986) Unpublished data. In: Olive DL and Haney AF (eds). Endometriosis associated infertility: a critical review of therapeutic approaches. *Obstetrics and Gynecologic Surveys.* **41**:538–55.

28 Feste JR (1989) CO_2 laser surgery treatment for endometriosis for stages I through IV. Presented at the International Symposium on Endometriosis, Houston, Texas, April.

29 Nezhat C (1989) Video laseroscopy in the treatment of endometriosis. In: Studd JWW (ed). *Progress in Obstetrics and Gynaecology.* Churchill Livingstone, Edinburgh. **19**:293–303.

30 Lichten EM and Bombard J (1987) Surgical treatment of dysmenorrhea with laparoscopic uterine nerve ablation. *Journal of Reproductive Medicine.* **32**(1):37–42.

31 Tjaden B, Schlaff WO, Kimball A, Rock JA (1990) The efficacy of pre-sacral neurectomy for the relief of mid-line dysmenorrhoea. *Obstetrics and Gynaecology.* **76**:89–91.

32 Andebert AJM (1993) Laparoscopic ovarian surgery and ovarian torsion. In: Sutton CJG and Diamond M (eds). *Endoscopic Surgery for Gynaecologists*. WB Saunders, London. pp.134–41.

33 Sutton CJG and McDonald R (1990) Laser laparoscopic adhesiolysis. *Journal of Gynecologic Surgery*. 6:155–60.

34 Lundorff P, Hahlin M, Kiallfelt B, Thorburn J, Lindblom B (1991) Adhesion formation after laparoscopic surgery in tubal pregnancy: a randomised trial versus laparotomy. *Fertility and Sterility*. 55:911–15.

16

Operative Endoscopic Management of Leiomyoma Uteri

JEAN B. DUBUISSON, FABRICE LECURU and L. MANDELBROT

Introduction

The indications for operative hysteroscopy have increased greatly over the past few years, especially for submucous myomas, with the development of electrosurgery and the Nd:YAG laser. Operative laparoscopy also has an increasing number of indications, particularly for interstitial and subserous myomas[1–4].

Between 1st January 1990 and 1st May 1992, we performed 191 laparoscopic myomectomies in 95 patients. During the same period, 144 myomectomies were performed by laparotomy in 13 patients without prior attempts at laparoscopy, and one myomectomy was performed by laparotomy after failure by laparoscopy, because of the absence of cleavage between the tumour (adenomyosis) and the myometrium. In this chapter we report our techniques and short-term results. In selected cases, with the advantages of laparoscopic surgery, laparoscopic myomectomy appears to be a safe technique.

Technique and prerequisites

Procedures are usually performed under general anaesthesia. The bladder is drained and a Foley catheter is left in place throughout the procedure. A cannula is introduced into the uterine cavity to allow mobilization of the uterus. Laparoscopy is performed transumbilically using a 10 mm endoscope with video enhancement. The following instrumentation is used:

- atraumatic grasping forceps
- monopolar hook
- needle holder and suture forceps

- scissors
- bipolar forceps
- pelvicleaner.

In some cases, we also used Semm's myoma enucleator for the thermo-coagulation[5].

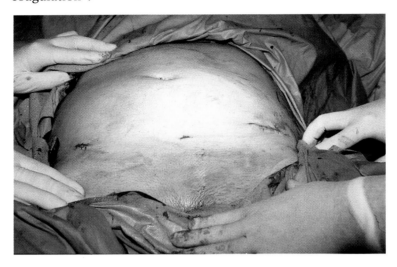

Figure 16.1: Puncture sites located 4 finger breadths above pubic line and 2 finger breadths medial to iliac spines.

The instruments are introduced through three suprapubic puncture sites (5/10 mm in diameter). Myomectomy is performed according to the principles of atraumatic infertility surgery in all cases: magnification, meticulous haemostatis and irrigation with saline solution. However, we do not use vasconstrictive agents. Many investigators report blood loss at the operative site with such agents (dose: 1 amp in 30 cc saline).

For pedunculated myomas, the pedicle is coagulated and transected at its junction with the uterus. The use of endoloops or extracorporeal ties may also be employed to obliterate the vascular pedicle. We use the same technique for subserous myomas when the implantation surface is small ($\leqslant$ 1 cm^2). For subserous myomas with a large implantation surface and interstitial myomas, the uterus is incised at the site of myoma with the hook. Cautery or laser are especially useful, as a dual-effect Nd:YAG laser fibre allows cautery and coagulation effects within the same fibre. Traction and counter traction are useful especially when used in conjunction with a myoma drill or screw. Two grasping forceps and the pelvicleaner are used to remove the leiomyoma from its capsule. Blood vessels are coagulated before section. The myomectomy does not necessitate the opening of the uterine cavity except in cases of submucous myomas.

In cases of deep interstitial myoma, it may be useful to colour the uterine cavity by instillation of methylene blue with a uterine cannula to prevent the

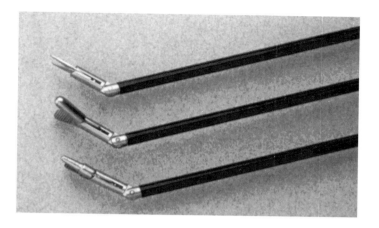

Figure 16.2: Roticulated scissors, dissectors and graspers aid in tumour enucleation.

opening of the uterine cavity. At sites of serosal incision for myomas less than 3 cm and at sites with a raw surface of less than 1 cm², the edges are irrigated and complete haemostatis is achieved. Where deep subserosal or interstitial myomas have left a large gap in the myometrium, or if the serosal incision is more than 3 cm, the edges are reapproximated with sutures. Usually we close the uterus in one layer with interrupted or running 3-0 Vicryl sutures. The distance between each suture is 1 cm. In one case, an intraligamentous myoma (130 mm in diameter) was removed. The technique consists of coagulation and section of the round ligament, and identification of the ureter before myomectomy.

Myomas less than 20 mm may be removed through the secondary puncture sites or pulled through the trocar cannula after enlargement of the skin incision (20 mm) with a single tooth tenaculum. Myomas larger than 20 mm are brought to the suprapubic incision and pressed on the peritoneum to prevent loss of carbon dioxide. They are then fragmented under laparoscopic control, using a small blade or laser passed through the incision. Extraction through a posterior colpotomy is also a possibility, but this lengthens the duration of the operation and may be cumbersome with loss of pneumoperitoneum. In cases of voluminous myomas (> 80 mm in diameter), a transversal suprapubic incision of 40 mm may be performed for the extraction of myomas after fragmentation. In these cases, the uterine incision may be closed transparietally, using a classic needle holder placed through the suprapubic incision under laparoscopic control. In all cases, at the end of the procedure, the peritoneal cavity is irrigated with saline solution. A somewhat smaller tissue extraction system has been described elsewhere in this text. The trocar sleeves of 15 or 20 mm diameter are introduced through which are passed extraction tubes with a serrated sharp edge on the distal end.

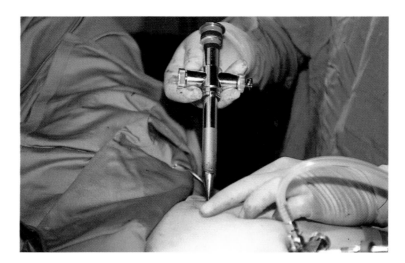

Figure 16.3a: Large cannula (15/20 mm) require significant effort. Insert with extreme caution.

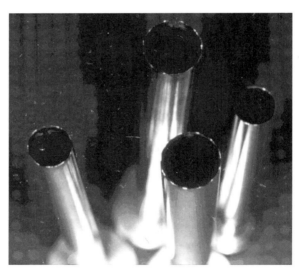

Figure 16.3b: 'Cookie cutter' serrated tissue extraction tubes.

Using a claw forcep the myoma is pulled up towards the serrated end, and with a twisting motion by the operator, a large core of tissue is cut and retracted up into the tube.

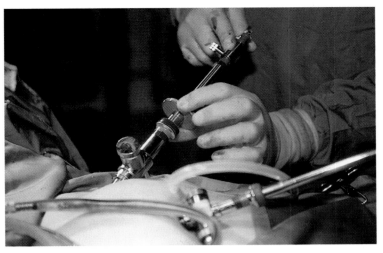

Figure 16.3c: Tissue is kept against distal serrated tube as twisting motion 'cores' the sample.

The inner extraction tube is then removed from the sleeve and the tissue sample obtained.

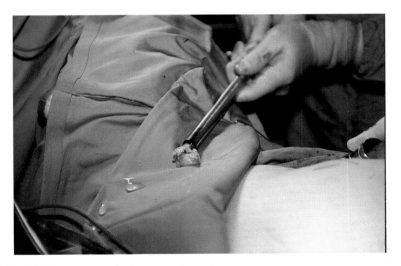

Figure 16.3d: Fibroid tissue removed via extraction tube.

This 'cookie cutter' technique is extremely useful but caution is advised as the distal sharp end may be traumatic to surrounding structures if the operation uses this system indiscriminately. Alternative methods of extraction include the use of a larger 33 mm trocar cannula (Ethicon Ltd) (*see* Figure 16.4) to allow larger chunks of fibroids to be removed under laparoscopic guidance. The editor's experience with large trocars demonstrates that this technique is feasible and that the majority of patients may go home later the same day, despite the larger abdominal incisions[6]!

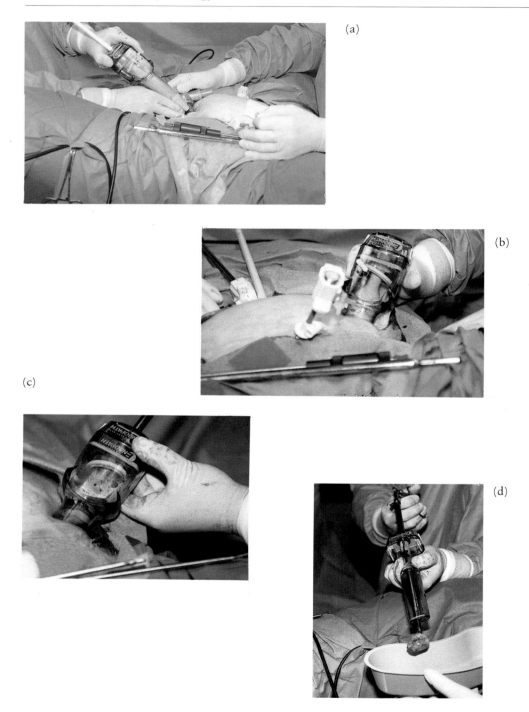

Figure 16.4: a 33 mm cannula inserted via guide rod. **b** Cannula remains stationary with fascia threads. **c** As tissue is removed, it can be visualized within the cannula. **d** 33 mm extraction tube and specimen.

In our series, the mean age was 35.5 years (range 26–50). Sixty-one patients were treated with a depot Gn RH-a for two or three months because of bleeding (eight cases) or the size of the myomas (53 cases). Unfortunately, prolonged use of GNRH tends to soften the myoma tissue and makes the extraction process difficult. As a consequence, some authors have returned to the oral use of danazol which still creates devascularization of the myoma but does not interfere with the tumour capsule. These medications are effective and economical.

We observed no complications (and no transfusions were necessary). On occasion the large amount of force required to insert the large cannula and trocar may lead to significant ecchymosis postoperatively.

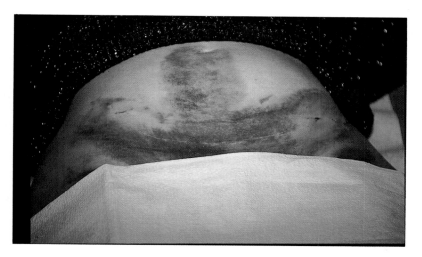

Figure 16.5: Postoperative ecchymosis from large trocars.

Although of some concern to the patient, this discoloration disappears completely. The length of hospitalization postoperatively was two or three days. Follow-up laparoscopy was performed in 13 cases, and no adhesions were noted in 11 cases. So far 10 patients have delivered normally and one has had two late abortions without complications.

Discussion

Preoperative evaluation is crucial for determining operative strategy, according to the number, size and localization of myomas. Lesions within the uterus should be diagnosed by hysterosalpingography or hysteroscopy. Hysteroscopy should be performed systematically before laparoscopy, as it allows the identification of deep interstitial myomas that can be treated by laparoscopy and submucous myomas that can be treated by hysteroscopy. Hysteroscopy may be used to diagnose submucous myomas associated with subserous or interstitial myomas. In these cases, ablation of submucous myomas may be performed during the same operation either by operative hysteroscopy or by laparoscopy. Small interstitial myomas, which may be palpated during laparotomy, can be overlooked during laparoscopy and should therefore be detected by preoperative ultrasound before any medical treatment[7]. Consequently, precise preoperative diagnosis will indicate whether laparotomy should be performed for voluminous or multiple myomas, although larger myomas are now being removed laparoscopically.

Myomectomy is generally performed by laparotomy. Myomectomy must be an atraumatic procedure, minimizing blood loss, and preventing fragilization of the uterus and postoperative pelvic adhesions. Advances in operative endoscopy have enabled myomectomy to be performed by laparoscopy. In our experience, the mean operating time is less than two hours. We have observed no complications. Voluminous and multiple myomas (> 100 mm in diameter or more than four in number) are contraindications for the novice endoscopist because of the risk of possible bleeding, difficulties in the extraction of myomas and a very lengthy operating time. In our series, however, myomas larger than 12 cm have been extracted in outpatient procedures. After deep interstitial or submucous myomectomy, closure of the myometrium and the serosa is recommended to prevent postoperative bleeding and fragilization of the uterus according to the same techniques as performed in laparotomy. In our experience, we have observed no uterine rupture. The risk of adhesion formation after laparoscopic myomectomy with or without sutures seems to be low. The frequent use of second-look laparoscopy has confirmed these findings in a review of the world literature.

Conclusions

Operative laparoscopy has several advantages over laparotomy. The postoperative recovery is much shorter and more comfortable. However, these techniques require experienced endoscopic surgeons, and many limitations are due to the unavailability of the proper equipment for morcellation and because it is still a manual procedure. What is needed is a motorized 'shaver' or 'grinder' to fragment the fibroid tissue; until then, tissue extraction will still remain the limiting step for the laparoscopic approach.

Note: All photos courtesy of New Jersey Laser Institute.

References

1   Dubuisson JB *et al.* (1991) Myomectomy by laparoscopy: a preliminary report of 43 cases. *Fertility and Sterility.* **56**:827–30.

2   Nezhat C *et al.* (1991) Laparoscopic myomectomy. *International Journal of Fertility.* **39**:275–80.

3   Bruhat MA *et al.* (1977) Essai de traitement per coelioscopique de la grossesse extra-uterine. A propos de 26 observations. *Revue Française de Gynaecologie et Obstetrie.* **72**:667–73.

4   Murphy AA (1987) Operative laparoscopy. *Fertility and Sterility.* **47**:1–18.

5   Semm K and Mettler L (1980) Technical progress in pelvic surgery via operative laparoscopy. *American Journal of Obstetrics and Gynecology.* **138**:121–7.

6   Grochmal S and Connant C (1993) Outpatient Laparoscopic Myomectomy (8–12 cm): A Report of 112 Cases. Abstracts of World Congress of Gynecologic Endoscopy, San Francisco.

7   Fedele L *et al.* (1990) Treatment with Gn RH agonists before myomectomy and the risk of short-term myoma recurrence. *British Journal of Obstetrics and Gynaecology.* **97**:393–6.

Additional Reading

Nezhat C *et al.* (1994) Laparoscopically assisted myomectomy: A report of a new technique in 57 cases. *International Journal of Fertility.* **39**:39–44.

Carlson K *et al.* (1994) The Maine Women's Health Study: II Outcomes of non-surgical management of leiomyomas, abnormal bleeding and chronic pelvic pain. *Obstetrics and Gynecology.* **83**.

Rozenberg S *et al.* (1994) Bone mineral content of women with uterine fibromyomas. *International Journal of Fertility.* **39**:77–80.

17

Laparoscopic Management of Pelvic Pain

SAMUEL TARANTINO

Introduction

One of the common complaints of women seen in a clinical practice is chronic pelvic pain[1]. It accounts for approximately 10% of outpatient gynaecological visits, 10–30% of all laparoscopies, and 10–12% of all hysterectomies[1-3]. Although chronic pelvic pain is a common clinical presentation, it is often difficult to determine the aetiology[4-6]. Chronic pelvic pain without pathology has been reported in between 9 and 36% of surgical cases.

Pelvic sensory signals are modulated at the spinal cord in the brain, affecting the way in which pain is perceived. The perception of pelvic pain is not only influenced by the patient's pain stimuli, but by the patient's psychological profile. There appears to be a relationship between manifestations of chronic pelvic pain and cultural, social and psycho-sexual factors[7]. For example, it has been shown that rape victims suffer from a higher incidence of chronic pelvic pain. In investigating patients with pelvic pain, we must investigate both organic and psychological disturbances, both of which may be responsible for these symptoms.

Nerve fibres

Sensory pathways from the pelvis are derived from the lumbar and lower thoracic sympathetic ganglion and the superior, middle and inferior hypergastric plexuses[8]. The sensory input from the body of the uterus, the cervix and the proximal portions of the fallopian tube are transmitted through the afferent fibres, which follow sympathetic nerves into the spinal cord at the level of T10, T11, T12 and L1. These fibres become part of the uterine and cervical plexus, pelvic plexus, the hypogastric nerve and the superior hypergastric nerve. The superior hypogastric plexus is known as the presacral nerve. In order to identify the presacral complex, it is important to understand its anatomical location. The plexus is located posterior to the peritoneum in complex adipose and loose areolar tissue. It lies approximately anterior to the body of the fourth and fifth lumbar vertebrae. Most commonly it consists of two to four incompletely fused bundles and is usually on more than one anatomical plane. In 24 % of subjects, there is a complete fusion to form a single nerve[9]. The middle sacral vessels are usually located between the nerves and the periosteum. To the right of the hypogastric nerve plexus, we encounter the common iliac vessels and the right ureter. Superior to the presacral nerve is the bifurcation of the aorta and vena cava. Nerve fibres from the presacral nerve pass by the inferior hypergastric plexus downward laterally near the inferior portion of the ureteral sacral ligaments. These fibres then pass over the lateral surfaces of the rectum to join the pelvic plexus.

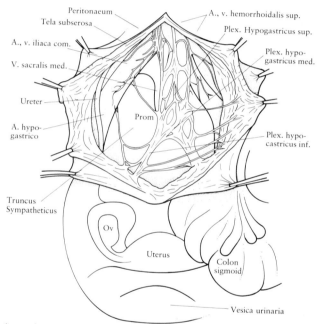

Figure 17.1: Anatomy of pelvic region.

The afferent fibres from the ovary travel with the ovarian vessel and enter the sympathetic nerve bundle at the fourth lumbar sympathetic ganglion. They then ascend with this sympathetic chain and enter the spinal cord at T9 and T10. The outer portions of the fallopian tubes and the upper ureters have similar innervation. The ovary and proximal fallopian tubes do not send any afferent nerve fibres to the hypogastric plexus.

The development of laparoscopic procedures

Recently two laparoscopic procedures, the presacral neurectomy and the uterosacral nerve ablation have been utilized to treat pelvic pain. In the past, both of these procedures have been performed by laparotomy, but with increasing expertise in operative laparoscopy, these endoscopic approaches are used with increasing frequency. The previously described anatomical relationships make presacral neurectomy and uterosacral nerve ablation potentially successful in the treatment of pelvic pain.

Presacral neurectomy for surgical management of chronic pelvic pain is controversial. Although most authors have found that pelvic pain is significantly diminished after the procedure, many doubt its efficacy because few prospective randomized clinical studies have been performed.

The first presacral neurectomy was described by Jaboulay and Ruggi in 1899[10-11]. At that time, the procedure was rarely performed; it was not until 1925 that Cotte popularized this procedure[12-13]. In 1964, Black reviewed the world literature and reported on 9 937 cases. He found a 70-80% relief of dysmenorrhoea after presacral neurectomy[14].

Lee and colleagues reported 50 patients with chronic pelvic pain and who had undergone presacral neurectomy[15]. They observed that 73 % of patients had at least a 50% subjective relief from dysmenorrhoea, while 77% experienced relief from dyspareunia. In both of these groups, the patients had been followed for an average of 2.5 years. Recently, Polan and DeChurney compared two groups of patients suffering from infertility and pelvic pain. One group had a laparotomy and presacral neurectomy, and the second group had laparotomy and cauterization of endometriosis. The presacral neurectomy group experienced a 70% and the control group a 20% relief of pain after a two-year follow-up. This study also demonstrated that adding a uterosacral nerve ablation did not reduce the complaint of pain further[16].

In a recent prospective study, Tjaden et al. observed that midline dysmenorrhoea was abolished in 100% of patients undergoing presacral neurectomy[17]. They studied 26 patients with stage III and IV endometriosis and who were experiencing moderate to severe dysmenorrhoea. The patients were assigned randomly either to a presacral neurectomy or a non-presacral neurectomy group. Neither group knew which procedure was being undertaken. The patients answered questionnaires before surgery and six months postoperatively. The six-month postoperative questionnaire revealed a significant difference between the two groups. The monitoring committee discontinued the study after evaluation of the first 26 patients because they felt that it was unethical to deprive patients of this treatment.

In the late 1960s and early 1970s presacral neurectomy began to lose favour because of the successful introduction of medical treatment for dysmenorrhoea. These drugs included non-steroidal anti-inflammatory agents, oral contraceptives, danazol, and most recently the gonadotropin-releasing hormone agonists. With more emphasis placed on the medical management of pelvic pain, fewer physicians were trained in the technique of presacral neurectomy, and the number of presacral neurectomies decreased. However, although many patients with pelvic pain are controlled with medical therapy, approximately 25% fail to respond.

Perez[18] was the first surgeon to describe the laparoscopic presacral neurectomy; recently Nezhat has also described his technique. Laparoscopic presacral neurectomy was developed in an attempt to perform this procedure without the disadvantages of laparotomy. There are several advantages to performing presacral neurectomy as an outpatient procedure: reduced cost, improved recovery time, and a potential for reduced adhesion formation.[5,9]

Technique

We have developed a technique for laparoscopic presacral neurectomy for visualization of the pelvis. The initial placement of the trocars for operative laparoscopy is as follows: a suprapubic 10 mm trocar, a 10 mm subumbilical trocar in the midline, and two lateral 5 mm trocars. The laparoscope is placed in the subumbilical trocar site and the pelvic structures are systematically visualized. When all the pelvic pathology is visualized and treated laparoscopically, the laparoscope is then placed suprapubically, which facilitates visualization of the presacral area. For adequate visualization of the presacral area, the patient is placed in a left lateral tilt position, which displaces the descending colon laterally. In addition, a 5 mm atraumatic grasper is used to restrain the colon in this position.

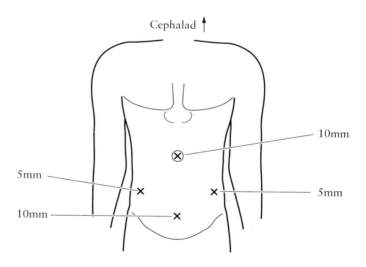

Figure 17.2: Presacral neurectomy trocar sites. The laparoscope is placed at the 10 mm suprapubic puncture for better visualization of the anatomy.

After identification of the aortic bifurcation, the peritoneum covering the sacral promontory is elevated and carefully incised, using sharp dissection. We use a pair of scissors in the 12 mm port, because we feel that the presacral peritoneum is best incised at this angle. The presacral peritoneal space is then completely opened using a vertical incision extending from the bifurcation of the aorta to the level above the sacral prominence. The advantage of the suprapubic approach is the ability to visualize the presacral area and the familiar anatomical relationship. The presacral peritoneum is then undermined using sharp and blunt dissection. The lateral 5 mm trocar sites are used for grasping the peritoneum and for elevation. The bifurcation of the aorta and the common iliac vessels are identified, as well as the right ureter. On the left, the inferior mesenteric super-haemorrhoidal vessels are also visualized. At all times these relationships must be noted in order to avoid serious complications. The middle sacral vein and artery must be identified and then either avoided or clipped during the presacral neurectomy.

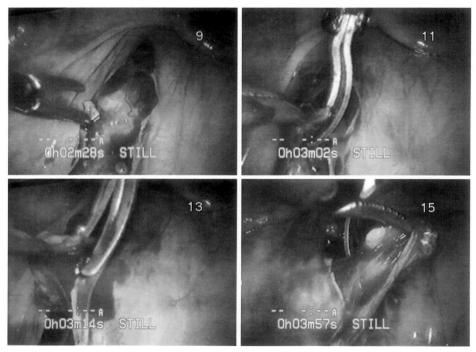

Figure 17.3: The retroperitoneal space has been incised (9) and sharp dissection is utilized to remove adipose tissue (11 and 13). The blunt dissection is then carried down further until the plexus is located (15).

The presacral fat pad is then encountered, and using sharp dissection the tissue is freed from both the presacral surfaces and the periosteum. Recently, investigators reported on a laparoscopically delivered ultrasonic aspirator to dissect away tissue on the presacral surfaces[19]. At this time, care must be taken not to traumatize the great vessels, the aorta or the middle sacral vessels inadvertently. We use bipolar cautery to desiccate the presacral plexus, and then sharp dissection to resect the nerve. Usually 2–3 cm of nervous tissue is excised and sent to pathology to confirm the identification of nervous tissue. The presacral area must then be thoroughly irrigated with Ringer's lactate solution, and the areas of bleeding identified and cauterized. We have been placing a piece of Surgicel in the presacral space, and then suturing or stapling the presacral area closed. We believe this accomplishes two goals: first, by applying pressure to the presacral area, we 3D tamponed small bleeding points. Second, we believe that this area is a raw surface which may allow adhesion formation.

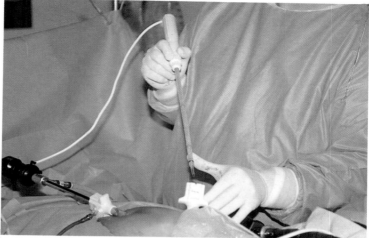

Figure 17.4: A 10 mm endoscopic ultrasonic aspirator may be utilized to skeletize and remove presacral fat and adventitia. Since the ultrasonic aspirator is fibrin sparing, damage to surrounding vessels and intact nerve tissue is prevented.

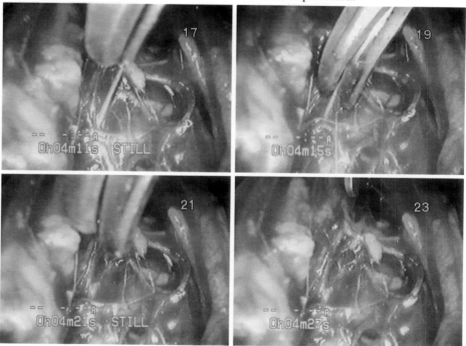

Figure 17.5: After skeletization of the presacral nerve group (17), the nerves are severed (19, 21) sharply and there is minimal bleeding encountered with the plexus completely visible (23).

The presacral neurectomy has been shown to be efficacious in many studies. Although a large prospective control clinical trial has not been performed, most studies have shown impressive results. A major consideration in the success of the presacral neurectomy is the physician selection of the patient

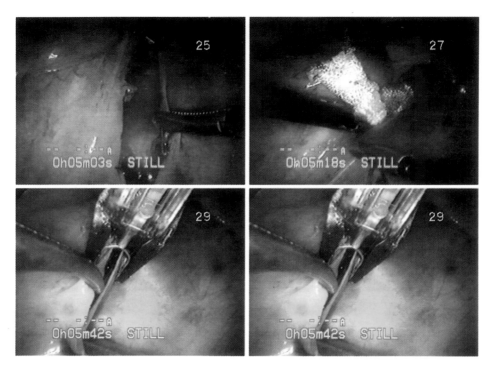

Figure 17.6: Upon completion of irrigation of the operative site, the peritoneal edges are identified (25). Surgicel (optional) is placed into the retroperitoneal space (27) and closure is achieved with clips (29).

population. Prior to surgery, an extensive evaluation of all related systems should be undertaken. Urological, gastro-enterological and orthopaedic causes of pelvic pain should be ruled out. All patients, especially those who did not demonstrate pelvic pathology, should have psychological assessment. Patients with chronic pelvic pain and psychiatric disorders are less likely to benefit from this surgical procedure.

As would be expected from the neural anatomical relationships, midline pelvic pain is most likely to benefit from a presacral neurectomy. The pain of central origin, probably originating in the uterus or cervix, is most amenable to presacral neurectomy. Pain of adnexal origin is unlikely to respond to presacral neurectomy, because these nerve fibres traverse the infundibulo–pelvic ligaments. Complete denervation of the presacral nerve is essential. The presacral nerve complex has individual anatomical variations. There must be attention to adequate dissection and resection of the complete nerve plexus. A failure to resect the presacral nerve complex fully will lead to a surgical 'failure'.

Complications

Complications with presacral neurectomy are uncommon. Care must be taken to avoid damage to the middle sacral vessels during dissection of the presacral fat pad. Either identification and ligation or avoidance is mandatory. At all times attention must be paid to the aorta and vena cava, right ureter and mesenteric vessels. One must also avoid deep dissection, inferiorly near the sacral hollow. These areas contain many large venus plexuses and profuse bleeding could ensue if these plexuses are interrupted. Fastidious haemostasis must also be maintained prior to terminating the presacral neurectomy. Periosteal venus bleeding usually responds to Surgicel or bipolar electrocautery.

Postoperative complications are rare. There have been reports of acute urinary retention for short periods without sequelae. Reports of urinary urgency, constipation, vaginal dryness and painless labour have also been described[15,20]. Although not well studied, presacral neurectomy does not appear to have adverse effects upon fertility[21].

Presacral neurectomy appears to be an appropriate treatment for a subset of patients with chronic pelvic pain. Physicians must perform extensive investigations to rule out all possible causes for pelvic pain. Laparoscopic treatment appears to have multiple advantages and may have equal success, but a well designed randomized clinical trial is needed to ascertain which patients will benefit.

Laparoscopic ureterosacral nerve ablation

The Doyle procedure was first described in 1955 as a surgical procedure designed to alleviate central pelvic pain[23]. At the time, the procedure was performed transvaginally and involved segmental resection of the ureterosacral ligament. The Doyle procedure was felt to be effective, because it would transect the afferent sympathetic fibres, which innervate the uterus at the proximal fallopian tubes. Transsecting these ligaments interrupts most of the uterine and proximal fallopian tubes and sensory fibres. Recently several authors have described laparoscopic ureterosacral nerve ablation or LUNA[24,25]. With the advent of operative laparoscopic techniques, this procedure is easily performed. Like other authors, we have utilized the Nd:YAG laser, KTP laser, and CO_2 laser with comparable results. The CO_2 laser is less than optimal for the LUNA procedure because the plume generated tends to be excessive, and its coagulation properties are poor. Fibre delivered laser energy (Nd:YAG) is preferable as it provides a more acceptable incision and source of coagulation.

Technique

Regardless of the cutting tool utilized, adherence to certain surgical techniques minimizes the risk of complications. When performing a ureterosacral nerve ablation, the ureterosacral nerve is transsected in the area where the nerve intersects the cervix. By using adequate uterine manipulation, the uterus is anteverted, placing the ureterosacral ligaments on

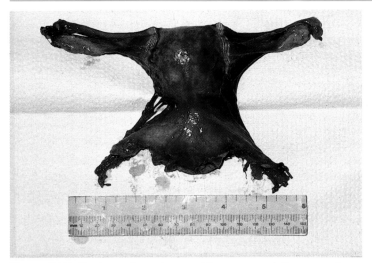

Figure 17.7: Extirpated specimen with uterosacral ligaments intact. Destruction of the ligament appropriately should be accomplished at the USL insertion at the cervix (photo courtesy of J. Wright, Chertsey, UK).

stretch. It is extremely important to realize that a significant distortion of the ureterosacral nerve ligaments may be a relative contraindication to the procedure; because the proximity of the ureter and the uterine vessels to this area is significant, anatomical distortion might place these structures in jeopardy.

When performing the LUNA, the goal is to transsect the ureterosacral ligaments completely. As discussed above, one must be concerned about

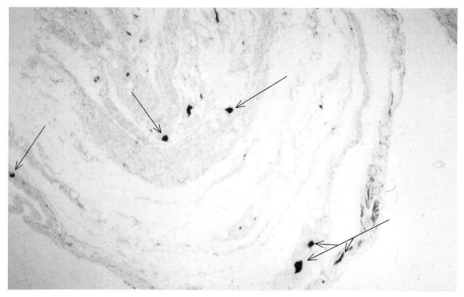

Figure 17.8: Cross-section of ureterosacral ligament with special nerve tissue stain. Note that the blue areas represent nerve fibres and are located throughout the entire ligament. Excision of a portion of the ligament will assure complete nerve fibre interruption.

extreme lateral transsection, which might damage a ureter, whereby extreme medial dissection could potentially damage the artery which runs along the medial aspect of the presacral ligament. If damage does occur to an artery along the ureterosacral ligament, bipolar cautery must be used instead of monopolar cautery. Use of monopolar energy could result in delayed thermal damage and postsurgical scarring. Although some surgeons recommend vaporization of the peritoneum between the ureterosacral ligaments, no one to date has shown that this improves outcome.

Literature describing the success of this procedure is scarce. Festi has recently reported a 70% relief of dysmenorrhoea after a one-year follow-up of women undergoing LUNA[25]. Lichten and Bombard reported a perspective study with a limited number of women which showed an 80% relief of pain after a one-year follow-up[24]. Unfortunately, to date there have been no well designed control studies investigating the efficacy of the laparoscopic ureterosacral nerve ablation.

Professional concerns

Over the past few years, some concerns have been raised about the LUNA procedure. Several surgeons have commented that LUNA might predispose patients to uterine prolapse. The ligamentive support of the uterus is primarily cardinal; ureterosacral ligaments appear to play a small role in uterine support. Ureterosacral nerve transsection, therefore, should not lead to uterine prolapse. Another frequently asked question concerning the LUNA procedure is whether this procedure can be repeated. A well performed LUNA procedure, with complete transsection of the ureterosacral ligaments should not be repeated if unsuccessful. If a well performed LUNA has failed, it is logical to assume that a repeat procedure would not improve results. In addition, scarring can occur with subsequent medial displacement of the ureters. This anatomical distortion could place the ureter in potential jeopardy if a repeat procedure were performed.

The LUNA procedure has been successful in relieving central pelvic pain. This is consistent with the neuro-anatomical relationship of the afferent nerve supply to the uterus and medial fallopian tubes. It should not be performed in a woman whose major component of pelvic pain is lateral. Laparoscopic ureterosacral nerve ablation can decrease the discomfort associated with midline pelvic pain. It is easy to perform, and in experienced hands has a low complication rate. Although well performed control studies are lacking, initial reports appear to support its use in selected patients.

References

1   Gidro FL and Eylarlt GT (1960) Pelvic pain and female identity. *American Journal of Obstetrics and Gynecology.* **79**:1184.

2   Magni G *et al.* (1986) Psychological profile of women with chronic pelvic pain. *Archives of Gynecology.* **237**:165.

3   Gross R *et al.* (1980–81) Borderline syndrome in incessant chronic pelvic pain patients. *International Journal of Psychiatry and Medicine.* **10**:79.

4   Kresch AJ *et al.* (1984) Laparoscopy; an evaluation of 100 women with chronic pelvic pain. *Obstetrics and Gynecology.* **64**:672.

5   Rapkin AJ (1986) Adhesions in pelvic pain; a retrospective study. *Obstetrics and Gynecology.* **68**:13.

6   Walker E *et al.* (1988) Relationship of chronic pelvic pain to psychiatric diagnosis in childhood sexual abuse. *American Journal of Psychiatry.* **145**:75.

7   Kerns RD *et al.* (1985) The West Haven–Yale Multidimensional Pain Inventory (WHYMPI). *Pain.* **23**:345.

8   Curtis AH *et al.* (1942) The anatomy of the autonomic nerves and the relationship to gynecology. *Surgery, Gynecology and Obstetrics.* **75**:43.

9   Bonica JJ (1953) *The management of pain.* Lea and Febiger, Philadelphia.

10 Jaboulay M (1899) Le traitement de la neuralgie pelvienne par la paralysie du sympathique sacre. *Lyon Med.* **90**:102–8.

11 Ruggi C (1899) *La simpaticectoma abdominale utero-ovarica come mezzo di cura di alcone lesini interne de gli organi genitali della donna.* Zanichelli, Bologna.

12 Cotte MG (1937) Resection of the presacral nerve and treatment of abstinent dysmenorrhea. *American Journal of Obstetrics and Gynecology.* **33**:1030–40.

13 Cotte MG (1949 Techniques of presacral neurectomy. *American Journal of Surgery.* **78**:50–3.

14 Black WT (1964) Use of presacral sympathectomy in the treatment of dysmenorrhea. *American Journal of Obstetrics and Gynecology.* **89**:16.

15 Lee RB *et al.* (1986) Presacral neurectomy for chronic pelvic pain. *Obstetrics and Gynecology.* **68**:517.

16 Polan ML and DeChurney A (1980) Presacral neurectomy for pelvic pain and infertility. *Infertility and Sterility.* **34**:557.

17 Tjaden B *et al.* (1976) The ethicacy of presacral neurectomy for the relief of midline dysmenorrhea. *Obstetrics and Gynecology.* **56**:89–91.

18 Perez JJ (1990) Laparoscopic presacral neurectomy; results of the first 25 cases. *Journal of Reproductive Medicine.* **35**:625–30.

19 Grochmal SA *et al.* (1993) Applications of the laparoscopic ultrasonic aspirator for advanced gynecologic operative endoscopic procedures. *Journal of American Association of Gynecologic Laparoscopists.* **1**:43.

20 Nezhat C (1992) A simplified method of laparoscopic presacral neurectomy for the treatment of central pelvic pain due to endometriosis. *British Journal of Obstetrics and Gynaecology.* **99**:659–63.

21 Malinak LR (1980) Operative management of pelvic pain. *Clinics in Obstetrics and Gynecology.* **23**:191.

22 Maltingly RF (1977) *Presacral neurectomy. Telinde operative gynecology*, 5th edn. J.B. Lippincott, Philadelphia. p.253.

23 Doyle JB (1955) Paracervical uterine de-innervation by transection of the cervical plexus for the relief of dysmenorrhea. *American Journal of Obstetrics and Gynecology.* **70**:11.

24 Lichten EM and Bombard J (1987) Surgical treatment of primary dysmenorrhea with laparoscopic ureteral sacral nerve ablation. *Journal of Reproductive Medicine.* **32**:37–41.

25 Festi JR (1985) Laser laparoscopy; a new modality. *Journal of Reproductive Medicine.* **30**:413–17.

18

Gynaecological Applications of Optical Catheters (Microhysteroscopy and Microlaparoscopy)

STEPHEN A. GROCHMAL

Introduction

I first learnt about optical catheters and their potential applications in gynaecology late in 1989. I was impressed by the concept of introducing small flexible catheters into tiny areas of the body. In gynaecology, exploration of the fallopian tube has always been elusive, and I thought that there might be some use for optical catheters in this area. It was not until I had obtained a working prototype of the optical catheter system that I began to understand how many potential applications there were in gynaecology, in diagnostic as well as operative procedures.

Since then I have treated over 2000 patients with this particular technology. I have seen how improvements in the technology and its design can benefit my diagnostic and operative techniques and also increase patient safety and comfort. The technology has been taken up by general surgeons and urologists[1].

History of the development of optical catheters

The fibreoptic transmission of light and images was first developed in the 1970s. The evolution of optical catheter technology began in 1985 in the research laboratories of Medical Dynamics in Englewood, Colorado. The initial problem stemmed from the fact that most small-diameter flexible endoscopes had several light-carrying fibres in their systems but generally did not supply enough illumination. Approximately half of the device was made up of the coherent image guide, and half was composed of the light transmission fibres. The challenge was to develop a new way of delivering light to the target site while keeping the diameter of the delivery device as small as was technically possible. This led to the development of the first laser optical catheter (Figure 18.1). It was composed of a control unit which had the camera and optics for coupling to the image guide and displaying an image on a television monitor. The light source was a very early infrared diode laser which was able to provide approximately 10–12 mW of output. This was a beautiful device. It delivered oceans of light, and a 0.5 mm catheter could be pointed at objects across a room and visualize them on a monitor extremely well. The light source put out light at 780 nm and was invisible. One could sit in a totally dark room and see on a television monitor a superb picture of anything the device was pointed at: pictures on the walls, furniture, people etc. The only problem was that the picture was monochrome. Later some of the initial problems were solved. There was a device which was still smaller in diameter than any flexible fibrescope (a coherent fibre bundle was obtained to carry the image but had only one light-carrying fibre which was the size of a human hair). The device had excellent illumination, and image quality, but there was still no colour.

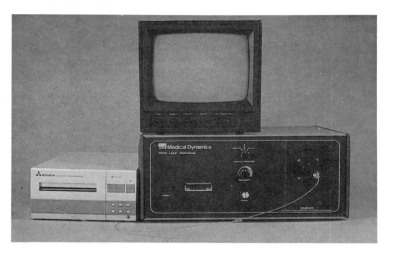

Figure 18.1: Laser optical catheter circa 1985 (photo courtesy of Medical Dynamics).

The work of Max Cohen of the Physics Department at Northwestern University in Chicago, Illinois, led to the next step forward. Dr Cohen was interested in how white light from a laser could be directed down a single fibre for the illumination of endoscopes. His initial experimentation was successful in demonstrating that this concept could be efficiently achieved. Now there was a single fibre with white light (a mixture of three outputs from a nitrogen laser — red/green/blue). His concept and developmental research were so unique that the technology was licensed and incorporated into the developmental research being performed at Medical Dynamics.

The combination of white laser light and the single fibre transmission technology led to the development of a wonderful device. It had all the advantages of the original laser catheter, but the picture was now available in colour. Through trial and error, some of the early difficulties were overcome with this new device in that laser speckle could finally be eliminated by the use of a simple diffuser which was placed at the end of the light fibre. As with all new technological advances, however, the major problem was cost. The price for a laser suitable for this type of device to deliver a white light output was still in the $40 000 range, which was not likely to decrease in the immediate future. It was a wonderful concept, and certainly a marketable one, but not practical because of cost.

In 1988, the decision was made to attempt to develop this device with a xenon light which would be more cost-effective. This required a redesign of the xenon light source so that the maximum amount of light was focused on a small bundle of fibres; there was also a light filter in the infrared range, which could stop infrared light from causing heat to build up and melt the fibres in the bundle. After much experimentation this was accomplished; with the focused light on the end of a light-carrying fibre, and the infrared light removed, the result was a very bright source of illumination. The technology relied upon an ability to couple the image fibres (coherent fibre) directly to a video camera with suitable optics, and to couple the light source directly to the light fibres in the fibrescope. This direct coupling technique prevented the losses that the inherent fibre had in the standard configuration scope. This led to the first telescope designed without an eye-piece.

With the eye-piece, the coupler and the camera now removed from the equation, this device could:

- be lightweight and extremely easy to manipulate
- deliver a plentiful amount of light to the target site, with no light loss due to multiple connections in the light 'train'
- provide better image quality because of the direct coupling to the camera optics
- offer smaller diameters than had been previously available
- provide greater lengths of fibre bundles possible because there was no coupling loss
- make greater lengths of fibre bundles possible because there was no coupling loss
- allow the use of ultraviolet and/or infrared light.

One could mate an infrared laser and Doppler unit to an optical catheter by utilizing only two light fibres, and produce an endoscope which provided an image as well as simultaneous measurement of (for example) capillary blood flow and tissue. This device could also be adapted to give readings of pressure, temperature and even pulse oximetry.

Optical catheters could also be used for fluorescence detection. Since there is no eye-piece, a source of ultraviolet illumination can be delivered through the endoscope to excite fluorescens and then display the fluorescens on a colour monitor. This would be helpful in locating sites of endometriosis within the abdominal cavity by first tagging the cells with tamoxifen. Preliminary work in this field appears to show promise but no definitive long-term clinical results have been available to date.

This fluorescence detection can be taken one step further. Cancer detection within the abdominal cavity can also be done by using various haematopor-phyrin derivatives such as photofrin II. These particular substances selectively localize in malignant cells and fluoresce a brilliant red when radiated at 410 nm of light. As the technology continues to be refined, it is certain that these two above-mentioned applications are only the beginning of what will be achieved with microtechnology in the future.

Optical catheters can now be manufactured in almost any configuration. Currently there are three categories.

1   Rigid catheters such as optical catheter laparoscopes and arthroscopes (Figure 18.2).

2   Flexible catheters such as ureteroscopes (0.5–1.5 mm in diameter – Figure 18.3). Optical catheters can be manufactured in a flexible format, down to 0.2 mm in size if applications require such technology.

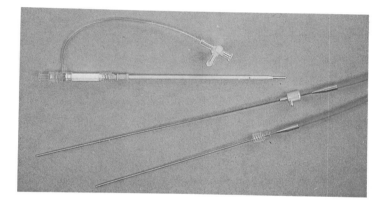

Figure 18.2: Rigid laparoscope and arthroscope (cladded) (photo courtesy of Medical Dynamics).

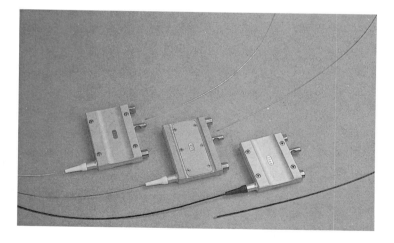

Figure 18.3: Flexible optical catheters (uncladded) 0.35 mm–0.75 mm (photo courtesy of Medical Dynamics).

3   Steerable devices, which can now be manufactured in a two-way or four-way deflection.

All of the above devices can be manufactured with irrigating and operating channels. The majority of these optical catheter devices are introduced into the operative site by an introducer set such as the one shown in Figure 18.4 as utilized in office arthroscopy. A second type of introducer set is the Verres needle for introducing into the abdominal cavity, and which is the basis for the micro-laparoscopic techniques (Figure 18.5). As development of this technology improves, and as the applications extend from the operating room to the office setting, development of specialized sterile disposable trays for office laparoscopy, hysteroscopy or arthroscopy will become available. These will include all the necessary draping, skin prep, irrigating tubing and distension medium for distending the particular body cavity for which the set will be utilized.

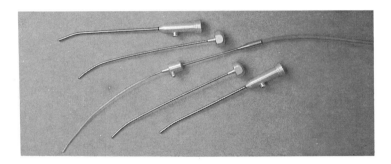

Figure 18.4: Arthroscopic rigid introducer set, later adapted for laparoscopic use (photo courtesy of Medical Dynamics).

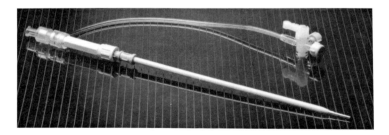

Figure 18.5: Adair/Verres needle cannula with proximal membrane valve and side arm tubing (photo courtesy of Medical Dynamics).

Since the original development of the optical catheters by Medical Dynamics, several other corporations have entered this new and exciting field. Some companies have tried to refine the optical catheter bundle without making any adjustments to the optical or electronic end of the fibrescope. As shown in Figure 18.6, a somewhat larger fibre bundle is attached directly to the eyepiece of a conventional digitized camera, which allows a larger image to be displayed on the video monitor, as well as improving the resolution of the

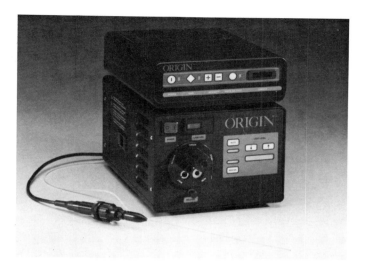

Figure 18.6: Fibrescope with conventional camera head attached (photo courtesy of Origin Medsystems, Inc.).

picture. More recently, optical catheters have been channelled down to steerable handles, through which distension medium can be pumped, and which can even provide an operating channel for office procedures (Figure 18.7).

It is possible that the near future will see fibres being reduced to 5 or 6 μm, as the technology of drawing smaller and smaller diameter fibres improves. Therefore optical catheters will have more fibres per bundle, producing higher resolution and an improved video image. New developments in the production of glasses and plastics will be utilized to provide better light transmission for these optical catheters, improving image quality overall.

Along with the developments in glasses and plastics will come the development of improved adhesives used in the manufacture of the fibrescopes, making them more durable and easier to process through soaking solutions and ethylene oxide sterilization systems. As laser manufacturers begin to provide diode lasers in the blue wavelength, we may see diode laser illumination with very inexpensive light sources. This would provide a white light diode laser for endoscopic illumination and significantly improve the amount of light transmitted through a fibre bundle.

Applications of optical catheters in gynaecology

Technical background

Although the original optical catheters were designed for arthroscopic use, I was always intrigued by their possible applications in gynaecology. Recent

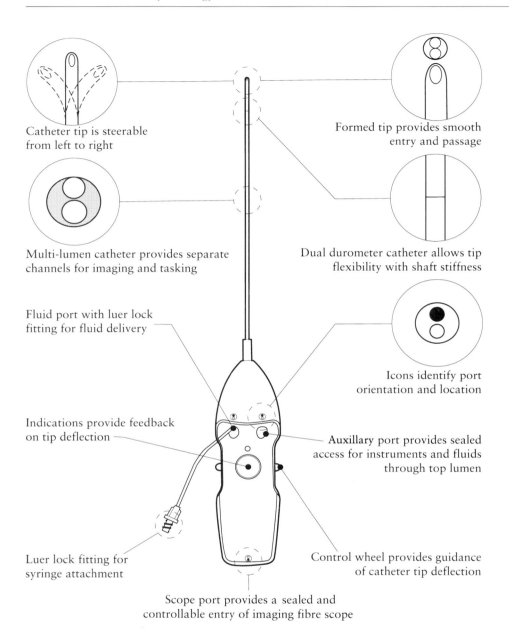

Catheter tip is steerable
from left to right

Formed tip provides smooth
entry and passage

Multi-lumen catheter provides separate
channels for imaging and tasking

Dual durometer catheter allows tip
flexibility with shaft stiffness

Fluid port with luer lock
fitting for fluid delivery

Icons identify port
orientation and location

Indications provide feedback
on tip deflection

Auxillary port provides sealed
access for instruments and fluids
through top lumen

Luer lock fitting for
syringe attachment

Control wheel provides guidance
of catheter tip deflection

Scope port provides a sealed and
controllable entry of imaging fibre scope

Figure 18.7: Schematic of steerable catheter with features (illustration courtesy of Catheter Imaging Systems, Inc.).

technological advances have now allowed the bundling of up to 15 000 plastic fibres into one small optical package. In gynaecology, these optical catheters may or may not be metal cladded (Figures 18.2 and 18.3).

The original arthroscopic cladded bundle fibres were utilized in our initial laparoscopic and hysteroscopic studies. Since our initial investigation, technology has provided us with longer optical catheters, which allow us to explore deep into the pelvis, especially in the cul-de-sac and/or in the high reaches of the uterine cavity near the cornua.

The optical catheter system consists of an electronic console which contains a xenon light source (300 W), as well as the focusing and telescopic camera lenses of a conventional digitized chip camera. These two elements are housed in the one console, which by patented technology allows both functions to be combined and channelled into the fibre bundle of the catheter (*see* Figure 18.8). Additional features of the console include an automatic white bounce capability as well as continuous auto-light adjustment and light intensity modifications. In the console is a separate motorized unit which allows a zooming effect or magnification of the image size which can be displayed on the video monitor, as well as a colour bar generator and other optical enhancements such as adjustable focus and adjustable light intensity. The entire system, which includes the camera optics as well as the light source (xenon), transmits into the optical fibre bundle via a connecting block, to which any of the various diameters of the optical catheters, cladded or uncladded, are attached.

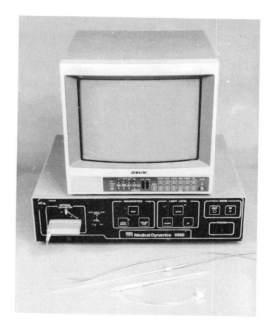

Figure 18.8: Optical catheter control unit with catheter attached via connecting block (photo courtesy of Medical Dynamics).

Optical catheters currently available range in size from 0.35 mm to 1.6 mm in outside diameter (*see* Figures 18.2 and 18.3). The distance from the insertion of the fibre bundle into the connecting block to the proximal end of the cladded portion of the catheter is approximately 2 m. The outside diameter of this vinyl-cladded fibre bundle is approximately 2.7 mm. Therefore the fibre cladded bundle is all that exists between the patient and the equipment itself. This lends itself nicely to working in areas where sterile conditions are required and where conventional endoscopes and light cable systems would be too bulky.

Operation of the entire unit is easy. Once power-up has been accomplished, an automatic white balance is set, and the light intensity and focus are adjusted. The system continues to adjust focus and light intensity automatically.

Entrance into the abdominal cavity for laparoscopic use, and/or into the endocervical canal for hysteroscopy, requires the use of a special cannula system. For laparoscopy, a flexible silastic Adair cannula, with an outside diameter of 2.7 mm, is placed over a standard conventional 150 mm Verres needle (Figure 18.5). The end of the flexible cannula locks in place at the proximal end onto the Luer lock of the Verres needle. In the case of laparoscopy, once the umbilical incision has been made, the Adair/Verres needle cannula is inserted through the abdominal cavity, and proper confirmation of Verres needle placement is made by passing the optical catheter down through the cannula itself (*see* Figure 18.9). This is obviously useful where there may be obstruction below the umbilicus. Once proper location is confirmed, the Verres needle portion of the cannula system is withdrawn, and a one-way membrane valve is attached to the proximal end of the flexible Adair cannula. To the side of this valve system is attached a side arm tubing, through which CO_2, or fluid distension medium in the case of hysteroscopy, can be channelled.

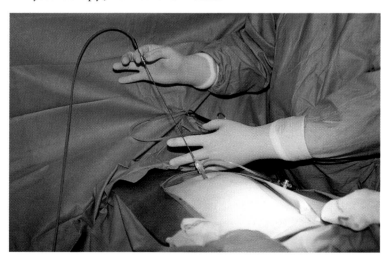

Figure 18.9: Upon insertion of Adair/Verres cannula the microlaparoscope is advanced to confirm proper cannula location (photo courtesy of N.J. Laser Institute).

It has been my experience, when using these microendoscopic techniques for laparoscopy, especially when patients are under intravenous sedation, that an intra-abdominal pressure of 8–10 mm should be utilized, with a maximum volume of CO_2 of approximately 1.5–3 L. In laparoscopy, once 0.5 L of gas has been slowly instilled into the abdominal cavity, one can begin to carry out laparoscopy immediately[3]. The flexible cannula which was placed through the umbilical incision acts as a trocar for the cladded optical catheter. I have found that the cladded optical catheters work especially well for microlaparoscopic use since they are semiflexible and are rigid enough to be manipulated through the cannula and into and around the entire pelvic and abdominal cavities.

Although the microendoscope is inside the Adair cannula, insufflation can continue around the catheter so that proper levels of distension can be achieved within a short period. Upon completion of the insufflation of the abdominal cavity, diagnostic or operative laparoscopy can commence.

Laparoscopic applications

As with any new technology, there are always various ways of describing the devices. In this chapter I refer to the optical catheters as either microendoscopes, microlaparoscopes or microhysteroscopes. This section deals specifically with applications of this technology in laparoscopy, ie microlaparoscopic applications.

I have utilized the microlaparoscope in almost all procedures where conventional laparoscopy would currently be the standard choice. It is especially useful for diagnostic procedures, and in the last three years I have performed numerous operative procedures under the surveillance of the microendoscopic video image. It should be noted that this small 1.6 mm laparoscope can be manipulated easily due to its semiflexible configuration within the abdominal cavity. However, it is important to remember that the optical fibre bundle cannot provide a very large panoramic view of the entire pelvic or abdominal target site, nor can it provide an ocean of illumination over a large distance from the target site. Therefore the surgeon must be no further than 4 cm away from the area under visualization, and must learn to perform an organ by organ assessment of the patient very slowly. It takes some practice to become accustomed to working closer to the operative site, as well as to readjust your eyes to a much smaller image size on the video monitor. Thanks to the use of digital technology, the image size of the monitor can be increased to fill an 8 inch diameter circle on the monitor screen (*see* Figure 18.10).

I was intrigued by the possible application of this microtechnology in gynaecology because it was apparent to me that it could be used in conjunction with intravenous sedation techniques or perhaps with local anaesthetic agents to the skin surface. This could be an advantage, especially in patients who for certain reasons may require repetitive laparoscopies. The technique and preparation which I employ is as follows.

All patients undergoing microlaparoscopy are prepared in the same way as if they were undergoing conventional laparoscopy. The findings at the time of the microlaparoscopy may reveal pathological situations which require a larger, more conventional laparoscopic approach. Therefore all patients undergoing this procedure should also give their consent for possible laparoscopy. All patients are treated interoperatively with an indwelling

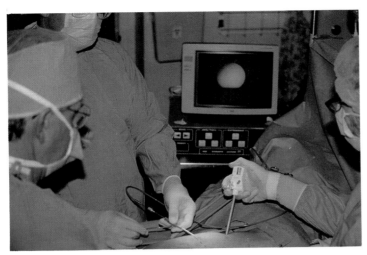

Figure 18.10: Adequate enlarged video image is obtained while 3 mm trocar is inserted under visual guidance (photo courtesy of N.J. Laser Institute).

Foley catheter; the night before surgery, administration of an antibiotic is routine, as is cleansing of the lower bowel via enema on the morning of surgery. Once the patient is on the operating table, intravenous sedation is initiated. A combination of medications including fentanyl, propofol and Versed is administered in incremental dosages until an adequate level of sedation and elimination of pain is achieved. Continuous administration of nasal oxygen to maintain the oxygen saturation at the 99–100% level is critical, as is continuous monitoring of the patient's level of sedation. Advantages of these medications are that a good level of anaesthesia can be achieved, as well as successful elimination of postoperative emesis and a very good amnesia effect during, before and after the operative procedure.

Generally 0.25–0.5% bupivacaine can be utilized for local anaesthesia at the level of the skin incisions. The longer-acting effect of this medication is useful, especially if the procedure should become an operative one. With this type of combined medication, patients can remain under intravenous sedation for between one and four hours of surgery. All patients are discharged within two hours postoperatively with minimal side-effects from the surgical experience. Administration of the local anaesthetics at the level of the skin should be carried down to the preperitoneal layer whenever possible. This can easily be achieved once the microendoscope is in the umbilical region, since visualization of the needle tip administering the local anaesthetic can be seen bulging just above the peritoneal surface on the video monitor.

With the microendoscope in the umbilical port, transillumination and direct insertion techniques can be utilized with the optical catheter. For this purpose, the autoillumination circuit is bypassed and the light source positioned manually in order to transilluminate the abdominal wall. I have found that small 3 mm trocars (US Surgical – Figure 18.11), and/or the Wolf 3 mm diagnostic cannula probe, can be utilized for secondary and tertiary puncture sites. I have also utilized Adair/Verres needle cannulae as secondary

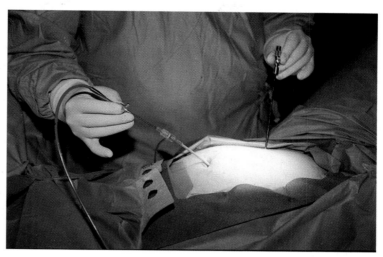

Figure 18.11: The operator performs diagnostic microlaparoscopy with secondary 3 mm cannula probe after local skin infiltration and IV sedation (photo courtesy of N.J. Laser Institute).

trocar sites using a Touey-Borst valve at the tip of the cannula to act as a trocar valve. This allows the passage of instruments up to 3 mm in diameter. For the operative procedure, I have on occasions utilized hysteroscopic biopsy forceps and scissors.

By utilizing a small amount of local infiltration of bupivacaine into the subcutaneous tissue and abdominal wall, I have found that the majority of patients can tolerate the insertion of the secondary trocar sites. With the passage of the secondary trocar sites, fibre-delivered laser energy can also be passed into the abdominal cavity for the operative procedures (*see* Figure 18.12).

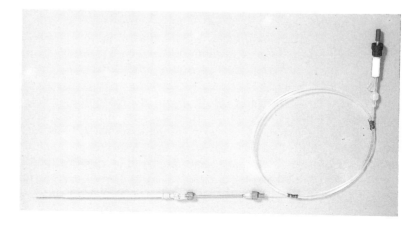

Figure 18.12: Adair cannula utilized as secondary trocar for laser fibre (photo courtesy of N.J. Laser Institute).

Some investigators have reported that, in patients undergoing tubal ligation under intravenous anaesthesia, a small endoscopic needle cannula can deliver small amounts of lidocaine or other anaesthetic, which can be dripped onto the serosal areas of the fallopian tubes. This makes the manipulation of the tube more comfortable for the patient, and placement of either a fallopring or cauterization of the fallopian tubes is performed with more comfort.

During microlaparoscopy, it is not necessary to have a fully distended abdominal cavity. Therefore the need to distend to cavity 4–5 L of CO_2 distension is not required, and overdistension of the abdominal cavity causes discomfort for the patients, especially when they are under intravenous sedation. I have found it easier to initiate insufflation of the abdomen once proper confirmation of the Adair cannula has been made visually with the optical catheter, and to instill 0.5–1.5 L of CO_2 gas. Placing the patient in a modified Trendelenburg position is also useful for manipulating the bowel away from the pelvic brim in order to visualize the uterus, tubes and ovaries more clearly. In cases where the optical catheter (microlaparoscope) is utilized for initiating the laparoscopic procedure, especially in patients who may have questions of subumbilical adhesions, the procedure can be carried out with a much larger amount of CO_2 distension as the optical catheter portion of the procedure will be replaced by conventional laparoscopic instrumentation requiring a larger pneumoperitoneum.

Surprisingly, patients under intravenous sedation can easily tolerate the 1.5 L of pneumoperitoneum, and do not mind manipulation of the internal organs, even if lidocaine drip is not utilized as part of the procedure. There is adequate distension for visualization of any pathology except for evaluation of very large tumours such as fibroids, and video documentation can easily be achieved satisfactorily. I prefer to use Sony high-8 video cassettes for all of my documentation, especially with microlaparoscopy, due to the smaller image size which can be achieved. I also prefer to utilize the image size at its minimal zoom setting which increases the clarity and resolution of the video picture. When one zooms the image up to a larger field of view on the monitor, one begins to lose some resolution; the picture becomes less crisp, and the edges of the video image become somewhat blurry. This is due to the enlargement of the microfibres which are utilized within the optical bundle of the catheter system. However, recent advances in digital technology are bringing improvements.

Once the microendoscope is in the umbilicus and the secondary and tertiary trocar sites have been established, one can proceed with laparoscopy in the usual fashion. I have found that, for simple diagnostic or second-look laparoscopies after previous laparoscopic surgery, the use of the 3 mm blunt probe from Wolf makes it easier to manipulate the organs for inspection. At other times, I may choose to utilize a 5 mm trocar site in the left lower quadrant, and use atraumatic 5 mm grasping forceps for manipulation of the organs or to obtain biopsies or simple lysis of adhesions. The microendoscope can also be swung up into the right upper quadrant in order to visualize the gallbladder and more cephalad organ structures. This has attracted the interest of general surgeons, many of whom now utilize the microendoscope to explore the common bile duct, which they can incise using an operating cannula sheath, and then advance a smaller 0.35 or 0.5 optical catheter to explore the entire duct system. Many surgeons have also found the use of this

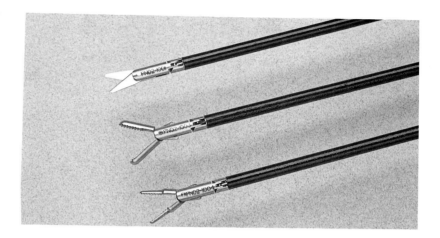

Figure 18.13: Prototypical 3 mm instrumentation for microtechniques (photo courtesy of Richard Wolf).

system advantageous to patients who develop postoperative pain and discomfort subsequent to laparoscopic cholecystectomy where adhesions may be suspected. Placement of the optical catheter through the umbilicus or in the right upper quadrant can be done on an outpatient basis to rule out any complications that may have arisen from the surgery.

As mentioned previously, it is necessary to perform an organ by organ assessment of the pelvis. Because there is less illumination than with a 10 mm laparoscope, it is necessary to remain approximately 4 cm away from the tissue surface. This is somewhat frustrating to the novice who is using this equipment for the first time; with practice, however, a visualization technique is easily accomplished and the image can be readily interpreted. Warming of the catheter just prior to insertion down the Adair cannula, and relocation of the CO_2 insufflation site through a secondary trocar port, prevent fogging of the distal tip of the microendoscope and improve the video image drastically.

Upon completion of the procedure, removal of the cannula-type trocar requires minimal suture closure. Generally sterile adhesive tape is all that is required. With the procedure as described above, most patients can undergo a second-look microlaparoscopy, and perhaps lysis of adhesions, under intravenous sedation as an outpatient, in no more than two or three hours. Many patients return to their usual routine that same day[3].

Gynaecological procedures with microendoscopy

Patient selection is critical, because not all patients tolerate intravenous sedation well. As always, one should bear in mind that severe pathological conditions are managed more appropriately by conventional laparoscopy or other open surgical techniques.

Table 18.1 lists many procedures which can be done successfully using the optical catheter technology in conjunction with intravenous sedation.

Diagnostic	Operative
Initial controlled abdominal wall entry	Chromotubation adhesiolysis (pelvic, abdominal)
Confirmation of pneumoperitoneum	Tissue biopsies
Diagnostic evaluation of:	Tubal ligation
• acute abdominal pain	Coagulation of endometriosis
• acute pelvic trauma	Aspiration of ovarian cysts
• suspected appendicitis	Salpingotomy
• ectopic pregnancy	Incidental myomectomy (1–2 cm)
• acute salpingitis	Oocyte aspiration/collection
Second-look laparoscopy for:	GIFT procedures
• endometriosis	Distal fimbrioscopy
• adhesions	
• tuboplasty	
• fimbrioscopy	
• evaluation of complications after conventional open surgery	

Table 18.1: Procedures which can be performed under intravenous sedation on an outpatient basis.

Obviously these are all procedures that are possible in an outpatient facility, where conventional laparoscopy can also be performed; the difference is patient comfort and the ability of patients to return to a normal activity level in a shorter period of time. I have seen patients return to work that same evening with very little discomfort or pain. One of the greatest benefits of these techniques is the patient's willingness to undergo surgery. Many patients have undergone significant numbers of laparoscopies for various reasons, and the thought of another conventional laparoscopic procedure with general anaesthesia and large puncture sites may be unacceptable. When patients are shown the size of the microinstrumentation, they are more willing to undergo these procedures in the knowledge that they can be performed satisfactorily with intravenous sedation techniques. Of course, every patient is told that there is always the possibility that more major conventional laparoscopy may be necessary, depending on the findings at the time of surgery. However, having performed these procedures since 1989, I can safely say that a competent endoscopic surgeon can easily perform these procedures with microtechniques under intravenous sedation without any difficulty.

I would recommend that physicians beginning to use this technology should start with diagnostic laparoscopy and perhaps simple operative procedures such as adhesiolysis and tubal ligation[4]. This should be done until the physician is comfortable working with the decreased image size and small instrumentation.

As with all new technologies, one problem is the lack of proper instrumentation. I mentioned earlier that I have been using hysteroscopic instrumentation through small cannulae. This is satisfactory, but certainly not as comfortable as if we had specifically designed instruments. As more and more procedures are completed, I am sure that proper instrumentation will evolve. If it is suspected that a significant amount of surgery may have to be done, then a 5 mm trocar site and 5 mm instrumentation are probably the most appropriate size to utilize in conjunction with the optical catheters.

Recently this technology has been used for more and more in-office procedures. The surgeon, of course, must be skilled in endoscopic surgery, and must also be able to call upon the skills of an adequately trained surgical assistant (former operating room nurse, nurse anaesthetist or physician's surgical assistant) and an anaesthesiologist and/or nurse anaesthetist, well versed in the application of intravenous sedation techniques. The gynaecologist who considers laparoscopy in an office setting should be familiar with the management of critical care situations, including cardiac arrest, and should have the necessary instrumentation and equipment for handling emergencies of this magnitude. Therefore the concept of in-office laparoscopy should not be taken lightly. Intravenous sedation techniques will be required for these types of procedures, and the proper monitoring equipment can be either rented or purchased. It is unusual for the gynaecologist to consider performing laparoscopy in the office, but after all we are already performing hysteroscopy in the office with excellent results.

My own experience with in-office laparoscopy currently consists of approximately 413 patients[5]. The level of awareness of potential complications associated with anaesthesia reactions, and/or inadvertent complications associated with laparoscopic procedures, even though diagnostic, certainly reaches a new height when they move from an outpatient surgical centre to your office. Obviously special liability requirements need to be addressed, and there must be emergency back-up systems for transporting patients to a hospital facility should a complication arise. Most of the procedures to date have been for pelvic pain, evaluation of follicular development or follicular harvesting techniques. Many reproductive centres are performing more of their GIFT/follicle aspiration techniques in an outpatient office setting. I feel that microlaparoscopy lends an additional sense of security that cannot be achieved with ultrasound.

Table 18.2 lists the procedures which I feel can be successfully achieved in an in-office setting with a very high margin of safety.

Diagnostic	Operative
Pelvic pain	
Chromotubation	Adhesiolysis
Unruptured ectopic (<6 weeks)	Tubal ligation
Fluorescence of endometriosis (investigational)	Follicle collection

Table 18.2: In-office microlaparoscopic procedures.

Complications associated with these procedures have been limited to vasovagal responses from anaesthesia ecchymosis of the mid-abdomen from countertraction during insertion of trocars, and moderately severe complaints of shoulder pain from diaphragmatic irritation of retained carbon dioxide gas. Proper patient selection is paramount for a successful outcome. It cannot be overemphasized that these in-office applications should be the last step for the gynaecologist after he has mastered these techniques in an operating room/outpatient surgical centre setting.

As this application becomes more popular around the world, and data are collected from colleagues already performing these procedures in consultant rooms or in their own in-office surgical suites, specific guidelines are likely to become established.

Microhysteroscopy

With the arrival of microlaparoscopic techniques in 1989, I was intrigued by the possibility that this optical catheter technology could be utilized for hysteroscopy. If the Adair cannula could be inserted into the umbilicus under intravenous sedation with minimal discomfort to the patients, then it would seem reasonable to assume that it could be inserted through the endocervical canal with minimal discomfort as well. This, in fact, turned out to be the situation as the Adair cannula's outside diameter is approximately 2 mm, which can be used in the same fashion as a larger 3, 4 or 5 mm standard hysteroscope. Used as a diagnostic tool, the advantages of the microhysteroscope are several. Since it is small, it can be passed through the endocervical canal and into the uterine cavity more easily than a conventional hysteroscope. Due to its smaller diameter, it is not necessary to dilate the cervix prior to insertion. This makes the use of the scope more acceptable to patients and less threatening (Figure 18.14).

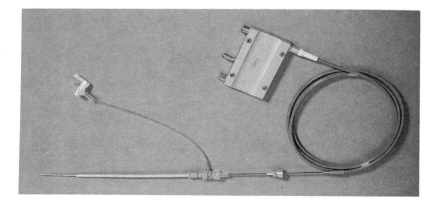

Figure 18.14: The Adair cannula is utilized for diagnostic hysteroscopy. Distension medium is fed via gravity through the side arm tubing (photo courtesy of Dr Grochmal).

As in-office hysteroscopy becomes a regular part of the gynaecologist's armamentarium, this microendoscopy system for hysteroscopy may replace the more commonly practised endometrial biopsies as a hysteroscopic directed biopsy could be performed as easily as a standard endometrial biopsy (blind procedure), leading to perhaps more accurate diagnosis and sampling of appropriate abnormal tissues. The same technology for microhysteroscopy is utilized as it is the same optical catheter that one would use for endoscopic intraperitoneal applications. Especially in the case of in-office hysteroscopy, where there is a limited amount of space, the small, long light-carrying bundle is certainly acceptable, and its ability to be cold-sterilized makes this an ideal instrument for in-office use. Because the metal cladded optical catheters are semi-rigid, they can be shaped in order to reach difficult areas within the confines of the uterine cavity (Figure 18.15).

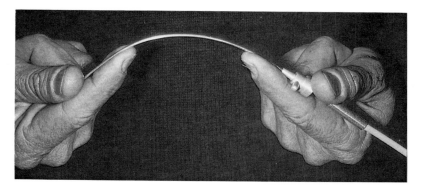

Figure 18.15: Metal cladded catheters are malleable (photo courtesy of Medical Dynamics).

Recently, new developments with steerable optical catheters as shown in Figure 18.7 have allowed the physician to steer his way into the uterine cavity and the tubal ostia. Operating channels within these steerable scopes allow biopsy forceps and other instruments to be passed freely so that small operative procedures can be performed. Again, as the technology improves, so will our ability to manipulate and utilize these miniature instruments within the confines of the uterine cavity. Since the uterine cavity is relatively small, visualization with these optical catheters is excellent, and provides an optimal field of view with adequate illumination on the video monitor. Considering its small outside diameter, optical catheters approach the excellence of visual resolution that can be achieved with the larger rod lens hysteroscope.

Uterine distension

The choices for uterine distension with optical catheters are limited to carbon dioxide and liquid media. The use of the optical catheter with a contact hysteroscopic technique has proven unsatisfactory. Although many hysteroscopists prefer a gas medium for distension of the uterine cavity, I have achieved the best results within a liquid medium. Saline is simply the cheapest and safest, and provides a more than adequately clear field of view. It is not necessary to use glycine or other electrolyte-poor solutions, as currently there are no electrical application instruments being developed for use in conjunction with optical catheters. The use of hyskon is futile as it is too viscous to be accommodated within the Adair cannula. In all the microhysteroscopies performed to date, we have not experienced any untoward effects from the use of saline as the distension medium.

Successful distension of the uterine cavity with saline can generally be achieved with a gravity flow system. This is accomplished by hanging the bag of saline above the level of the examining or operating table, perhaps on an intravenous pole. Large disposable tubing, such as that used for TURP procedures, affords a larger flow of fluid from the saline bag into the Adair cannula. For diagnostic hysteroscopy, the silastic portion of the Adair/Verres needle cannula system is utilized for the introducing sheath. The one-way membrane valve with side-arm tubing is attached to the proximal end of the Adair cannula. The side-arm tubing is then attached to the larger TURP tubing and is used to introduce the liquid distension medium. The one-way membrane valve also allows passage of the cladded optical catheter through the cannula and eliminates back flow of distension medium.

With experience and practice, this system will adequately serve the majority of needs for diagnostic hysteroscopy. There are, however, patients with larger uteri or intracavitary pathology (fibroids, polyps, septums) that require more pressure to achieve adequate distension. A simple solution to this problem can be the use of a hand-held pressurized syringe (Figure 18.16), which can be placed in between the tubing from the saline bag and the Adair cannula. By activating the pistol grip of the syringe, an increase in intrauterine pressure can be achieved. Unfortunately, these systems do not allow for an adequate measurement of intrauterine pressure.

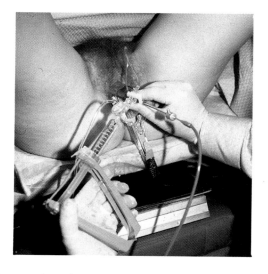

Figure 18.16: A Rochester type syringe is used to improve fluid distension and visualization during microhysteroscopy (photo courtesy of Dr Grochmal).

To control intrauterine pressure for uterine distension, a uterine pump is applied to the existing Adair cannula. The hysteroscopic pump can be used to distend the cavity to a safe intrauterine pressure of no greater than 80 mmHg, and to allow continuous inflow and outflow of the distension medium. This adequate distension of the uterine cavity is especially critical as overdistension of the uterine cavity can lead to a fluid overload syndrome. Although this is uncommon for a diagnostic in-office or outpatient hysteroscopic procedure, the potential for fluid overload is present during operative procedures. This same risk carries over into the microhysteroscopic applications as well. The constant distension irrigation system pump maintains safe intrauterine pressure and decreases the risk of fluid overload, particularly if the procedure is prolonged.

For operative procedures, however, it has been my experience that the pump improves the ability of the surgeon to work quickly within the uterine cavity. If a pressure pump is utilized for diagnostic hysteroscopy, it is necessary to use a T adaptor between the pump tubing and the side-arm tubing of the Adair cannula. This will allow for adequate flow of fluid to be passed through the Adair cannula while allowing monitoring of the intrauterine pressure. With the use of a multi-channel operating sheath, the T adaptor is placed on the inflow port of the operating sheath (Figure 18.17).

Figure 18.17: Rigid operating sheath with channels for optical catheter and biopsy forceps including two side channels for irrigation (photo courtesy of N.J. Laser Institute).

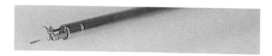

Smaller irrigating pressure pumps for uterine distension are currently being developed to address the needs of the optical catheter and small rigid hysteroscopic systems. These will eventually find their way into the in-office setting as more physicians utilize this technology for procedures other than diagnostic ones.

There are only two cannula systems which can be used as operating sheaths for invasive hysteroscopic procedures. As shown on Figure 18.14, this multi-port operative channel has an outside diameter of 4.9 mm and includes a 1.6 mm channel for the optical catheter and a 1 mm operating channel. This 1 mm operating channel can accommodate flexible biopsy forceps or scissors (Figure 18.18). Laser fibres up to 800 μm can also be passed through the operating channel. Currently there are no electric energy loops or scissors for these miniaturized systems. This operating sheath also has an inflow and outflow port through which the fluid can be channelled for uterine distension. As in the case of diagnostic hysteroscopy, adequate distension with this operating sheath can be achieved via a gravity or pressurized syringe system. As more aggressive operative procedures have been undertaken, I have found the need to distend the uterus more efficiently, and recommend the previously mentioned set-up for the CDIS pump.

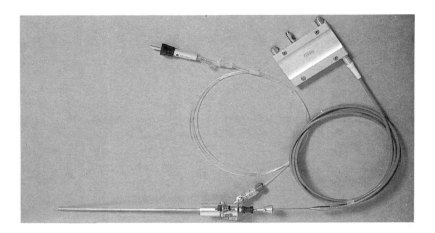

Figure 18.18: 4.7 mm OD operating sheath with Nd:YAG laser fibre inserted (photo courtesy of Sharplan Lasers).

Rigid and flexible systems

This operating sheath is a rigid system. As shown in figure 18.7, the CIS flexible and steerable catheter system may have more advantages over a rigid system. Easier acquisition of the cornual aspects of the uterus and the inner portions of the fallopian tubes can be achieved thanks to the steerable nature of the optical catheter. Proponents of rigid glass rod hysteroscopes are working to miniaturize the outside diameter of their systems without compromising visual acuity. A shown in Figure 18.19, this prototype has an outside diameter of 5 mm, yet it still gives the surgeon an excellent field of view as well as an operating channel.

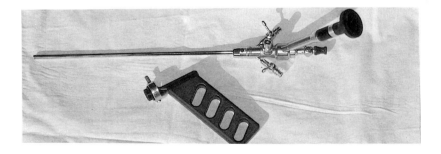

Figure 18.19: Offset rigid glass rod lens hysteroscope with OD of 5 mm. The handle is detachable. Includes operating port. (photo courtesy of Richard Wolf).

Anaesthesia

Requirements for anaesthesia are minimal. Due to the small size of the Adair cannula, a paracervical block is sufficient. For diagnostic hysteroscopy, infiltration of the cervix at 12 o'clock for placement of a tenaculum is all that is required. A complete cervical block can be used for more aggressive procedures, especially when a larger operating cannula is utilized. Here, infiltration at the 12, 3, 6 and 9 o'clock positions of the cervix appears to be satisfactory. A small 25 gauge needle causes minimal discomfort to the patient. Short-acting local anaesthetics can be utilized: however, some physicians prefer a longer-acting block with agents like bupivacaine.

Instrumentation

Adair cannulae are available as sterile disposable items, so there is a minimal amount of sterilization required for the optical catheter system. A list of the required equipment is shown in Table 18.3.

1.6 mm optical catheter
Adair cannula with side-arm tubing
Saline bag, 250 cc
TURP tubing
25 gauge needle with Tubex syringe
Needle extender (optional)
Single tooth tenaculum
Vaginal speculum
Receptacle to receive outflow distension fluid

Table 18.3: Equipment necessary for in-office hysteroscopy.

Diagnosis of abnormal bleeding
Management of cervical stenosis
Hysteroscopic directed endometrial biopsy
Excision of uterine polyps
Evaluation of endocervical canal in conjunction with colposcopy
Excision of small uterine septum
Transection of uterine septum
Endometrial laser ablation
Proximal tuboscopy
Hysteroscopically assisted laser tubal sterilization (HALTS) (investigational)

Table 18.4: Applications of microhysteroscopy.

Table 18.4 shows that any procedure that can be done with conventional hysteroscopy can also be performed successfully utilizing micro-optical catheter techniques. Diagnostic hysteroscopy, for instance, is a quick and simple procedure which causes minimal discomfort to the patient. In cases of cervical stenosis which have been diagnosed at the time of conventional hysteroscopy, I have found the optical catheter to be useful. In these situations, passage of the optical catheter into the partially dilated endocervical canal can often lead to a diagnosis of a cervical fibroid or false channel created at the time of the attempted cervical dilatation. This has helped to avoid unnecessary perforation or further development of a false channel.

A hysteroscopically assisted endometrial biopsy is often more satisfactory than blind endometrial biopsy as the physician can not only visualize the uterine cavity and its topography, but also take a more specific biopsy of any areas that appear to be suspicious[6]. This can be accomplished with an operating channel and small 1 mm biopsy forceps (*see* Figure 18.20). Due to the small basket at the tip of the forceps, multiple bites are necessary in order to obtain an adequate sample for analysis.

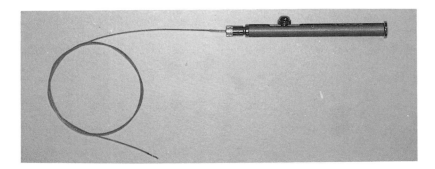

Figure 18.20: 1 mm flexible biopsy forceps (photo courtesy of N.J. Laser Institute).

Utilizing the same operating channel for endometrial biopsies, polyps and uterine synechiae can be incised and removed with the use of small scissors through the operating channel. In some instances, physicians have utilized a small Nd:YAG laser with fibre delivery system to incise, vaporize or cut polyps, adhesions, and even small leiomyoma. For these procedures, some preoperative sedation with an anti-prostaglandin medication and anaesthesia block of the cervix is needed to eliminate any patient discomfort. These procedures have been successfully carried out within an office setting under proper circumstances. The guidelines for in-office hysteroscopic surgery apply as for microlaparoscopy.

Endometrial laser ablation can be performed successfully in an outpatient surgical setting via microlaparoscopy; however, no distinct advantage is really noticed as these procedures are successfully carried out under intravenous sedation techniques with conventional-sized hysteroscopes/resectoscopes. Some patients who have undergone long-term follow-up studies in our institution have developed residual patches of endometrium many years after the endometrial ablation. In these patients, we have successfully ablated and vaporized the residual patches within the office setting.

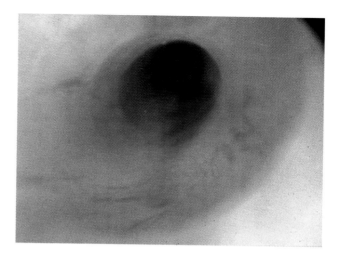

Figure 18.21: View of tubal ostium via 0.5 mm optical catheter (photo courtesy of Dr Grochmal).

Exploration of the proximal end of the fallopian tube (Figure 18.21) to rule out tubal isthmica nodosum can be achieved with the micro-system. In conjunction with the operating channel, Novy cannulae may be snaked through the proximal end of the fallopian tube, and a smaller optical catheter threaded through the interior portion of the Novy cannula (Figure 18.22).

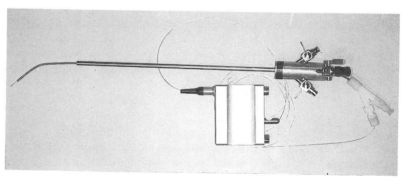

Figure 18.22: Optical catheter and Novy 5.5 French Catheter Guide in operating channel of rigid sheath (photo courtesy of Dr Grochmal).

Once this has ben achieved, injection of saline through the outer cannula will distend the tubal lumen, and a retrograde tuboscopy can be carried out via the smaller optical catheter within the Novy cannula (Figure 18.23). As catheter technology improves and steerable catheters can be manufactured at very small diameters, cannulization to the distal portion of the fallopian tube, allowing complete visualization of the entire tubal lumen surface will be possible.

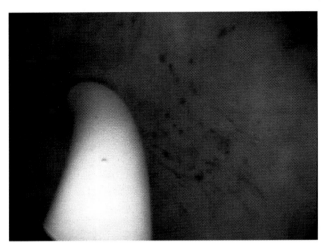

Figure 18.23: Novy Catheter as seen via 1.6 mm optical catheter in left tubal ostium (photo courtesy of N.J. Laser Institute).

The future

There are several techniques that may in the future benefit from the use of optical catheters. For instance, in the area of fertility, very small optical catheters are being used to scan the zona pellucida for areas of defect within the wall. In some reproductive centres, drilling of the zona is done under optical catheter surveillance. Traditional amniocentesis procedures may give way to the passage of small optical catheters down into the amniotic cavity to observe the fetus. This may lead to the use of catheters for the diagnosis of intrauterine anomalies that may not be clearly identified by ultrasound techniques. Perhaps this may also lead to a new area of expertise for maternal fetal specialists in intrauterine surgical procedures, and allow minimally invasive procedures to be performed on the fetus itself.

Preliminary studies show that a small laser fibre can be directed into the fallopian tube, via optical catheters, and an adequate sterilization effect can be achieved. Perhaps this procedure may eventually find itself into the physician's office, saving millions of health-care dollars around the world. The ease of this procedure will certainly be attractive to those third-world countries where population control has become an important issue. Our own preliminary work in London has demonstrated low failure rates after a three-year follow-up[7].

Miniaturization of the technology certainly gives the gynaecologist access to the pelvic cavities of young female children who would in other circumstances not be candidates for laparoscopy. Our urological colleagues have already shown that microlaparoscopy appears to be ideally suited for paediatric urology. Until recently, laparoscopy in paediatric urology was only diagnostic, yet now this technology provides a satisfactory field of view in children, and can be utilized for the evaluation of undescended non-palpable testes. With the use of additional puncture sites, even first stage of Stevens-Fowler orchiopexy may be undertaken. Determination of intersex is also an emerging application for this technology. Evaluation of a young child's abdomen to rule out acute appendicitis or internal haemorrhage may bring this technology into the minor surgery suites of emergency rooms.

Optical catheter technology may in the future be applied to another area which has remained a blind procedure in laparoscopy. The last remaining step that is still not done under direct visualization is the placement of the Verres needle. Within a short period of time, prototypes will become available which will combine the Verres needle and the optical catheter. With this combination, it will be possible to insert the Verres needle down through the layers of the abdominal wall and reach the preperitoneal space under direct visualization. Entrance into the peritoneal cavity may then be done under direct visualization, thus avoiding the need for the more cumbersome techniques using Hassan trocars or open minilaparotomies. Prototypes with various configurations of needle cannula systems are currently being utilized in neurosurgery, arthroscopy and in rheumatology for the study of carpal tunnel syndrome. This visual-Verres, as I have come to call it, will soon perhaps obviate the current system of Verres needle entry.

References

1 Grochmal SA and Curlik MR (1994) Microlaparoscopy in urologic surgery. In: Gomela L *et al.* (eds). *Laparoscopic Urologic Surgery*. Raven Press, New York. pp 91–95.

2 Grochmal SA (1993) Gynaecology. In: Rosin D (ed). *Minimal Access Medicine and Surgery*. Radcliffe Medical Press, Oxford. pp 165–6, 180–2.

3 Grochmal SA and Lomano J (1992) New microlaparoscopic technique reduces scars and recuperation time. *Clin. Laser.* 1:125–6.

4 Dorsey JH and Tabb CR (1991) Minilaparoscopy and fibreoptic lasers. *Obstetrics and Gynecology Clinics of North America*.

5 Grochmal SA *et al.* (1994) *In-office laparoscopy with optical catheters: Report of initial experience in 413 patients*. Abstract for American Association of Gynecologic Laparoscopists Meeting, New York.

6 Grochmal SA (1993) *Five year follow up of patients undergoing endometrial laser ablation: Report of 237 cases*. Abstract from American Association of Gynecologic Laparoscopists Clinical Meeting, San Francisco.

7 Weekes A *et al.* (1994) *Abstract in Proceedings of Operative Gynecology/ Endoscopy*. Symposium of New Advances in Gynecologic Endoscopy. University of Teikyo, Teikyo.

Part IV: Hysteroscopic Procedures

Uterine Distension Methods and Fluid Management in Operative Hysteroscopy

Hysteroscopy, Laparoscopy and In Vitro Fertilization

Operative Hysteroscopy with Electricity

Laser Endometrial Ablation

Endometrial Ablation with SideFire Laser Fibre

Hysteroscopic Surgery for Menorrhagia: Long-Term Outlook and Anxieties

Complications of Operative Hysteroscopy

19

Uterine Distension Methods and Fluid Management in Operative Hysteroscopy

RAY GARRY

It is essential for safe hysteroscopic surgery to maintain continuous crystal clear vision throughout the operative procedure. The uterine cavity is only a potential space, however, and the anterior and posterior walls of the uterus normally lie approximated. Without distension, nothing of the structure of the cavity can be seen with even the most sophisticated of endoscopic systems. Distension of the cavity is therefore an important prerequisite for safe and effective hysteroscopic surgery. Fortunately the cavity is accessible and readily distensible. This chapter discusses the various techniques which have been developed to distend the uterine cavity and the problems produced by such techniques.

The uterine cavity is surrounded by a layer of muscle 20 mm thick. A significant force is required to overcome the tone of this muscle, and to achieve adequate distension of the cavity, the medium must be infused under significant pressure. Adequate distension of the uterine cavity usually requires an intrauterine pressure (IUP) of more than 40 mmHg. Satisfactory distension can be produced with either gaseous or fluid media.

Distension media

Carbon dioxide

For diagnostic hysteroscopy, particularly in the outpatient or office environment, gaseous distension media are usually preferred. The use of the carbon dioxide was first described by Rubin in 1925 and it is now the most frequently used gas[1]. It is preferred because of its availability and convenience and is the least messy of the available agents. CO_2 infused under pressure tends to flatten the endometrium and to give excellent visibility. It has virtually the same index of refraction as air and excellent photographs can be obtained with this medium.

A continuous flow is necessary to replace gas lost through the tubes, around the hysteroscope and absorbed into the uterus. The rate of flow must be carefully controlled, because deaths have occurred from gas embolism. Intravasation can occur and bubbles of gas have been detected moving in the pelvic vessels during simultaneous hysteroscopy and laparoscopy[2]. The risk of gas embolism is proportional to the flow rate of the infused gas. Lindemann et al.[3] demonstrated in a series of experiments in dogs that flow rates below 200 ml min^{-1} were associated with minimal changes in pulse rate and breathing. Flow rates above 400 ml min^{-1} were associated with tachypnoea and arrhythmias and rates of 1000 ml min^{-1} were associated with death within 60 seconds. Physiological mechanism can cope with the transport of 150 ml of CO_2 per minute without risk of embolism or metabolic disturbances. Hulf et al.[4] showed no changes in electrocardiograms, PCO_2 or pH during CO_2 hysteroscopy with controlled rates of CO_2 flow. It is essential to use an infusion apparatus specifically designed for hysteroscopy. The maximum flow rate must be fixed at not more than 100 ml min^{-1} and a flow rate of 40 ml min^{-1} is usually adequate. Equipment designed for laparoscopy permits flow rates of 3000–9000 ml min^{-1} and must never be used for hysteroscopy.

Complications and safeguards

The principal disadvantage of CO_2 as a distension medium is the tendency for troublesome gas bubbles to form. These are particularly likely to occur when the gas mixes with blood and can obscure vision. These bubbles can usually be avoided with good technique. Blood and mucus should be carefully cleansed from the cervical os with a dry swab and detergent skin cleansing agents should be avoided. The hysteroscope should be advanced slowly under direct vision after creating a series of microcavities just ahead of the tip of the hysteroscope. The instrument can, in this manner, be kept in the centre of the canal and introduced into the uterine cavity without damaging the cervical mucosa which is the usual source of bleeding.

Most physicians use CO_2 hysteroscopy only for diagnostic purposes, because bleeding and smoke can seriously impair vision during surgical manipulations. Gallinat et al.[5], however, also uses CO_2 during Nd:YAG laser ablation of the endometrium. He believes this is safer than fluid distension of the uterus because CO_2 avoids the potentially serious risk of fluid overload and he has designed a closed-circuit system to filter out smoke and plume produced during the ablation.

High-viscosity fluids

Dextran 70 (Hyskon) has a molecular weight of 70 000 and is a mixture of 32% dextran in 10% dextrose. It is a thick viscous fluid which is electrolyte free, non-conductive, and biodegradable. It was first used as a distension agent for diagnostic hysteroscopy because it is optically clear and immiscible with blood[6]. It is also an ideal medium for operative hysteroscopic surgery because of its optical clarity, immiscibility with blood and because its consistency reduces the risk of extravasation into the uterine circulation[7]. A pool of static dextran will remain optically clear for longer than a similar pool of a low molecular weight fluid and in such circumstances may be the preferred agent.

However, dextran 70 is a difficult medium to work with. Its high viscosity makes continuous infusion difficult, and a laborious and labour-intensive system of intermittent instillation and extraction with large syringes is required. Some force is necessary for this instillation and unless specially modified tubing is used, accidental disconnection of the tubing with consequent spraying of the sticky material is quite common. When dextran 70 dries it sets solid. If the equipment is not immediately and thoroughly washed in hot water, switches and taps will jam and expensive equipment can be ruined. When used with instruments producing high local temperatures, dextran 70 can caramelize and the dark brown colour may impair vision as seen with laser endometrial ablation.

Dextran 70 is hydrophilic, and when infused into the circulation its high molecular weight pulls with it at least six times its own volume of fluid. Fluid overload and pulmonary oedema may occur. Cases of non-cardiogenic pulmonary oedema have also been described following the use of dextran 70 during hysteroscopy[8,9]. It is suggested that in such cases the dextran 70 may have a direct toxic effect on the pulmonary capillaries, resulting in extravasation and interstitial pulmonary oedema. Jedeikin et al.[10] described a case of disseminated intravascular coagulopathy and adult respiratory distress syndrome complicating dextran 70 hysteroscopy. Rare but potentially fatal anaphylactic reactions to dextran 70 have also been described[11]; the incidence of such life-threatening complications is between 0.069 and 0.008%.

Low-viscosity fluids

A uterine cavity distended with a stagnant pool of low-viscosity fluid will initially be clear but will soon become cloudy because of the accumulation of small particles of endometrial debris which are dislodged during hysteroscopic manipulation. As such fluids are also readily miscible with blood any oozing will further cloud the fluid and impair vision. If the fluid is repeatedly replaced and a continuous flow of the fluid under pressure is established, bleeding will be prevented by a 'tamponade' effect and the endometrial debris will be flushed out, thereby maintaining continuous clear vision. Under these circumstances clear fluids are the simplest, most convenient and cheapest media for hysteroscopy.

Dextrose

In their early cases of Nd:YAG laser ablation of the endometrium, Goldrath and colleagues[12] used 5% dextrose in water as the uterine distension medium but in several cases they observed dilutional hyponatraemia as an additional feature complicating fluid overload. As this substance has no clinical advantages over 0.9% sodium chloride solution, and has the significant additional risk of dilutional electrolyte disturbance, its use can no longer be recommended.

Glycine

When electrical energy is used inside the uterine cavity it is essential to use a distension fluid which is electrolyte free. 1.5% glycine has been widely used for this purpose by urologists during transurethral resection of the prostate. It is optically clear and non-haemolytic and does not conduct electricity. Excessive absorption of such an electrolyte-free solution can be associated with hyponatraemia and haemolysis. Magos et al. reported the systemic effects of the absorption of up to 4350 ml of glycine[13]. A fall in serum sodium to 107 mmol l^{-1} (normal 140 mmol l^{-1}) was noted in one case and this was associated with a significant rise in lactate dehydrogenase which is a marker of red cell breakdown. Glycine is metabolized in the liver and its breakdown can also be associated with an increase in ammonia radicals producing confusion, coma and death. Several deaths have occurred in Europe following intravasation of 1.5% glycine.

Sorbitol

Sorbitol is a non-conducting 3% sugar solution. It is optically clear and is being used as an alternative to glycine. It is hyperosmolar (165–180 mosmol) and excessive absorption can produce disturbances in blood glucose levels and diabetic features as well as overload and electrolyte disturbances.

0.9% Sodium chloride

Normal saline is optically clear and readily available. The concentration of electrolytes in this fluid approximate to that in blood and it is metabolically inert. Excess intravasation is not associated with major electrolyte or metabolic disturbances and any fluid overload can rapidly be reversed with diuretic therapy alone. Ringer's solution is even more physiological with additional potassium radicals added but is less freely available, and in practice offers only theoretical advantages over normal saline.

Summary of distension media

CO_2 is the most convenient and least messy of the distension media to use. It is useful for diagnostic procedures and is particularly suitable for outpatient and office investigations. Operative manipulations provoking bleeding and the production of smoke and bubbles during ablation impair vision and make CO_2 less suitable for operative hysteroscopy. Dextran 70 is difficult to work with and is associated with rare but serious complications. Sorbitol and glycine can both produce severe electrolyte and metabolic disturbances when absorbed in excess and are not recommended for routine use except when more physiological fluids are contraindicated. In practice this means that such fluids should only be used when electrical energy is being used inside the cavity during electroresection or rollerball ablation. In all other circumstances, 0.9% sodium chloride infused in a continuous manner is the distension fluid of choice.

Infusion systems

Hysteroscopes

When Goldrath and colleagues first attempted Nd:YAG laser ablation, they used a hysteroscope with an operating channel and a single channel which he used for infusion of the distending fluid. There was no outflow channel available and fluid could only escape around the barrel of the hysteroscope. To ensure that this occurred, it was necessary to dilate the cervix widely. Many difficulties encountered during hysteroscopic surgery are caused by using inadequate or inappropriately designed equipment. It is now clear that good operating conditions require the medium inside the cavity to be replaced at very frequent intervals and this can best be produced with a closed-circuit, continuous-flow system.

The uterine resectoscope is very closely modelled on the resectoscope used to perform transurethral resection of the prostate. Urologists have had many years in which to develop such a continuous-flow system. Many resectoscopes have a continuous-flow facility usually in the form of an outer sheath which surrounds the hysteroscope. With this arrangement, fluid is infused into the cavity down the central barrel of the hysteroscope and leaves via the outer sheath. It is essential that the inflow and outflow channels are completely separate, communicating only at the distal end of the hysteroscope barrel.

Endometrial ablation using the Nd:YAG laser was first described in 1981[12]. The early hysteroscopes used for this operation were slightly modified cystoscopes and were not specifically designed for the purpose. Many of the models still on the market are not suitable for laser hysteroscopy. Most operating hysteroscopes have at least two taps at the proximal end but in many instances these taps communicate in the common barrel. In these circumstances irrigation of the cavity is impaired. Hysteroscopes with completely separate fluid inflow and outflow channels are to be preferred. Such a hysteroscope has been designed by Baggish[7] and offers improved fluid circulation with consequent improved visibility (Figure 19.1). When a satisfactory continuous circuit is established inside the hysteroscope it is no longer necessary to dilate the cervix excessively, and indeed it is better to restrict dilatation to that which will ensure a watertight fit between the canal and the hysteroscope. Such a fit is facilitated if the outer barrel of the hysteroscope is round in cross-section. There seems little reason to continue to make hysteroscopes with an oval cross-section designed more to match the shape of the male urethra than the circular shape of both the cervical canal and the uterine dilators.

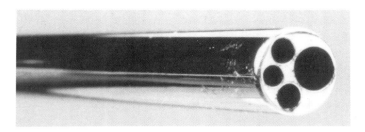

Figure 19.1: Weck–Baggish hysteroscope with an optic and three separate operating channels.

Fluid instillation

The potential cavity inside the uterus requires the application of pressure to separate the walls. The minimum pressure required to produce a satisfactory degree of distension is usually about 40–50 mmHg but can vary considerably. This can be achieved in various different ways.

1. *Syringes*. One or two large-capacity syringes can be used to maintain uterine distension. Such a system is labour-intensive and relatively uncontrolled, as neither the flow rate nor the pressure inside the cavity is known.

2. *Hydrostatic pressure*. A bag of infusion fluid suspended 60 cm above the uterus will enter the cavity with a pressure of about 45 mmHg. Varying the height of the bag over the patient will clearly alter this infusion pressure. This is a simple and inexpensive system for controlling the inflow pressure.

3. *Pressure cuff*. A suitably designed pressure cuff can be placed around the soft-walled infusion bag and the cuff inflated to a suitable level. Infusion rates can be varied by altering the pressure in the cuff.

4. *Simple pump*. The tubing from the infusion bag can be led through a simple roller pump. The rate of infusion can be altered by varying the speed of rotation of the pump. A constant flow of fluid for a given pump rate will be produced regardless of the outflow resistance.

5. *Pressure-controlled pump*. Various methods of limiting the pressure that a pump can produce have been devised. A compact regulating-compression apparatus which is favoured by Magos and others[13], and Hamou (Hamou Hysteromat, K. Storz, Tuttlingen, Germany) have developed a pressure-limited rotary pump which in a modified form is much favoured by the author (Figure 19.2).

It was soon appreciated that an inherent problem of infusing fluid into the uterine cavity under pressure was that a proportion of that fluid could be absorbed from the cavity into the systemic circulation. Goldrath *et al.*[12] reported several cases of pulmonary oedema and almost every subsequent worker has described similar complications. In a recent series of 859 cases of

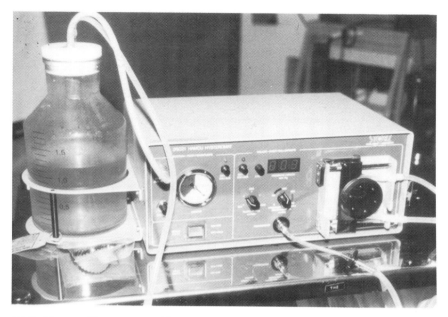

Figure 19.2: Hamou Hysteromat with a rotary pump connected to an integral pressure transducer.

endometrial laser ablation, there was a mean fluid deficit of 1350 ml[14]. In an earlier series Davis (1989) described a case in whom more than 12 l of fluid entered the circulation[15].

Minimizing fluid absorption

Various approaches to minimizing such fluid absorption have been proposed (Table 19.1). Goldrath *et al.*, because they only had available a hysteroscope with a single channel for fluid flow, found it necessary to recommend hyperdilatation of the cervix to allow fluid to escape from the cavity. This did provide the simplest form of safety valve to minimize the risk of excess IUP. Others have suggested that 'blanching' the surface of the endometrium rather than 'dragging' the laser fibre across and into the endometrium might minimize damage to the uterine vessels and hence reduce fluid absorption[16,17]. Baggish and Baltoyannis[18] (1988) advocated the use of the highly viscous dextran 70 which appeared to enter the circulation less easily. My colleagues and I believe that the use of a Hamou Hysteromat pressure-controlled pump can be associated with a marked reduction in fluid absorption[14].

Variable and constant rates of flow

Of the various systems for infusing fluid into the uterus, some deliver fluid at a constant rate of flow irrespective of the resistance inside the uterus. Syringes and simple roller pumps are examples of such a constant-flow, variable pressure system. Other systems provide a fixed head of pressure which results in a variable flow rate into the uterus depending on the resistance in the infusion circuit. Gravity feed and pressure-limited pumps are

Year	Authors	Cervical dilatation	Infusion	Outflow	Medium	Laser method
1981	Goldrath et al.[12]	Wide	Syringe	Free	Saline	Dragging
1987	Loffer[16]	Minimal	BP cuff	Free	Saline	Blanching
1988	Baggish & Baltoyannis[19]	Minimal	Syringe	Syringe	Hyskon	Dragging
1988	Lomano[17]	Wide	?	Free	Saline	Blanching
1989	Davis[15]	Wide	Pump	Free	Saline	Dragging
		Minimal	Gravity	Pump	Saline	Dragging
1989	Grochmal[16*]	Minimal	BP cuff	Suction	Saline	Dragging
1991	Garry et al.[14]	Minimal	Hamou pump	Free	Saline	Dragging

Table 19.1: Suggested methods for reducing fluid absorption during endometrial laser ablation.
* Personal communication

examples of this constant pressure-variable flow-rate system.

In general, the main advantage of a continuous-flow system is that excellent vision will be continuously maintained. Provided that the outflow channel remains patent such a system ensures that there will always be adequate flow to wash out debris and adequate pressure to maintain a tamponade effect and prevent bleeding into the cavity. The disadvantage of such a system is that the flow continues irrespective of outflow resistance and in some circumstances the intrauterine pressure levels can rise in an uncontrolled way and may become unacceptably high. This may result in excessive absorption of the distending medium into the systemic circulation.

The advantage of a continuously limited fixed pressure system is that fluid absorption will be minimized. The disadvantage of this system is that as the preset pressure level is approached the rate of flow gradually slows and the flow stops completely when the limit is reached. This slow or stagnant fluid pool rapidly clouds, and vision is soon impaired.

The ideal fluid distension system should be an amalgamation of both these systems. The pressure should be limited to prevent excess fluid absorption but set at a level just below the threshold at which absorption occurs. By maintaining the pressure at this highest possible level, the resultant flow of fluid should be maintained at a rate sufficient to flush out debris and maintain optimum visual conditions.

Factors influencing fluid absorption

The first 105 patients on whom we performed endometrial laser ablation in South Cleveland Hospital had uterine distension produced with a simple continuous-flow pump. The mean fluid absorption measured in this group was 1386 ml. In the next 92 cases the pump was replaced by a Hamou

Hysteromat with a preset maximum pressure level. Using such a continuous pressure system the mean absorption fell to 209 ml, a reduction of 85% in mean volume absorbed. We had demonstrated that control of the intrauterine pressure profoundly influenced the amount of fluid absorbed.

To investigate the factors influencing fluid absorption in more detail, we developed a system to measure intrauterine pressure directly. The pressure was measured by inserting a semi-rigid catheter down one channel of a Weck–Baggish hysteroscope (Linvatec, North Carolina, USA). This hysteroscope has two operating channels angled only slightly from the midline and with a three-way tap. One of these channels can accommodate both the path for fluid infusion and the fluid-filled catheter (Figure 19.3). The fluid in the recording catheter is maintained at a pressure of 300 mmHg so there is no flow into this catheter. The end of the catheter was connected to a pressure transducer and a pressure-monitoring system. Using this system we can observe the effects of varying intrauterine pressure on volume of fluid absorbed. We can also take X-ray hysterograms at specific intrauterine pressures and demonstrate visually the effect of such pressure changes.

Continuous-flow vs pressure-controlled pumps

In a prospective randomized trial, we used two different types of pumps. In

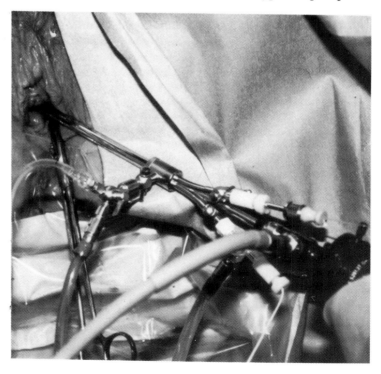

Figure 19.3: Weck–Baggish hysteroscope with a laser fibre in the left operating channel, a three-way tap for fluid inflow and a pressure-recording catheter in the right channel, and a three-way tap for reverse flushing on the outflow channel.

one group, in whom the fluid was infused with a simple continuous-flow pump, the mean volume of fluid absorbed was 1225 ml; while in the group in whom the IUP was directly measured and carefully controlled, the mean fluid volume absorbed was zero. The intrauterine pressure rose to a mean maximum value of 136 mmHg in the simple pump group and 70 mmHg in the pressure-controlled group[19]. We noted that fluid absorption appeared to occur in an 'all or nothing' manner, ie if the intrauterine pressure remained below a critical level no fluid absorption occurred, and if the pressure rose above that critical value, absorption occurred which seemed unrelated to any further increases in pressure. This critical level appeared to be related to the mean arterial blood pressure (MAP). This conclusion, based on our pressure studies, was confirmed by our hysterosalpingogram observations. X-rays taken at any pressure level below the MAP at the completion of an ablation showed the radio-opaque dye confined to the uterine cavity (Figure 19.4). X-rays taken at any level above the MAP showed dye freely entering the uterine capillaries and venous system, producing remarkably symmetrical venograms of the pelvic system (Figure 19.5).

We demonstrated that even small changes in uterine pressure would affect the passage of the radio-opaque dye. Pressures 5 mmHg below the MAP resulted in the dye staying in the cavity and values 5 mmHg above MAP resulted in the dye entering the venous system. The MAP under anaesthesia is usually around 75–85 mmHg and fluid absorption does not usually occur with IUP of that level. However, we demonstrated that in a patient with abnormally low MAP of 52 mmHg an IUP of 70 mmHg provoked a fluid deficit of 850 ml; conversely, in two hypertensive patients with MAP respectively of 130 and 135 mmHg, IUP levels of 120 mmHg were associated with no fluid absorption. We conclude that the MAP reflects the intrinsic resistance of the superficial layers of a given uterus to fluid intravasation.

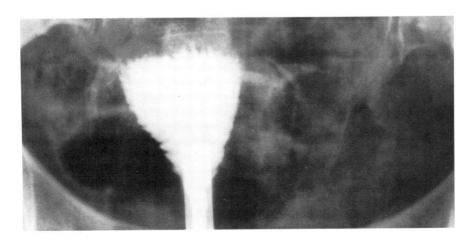

Figure 19.4: X-ray of the uterine cavity at the end of endometrial laser ablation with the uterine pressure set at 80 mmHg. Note the multiple irregularities caused by the laser furrows; at this pressure all the dye is retained inside the uterine cavity.

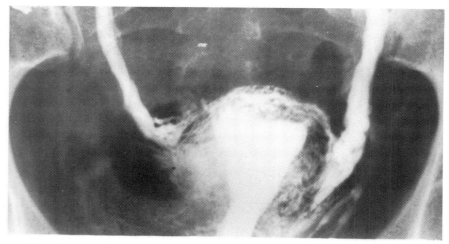

Figure 19.5: X-ray of the uterine cavity at the end of endometrial ablation with the uterine pressure set at 160 mmHg. Note that much of the radio-opaque material has left the cavity and is outlining the pelvic venous system, a typical finding in a 'high-pressure' absorption.

Maintaining IUP below that level is usually associated with zero fluid absorption.

Continuous-pressure monitoring

Once appropriate inflow and outflow rates are established, the IUP usually remains at a steady level. Like the MAP levels, it should be recorded at five minute intervals, and in the normal situation it should remain below the MAP. Continuous-pressure monitoring does, however, on some occasions demonstrate a sudden, unexpected and at times marked elevation in the IUP levels. The almost invariable explanation for such rises in pressure was complete or partial obstruction of the outflow channel by particles of endometrial debris (Figure 19.6). Such obstructions produce a reduction in outflow with a subsequent build-up of IUP. If recognized the obstruction can easily be freed by flushing with a syringe attached to the outflow channel. Such reverse flushing rapidly restores the uterine pressure to normal levels. We believe that, in an otherwise steady state, obstruction to the outflow channel is the principal cause of unexpected 'high-pressure' fluid absorption.

We feel that careful control of IUP prevents most but not all cases of excess fluid absorption. Using this system of direct pressure measurement and control in 23 consecutive cases of endometrial laser ablation we obtained zero fluid absorption in 21 cases. In one case, with an unusually large cavity containing a pedunculated fibroid, it was necessary to keep the IUP deliberately above the MAP to ensure adequate visualization, and in this case 1000 ml fluid deficit was noted. In the final case in this small series the procedure appeared to be technically uncomplicated; the IUP remained below the MAP and indeed fell as the procedure progressed. In spite of this, a fluid deficit of 1200 ml˙ was observed. An X-ray hysterogram taken at the

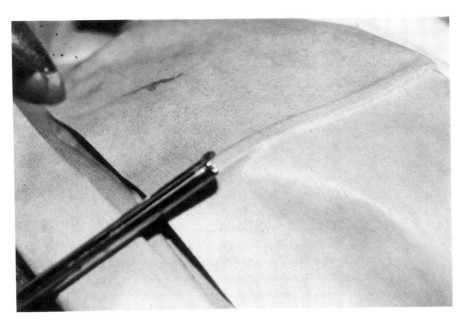

Figure 19.6: Particle of debris obstructing the outflow channel during an endometrial laser ablation.

completion of this procedure gave a clue to the cause of this 'low-pressure' absorption. The X-ray was taken at a pressure below the MAP but dye entered the uterine veins. The hysterogram was not, however, the typical symmetrical pattern and demonstrated only one side of the vascular tree (Figure 19.7). We have found that such asymmetrical venograms are consistently associated with cases of 'low pressure' absorption and they seem to demonstrate a direct communication between the uterine cavity and a major uterine vessel.

Laser biopsies

This uncommon 'low-pressure' absorption occurred unpredictably and was difficult to study until we started to take endometrial laser biopsies. During the development of this technique to take full-thickness endometrial biopsies with the YAG laser prior to endometrial laser ablation, we noticed that every time we took such a biopsy we observed the same type of 'low-pressure' absorption. This occurred even when pressure control and fluid management were otherwise satisfactory. X-ray hysterograms demonstrated that these biopsies penetrate deeply into the myometrium and can often be shown to enter major intrauterine vessels directly. As the pressure in the uterine veins is no more than 10–15 mmHg and the pressure in the cavity is in excess of 45 mmHg, fluid will inevitably be forced into the circulation from the cavity. We therefore suggest that this 'low-pressure' absorption is produced during endometrial ablation when the laser fibre or the resectoscope is taken too deeply into the myometrium, thereby producing a fistula between the large myometrial veins and the uterine cavity. It does not occur when tissue

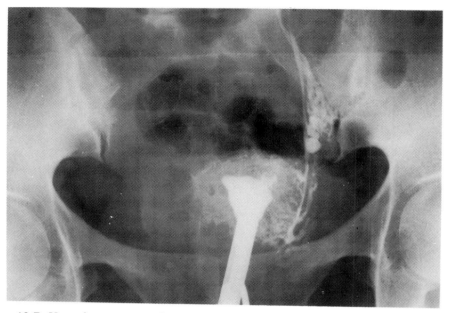

Figure 19.7: X-ray hysterogram of a patient with 'low-pressure' absorption showing an asymmetrical venogram demonstrated at an IUP of 75 mmHg.

destruction is confined to the superficial layers of the uterine wall. A good technique — removing sufficient but not too much tissue — will minimize the risk of this type of fluid absorption.

Summary

In summary, we believe that four main factors determine the amount of fluid absorbed from the uterine cavity during hysteroscopic surgery:

- the level of the intrauterine pressure
- the level of the mean arterial blood pressure
- the patency of the outflow channel of the hysterscope
- the depth of penetration of the uterine instruments.

The superficial layers of the uterine cavity seem to prevent ingress of fluid into the systemic circulation until the pressure in the uterine cavity exceeds a value equal to the MAP. When damage to the uterus is confined to the superficial layers, absorption is dependent on a simple pressure equation. If the MAP exceeds the IUP no absorption will occur. To ensure that this happens in practice, it is necessary to ensure that the level of the IUP is always lower than the MAP by limiting the infusion pressure. To avoid any resultant slowing and ultimate stagnation and consequent clouding of the fluid pool, it is necessary to ensure that the outflow channel remains patent at all times. To prevent direct entry into the major intramyometrial veins it is necessary to use correct techniques to restrict the depth of penetration of the laser fibre or the resectoscope. With good control of the factors mentioned above, other factors such as the size of the cavity, duration of the procedure, or state of the endometrium (ie thickness) do not seem to be important.

For optimal hysteroscopic surgery, it is important to use an operating hysteroscope with separate channels for fluid inflow and outflow and to establish a closed continuous-flow circuit with a watertight seal between the cervix and the hysteroscope. The intrauterine pressure should be measured and carefully controlled, complete patency of the outflow channel should be maintained, and a high fluid flow rate established. The laser fibre or the resectoscope wire should remove all the endometrium but should not penetrate too deeply into the myometrium. If these principles are followed, it is demonstrably possible to perform operative hysteroscopic surgery with continuous crystal-clear vision and minimal fluid absorption.

References

1   Rubin IC (1925) Uterine endoscopy, endometroscopy with the aid of uterine insufflation. *American Journal of Obstetrics and Gynecology*. **10**:313–15.

2   Donnez J (1989) Instrumentation. In: Donnez J (ed). *Laser operative laparoscopy and hysteroscopy*. Leuven: Nauwelaerts. pp.207–21.

3   Lindemann HJ *et al.* (1976) Der Einluss von CO_2-gas während der Hysteroscopie. *Geburtshilfe und Frauenheilkunde*. **36**:153–6.

4   Hulf JA *et al.* (1979) Blood carbon dioxide changes during hysteroscopy. *Fertility and Sterility*. **32**r:193–6.

5   Gallinat A *et al.* (1989) *The use of the Nd:YAG laser in gynecological endoscopy. Laser brief 14*. MBB-Medizintechnik, Munich.

6   Edström K and Fernström I (1970) The diagnostic possibilities of a modified hysteroscopic technique. *Acta Obstetrica et Gynecologica Scandinavica*. **49**:327–9.

7   Baggish MS (1989) Distending media for panoramic hysteroscopy. In: Baggish MS *et al.*, (eds). *Diagnostic and operative hysteroscopy*. Year Book Medical Publishers, Chicago. pp.89–101.

8   Zbella EA *et al.* (1985) Noncardiogenic pulmonary edema secondary to intra-uterine instillation of 32% dextran 70. *Fertility and Sterility*. **43**:479–80.

9   Leake JF *et al.* (1987) Noncardiogenic pulmonary edema: a complication of operative hysteroscopy. *Fertility and Sterility*. **48**:497–9.

10 Jedeikin R *et al.* (1990) Disseminated intravascular coagulopathy and adult respiratory distress syndrome: life threatening complications. *American Journal of Obstetrics and Gynecology*. **162**:44–5.

11 Borten M *et al.* (1983) Recurrent anaphylactic reaction to intraperitoneal dextran-75 for the prevention of postsurgical adhesions. *Obstetrics and Gynecology.* **61**:755–7.

12 Goldrath MH *et al.* (1981) Laser photovaporization of the endometrium for the treatment of menorrhagia. *American Journal of Obstetrics and Gynecology.* **140**:14–19.

13 Magos AL *et al.* (1991) Experience with the first 250 endometrial resections for menorrhagia. *Lancet.* **337**:1074–8.

14 Garry R *et al.* (1991) A multicentre collaborative study into the treatment of menorrhagia by Nd-YAG laser ablation of the endometrium. *British Journal of Obstetrics and Gynaecology.* **98**:357–62.

15 Davis JA (1989) Hysteroscopic endometrial ablation with the neodymium-YAG laser. *British Journal of Obstetrics and Gynaecology.* **96**:928–32.

16 Loffer FD (1987) Hysteroscopic endometrial ablation with Nd:YAG laser using a non-contact technique. *Obstetrics and Gynecology.* **69**:679–89.

17 Lomano JM (1988) Photocoagulation of the endometrium with the Nd:YAG laser for the treatment of menorrhagia. *Journal of Reproductive Medicine.* **31**:148–50.

18 Baggish MS and Baltoyannis P (1988) New techniques for laser ablation of the endometrium in high risk patients. *American Journal of Obstetrics and Gynecology.* **159**:287–92.

19 Hasham F *et al.* (1992) Fluid absorption during laser ablation of the endometrium in the treatment of menorrhagia. *British Journal of Anaesthesia.* **68**:151–4.

20

Hysteroscopy, Laparoscopy and In Vitro Fertilization
VITO CARDONE

Diagnostic and operative hysteroscopy

Introduction

Centres specializing in assisted reproductive technologies around the world are obtaining eggs and embryos of improved quality due to the appropriate management of ovarian stimulation and egg retrieval as well as improvements in sperm preparation and culture techniques. However, the implantation rate per embryo remains consistently low (average 10%).

Many centres are looking at a variety of techniques that may improve the quality of the embryo, thus increasing the chance of implantation. These techniques include blastocyst replacement and hatching. However, all agree that it is of the utmost importance to achieve perfect uterine and endometrial integrity before transferring embryos to the reproductive system.

Anomalies such as subacute or chronic endometritis, intra-uterine adhesions (Asherman syndrome), polyps, fibroids, and septa have all been implicated as possible causes of infertility and spontaneous abortions, theoretically causing a reduction in the implantation rate.

Diagnosis

Hysterosalpingograms are effective in diagnosing a number of uterine abnormalities but unfortunately there are high false-positive and false-negative rates (30.6 and 37.5 per cent respectively) compared with hysteroscopy[1]. Therefore a hysteroscopic approach is the most appropriate way of investigating the uterine cavity. Most series have contained cases of atrophy, endometritis, polyp, hyperplasia, submucous fibroid and adhesions, which were frequently not diagnosed by hysterosalpingogram, while all cases of septa, bicornuate, unilateral horn and deformed small uterine cavity were diagnosed.

As shown in Table 20.1, anywhere between 10 and 36% of all hysteroscopies done prior to in vitro fertilization (IVF) will have a definite uterine or endometrial anomaly which may interfere with the success of the procedure. As Frydman and colleagues have shown, at least 10% of hysteroscopies are abnormal[1], even in cases of completely normal gynaecological history and examination or a normal hysterosalpingogram.

	Number of patients	Uterine cavity or endometrial abnormalities	%
Frydman et al.[1]			
Group I: abnormal history and physical or hysterosalpingogram	102	37	36
Group II: normal hysterosalpingogram or gyn history and exam	78	8	10
Dicker et al.[2]	284	54	19
Goldenberg et al.[3]	224	32	14
Seinera et al.[4]	332	77	23

Table 20.1: Percentage of uterine or endometrial lining abnormalities found at hysteroscopy.

Anomalies

Most of these findings are surgically or medically correctable. The anomalies most frequently found are adhesions, submucosal fibroids and polyps (Table 20.2). These, as well as uterine septa, can usually be treated easily by operative hysteroscopy. Laser, resectoscope, microscissors and various forms of coagulator can be used to break down adhesions and excise a polyp, myoma or a septum. Endometritis can usually be corrected by a long course of antibiotic therapy. We most often use a broad-spectrum antibiotic such as doxycycline for at least one month. Atrophy or hypoplasia of the endometrium can be treated with high oestrogen supplementation such as Estradiol 2 mg twice daily or Premarin 2.5 mg once daily, day 1–25 of the cycle. However, the indication of hysteroscopy (diagnostic or operative) to be performed prior to entering an IVF cycle is still controversial. More and more centres are incorporating hysteroscopy at different levels in their diagnostic and therapeutic modality.

Type of abnormalities	Frydman et al.[1]	Dicker et al.[2]	Goldenberg et al.[3]	Seinera et al.[4]
Patients (N)	180	284	224	332
Submucosal myoma	3	12	1	6
Adenomyosis	3	2	–	3
Polyp	5	12	10	20
Endometritis	4	–	7	–
Adhesions	8	15	9	10

Malformation
    Uterine septa
    Bicornuate
    Unilateral
    Deformed sm cavity
	10	6	5	19

Atrophy (hypoplasia)	4	–	–	11
Hyperplasia	–	7	–	8

Table 20.2: Frequency and type of anomalies found at hysteroscopy.

Procedures prior to IVF

At our centre, a hysterosalpingogram is mandatory before IVF. If there is any evidence of abnormality in the uterine cavity, a hysteroscopy is also performed. If a patient with a normal hysterosalpingogram fails to get pregnant after two or three attempts with IVF in which good quality embryos are transferred to the uterus, and no other reasons for failure can be found (ie regarding hormones, sperm or culture), a hysteroscopic evaluation is done. This protocol may change with the availability of office hysteroscopy which can be performed simply under local anaesthesia or without anaesthesia altogether. Hysteroscopy should possibly be done on all patients undergoing IVF. In patients where there is no need to evaluate the tubal integrity, a hysteroscopy may replace the need for a hysterosalpingogram. Due to the many significant medical findings that a hysteroscopy can show the physician, we have incorporated hysteroscopy with all of our operative or diagnostic laparoscopies and are prepared to correct any abnormality that is seen at this time.

Hysteroscopic gamete intrafallopian transfer

Conventional intrafallopian transfer is done with the assistance of laparoscopy. When general anaesthesia or the presence of pelvic adhesions makes laparoscopy impossible, this can be done with the assistance of hysteroscopy or ultrasound. Two different approaches in recent years have been used to place the gametes or embryos in the fallopian tube, with ultrasonic guidance or hysteroscopic guidance under minimal or no anaesthesia. The latter procedure assures us of tubal ostia visualization and therefore we are confident that the gametes or embryos are placed in the tube. Hysteroscopic guidance also appears to be consistently technically successful: Seracchioli *et al.*[5] succeeded in performing this procedure in all 50 patients he attempted. The clinical pregnancy rate also seemed to be acceptable (26% per transfer).

This technique is more traumatic for the endometrium and cervix, and the data are very limited at present. However, it appears to be a promising alternative to IVF and conventional tubal transfer requiring laparoscopy in selected cases.

Diagnostic or operative laparoscopy

Diagnostic or operative laparoscopy can be done to retrieve eggs for a number of reasons:

- for immediate use (gamete intrafallopian transfer – GIFT)
- for further use, cryopreservation of embryo or oocytes
- for IVF or zygote intrafallopian transfer (ZIFT) in the same cycle.

In the early days of IVF in humans, laparoscopy was the only approach for retrieving eggs. It was therefore imperative for the gynaecologist performing the egg retrieval to have a knowledge of the pelvis especially with regards to the accessibility of the ovaries. It was also important to appreciate if there was a possibility of harvesting the eggs, before subjecting the patient to ovarian stimulation, monitoring, general anaesthesia and laparoscopy. Therefore, many groups made it mandatory to perform a diagnostic laparoscopy before the patient was allowed in an IVF cycle.

Many of these patients had undergone a purely diagnostic laparoscopy with chromotubation to inspect the pelvis for pathology and to appreciate tubal integrity in their initial infertility investigation. In a patient with poor ovarian accessibility, surgery and ovarian suspension was recommended prior to the IVF cycle. In this context, and in order to avoid almost back-to-back laparoscopies, it was suggested that both diagnostic and oocyte retrieval procedures should be combined.

In addition, the introduction of microlaparoscopic techniques, described elsewhere in this text, may improve our ability to perform repeated oocyte retrieval in association with frequent diagnostic or operative procedures.

Combining procedures

To eliminate one step, the patient underwent ovarian stimulation and laparoscopic egg retrieval in the same cycle without worrying about ovarian accessibility. This was adequate in the majority of cases; however, in 2–10% of patients (depending on the series reported) the ovaries were not accessible, ruling out egg retrieval. This approach prevented most patients from undergoing repeated laparoscopies, while in the small percentage of patients where the ovaries were obscured, either a laparotomy was performed at a later date or laparoscopic adhesiolysis with egg retrieval was performed at the same setting[6]. The adhesiolysis was done by blunt and sharp dissection using unipolar, bipolar or thermo-coagulation. This is usually successful in at least partly freeing the ovaries so that some of the follicles can be visualized and aspirated. This is definitely recommended practice today when egg retrieval is contemplated through laparoscopy and the ovaries are inaccessible[3].

With the advent of ultrasound-guided egg retrievals, the need to evaluate the accessibility of the ovaries became obsolete. Successful egg retrievals can be accomplished by abdominal, vesical or vaginal routes under abdominal or vaginal ultrasound guidance. Currently, laparoscopy for the sole purpose of egg retrieval has become very rare and laparoscopy is done only in circumstances where it is combined with GIFT or ZIFT.

Advantages of combining procedures

In recent years, the idea of doing IVF, GIFT or ZIFT in the same cycle as the initial laparoscopy evaluation has been proposed. There are a number of advantages in combining the initial diagnostic laparoscopy with ovarian stimulation and egg retrieval. This would be less expensive since egg retrieval adds only a few minutes to the operative time which would prevent two different operative sessions. It would eliminate the need for one laparoscopy, in cases of GIFT or ZIFT, and for a separate egg retrieval procedure in IVF, thereby reducing the need for anaesthesia. This would also give us an idea of the sperm and egg interaction, as well as the quality of eggs, and the ability of the gametes to fertilize very early in the infertility investigation. The eggs obtained can be transferred immediately into the tubes, if the tubes are known to be patent and normal, and the excess placed into in vitro culture and the developing embryos cryopreserved. The eggs could also be put in culture and the embryos transferred in the same cycle or cryopreserved for transfer in a natural cycle. All of these procedures are feasible and would give the patient a chance of pregnancy early in the evaluation period.

Experience

Wentz attempted this as early as 1982. She timed the laparoscopy in relation to an unstimulated cycle with minimal monitoring. However, the yield of eggs and embryos was extremely low and no pregnancy resulted[7]. Frydman and colleagues used either a birth-control pill or a progestogen to programme the retrieval and the diagnostic laparoscopy artificially at a convenient time and then cryopreserved the embryos obtained. Unfortunately the pregnancy rate was quite low[8].

Barad and colleagues selected patients who had had normal infertility evaluation, including a normal hysterosalpingogram, but no previous laparoscopy. They underwent ovarian stimulation with conventional monitoring, appropriately timed for GIFT. The egg retrieval was done before transferring the gametes. They obtained a very reasonable pregnancy rate, 10 pregnancies out of 25 cycles, with an ongoing rate of 32% per cycle (including two miscarriages)[9].

Two recent reports have compared results of combining IVF and screening laparoscopy with results in patients who had previous diagnostic laparoscopy and then IVF and obtained very similar results in both groups, so it seems that adding diagnostic laparoscopy in the IVF cycle does not seem to affect the result of IVF[10,11].

Disadvantages of combining procedures

However, many disadvantages exist in combining procedures. These include removal of some of the diagnostic accuracy of the laparoscopy; assessment of tubal patency and normality cannot be done in most cases since the injection of dye may disturb the uterine or tubal environment, making either the transfer of gametes or the embryo inadvisable. Many centres now recommend doing a hysteroscopy as a prerequisite to IVF; it would be most convenient to do it in conjunction with a diagnostic laparoscopy, but this may not be possible if you are planning a uterine transfer[1–4].

Many patients do not require IVF or GIFT after their diagnostic procedure: controlled ovarian stimulation and intrauterine insemination (IUI) have been very successful for unexplained infertility patients before they are placed into more complex treatment such as IVF or GIFT. Medical or surgical treatment of endometriosis, excision of cysts, lysis of adhesions and microsurgery may be successful and eliminate the need for assisted reproductive technologies altogether[15].

In Barad *et al.*'s group, where all of the investigation including the hysterosalpingogram was normal, 12 of the 25 patients (48%) had some pelvic pathology that could have benefited from an operative laparoscopy[9].

Other modalities

Is it possible to perform a reconstructive operative laparoscopy in conjunction with IVF or GIFT without interfering with the chances of success? This is still very controversial: Gindoff *et al.*[12] obtained very adequate and comparable results in patients undergoing the combined procedure and those who did not. For some patients, IVF results did not seem to be affected, even when laparoscopy was done for reconstruction[13,14]. However, Damewood and Rock[16] encountered no pregnancies in 39 cycles of combined operative laparoscopy for endometriosis and IVF. All of these authors do report subsequent spontaneous pregnancies after this combined cycle.

Conclusion

There seem to be very few indications for the use of combined diagnostic or operative laparoscopy with IVF or GIFT. We usually subject our patients to diagnostic laparoscopy and diagnostic hysteroscopy as part of our infertility evaluation. To avoid repetition of surgical procedures, it is important to be able to perform the necessary reconstructive procedures both through the hysteroscope (ie lysis of adhesions, metroplasties etc) and the laparoscope (ie lysis of adhesions, excision of endometrioma etc) at the time of the surgery. This may necessitate having all the surgical equipment required for these procedures available routinely (Table 20.3). Following this, the patient is treated medically if indicated (as in cases of diffuse endometriosis), or subjected to controlled ovarian hyperstimulation and IUI (in cases of unexplained infertility) or simply left an adequate number of cycles for pregnancies to occur spontaneously (in cases where reconstructive surgery was done). The only exception that we have made to this has been in patients where we want to speed up the investigative and therapeutic process. This can be true in older patients where we wish to shorten the time required for investigation and be as aggressive as possible.

Excision of uterine septum	Hysteroscopy
Excision of intrauterine adhesions	Hysteroscopy
Excision of uterine polyps	Hysteroscopy
Excision of adenomyosis	Hysteroscopy
Removal of fibroids	
Submucous	Hysteroscopy
Subserosa	Laparoscopy
Excision of endometrioma	Laparoscopy
Excision of pelvic adhesions	Laparoscopy
Excision of ovarian cysts	Laparoscopy

Table 20.3: Uses of operative endoscopy in preparing for assisted reproductive technologies (ART).

Our approach will not only prevent a number of patients from being subjected to more aggressive technologies unnecessarily, but also will prepare the pelvis to go through IVF or GIFT if necessary under the most favourable circumstances. Many of the findings can interfere with the response to stimulation (ie adhesions, ovarian cyst), to fertilization (ie endometriosis) or implantation (submucous fibroids, polyps) if not corrected before the patient goes through assisted reproductive technologies.

References

1   Frydman R *et al.* (1987) Uterine evaluation by microhysteroscopy in IVF candidates. *Human Reproduction.* **2**:481–5.

2   Dicker D *et al.* (1990) The value of hysteroscopy in elderly women prior to in vitro fertilization – embryo transfer (IVF-ET): A comparative study. *Journal of In Vitro Fertilization and Embryo Transfer.* **7**:267–70.

3   Goldenberg M *et al.* (1991) Hysteroscopy in a program of in vitro fertilization. *Journal of In Vitro Fertilization and Embryo Transfer.* **8**:336–8.

4   Seinera P *et al.* (1988) Hysteroscopy in an IVF-ER program. *Acta Obstetrica et Gynecologica Scandinavica.* **67**:135–7.

5   Seracchioli R *et al.* (1991) Hysteroscopic gamete intra-Fallopian transfer: a good alternative, in selected cases, to laparoscopic intra-Fallopian transfer. *Human Reproduction.* **6**:1388–90.

6   Daniell J *et al.* (1983) The role of laparoscopic adhesiolysis in an in vitro fertilization program. *Fertility and Sterility.* **40**:49–52.

7   Wentz A *et al.* (1983) Combined screening laparoscopy and timed follicle aspiration for human in vitro fertilization. *Fertility and Sterility.* **39**:270–6.

8   Frydman R *et al.* (1986) Programmed oocyte retrieval during routine laparoscopy and embryo cryopreservation for later transfer. *American Journal of Obstetrics and Gynecology.* **155**:112–17.

9   Barad D *et al.* Gamete intrafallopian tube transfer (GIFT): making laparoscopy more than 'diagnostic'. *Fertility and Sterility.* **50**:928–30.

10 Irsigler U and Van der Merwe JV (1987) Diagnostic laparoscopy v. combined screening laparoscopy and timed follicle aspiration for in vitro fertilization. *South African Medical Journal.* **71**:20–2.

11 Shoham Z *et al.* (1990) Combined diagnostic laparoscopy and follicular aspiration for human in vitro fertilization. *Acta Obstetrica et Gynecologica Scandinavica.* **69**:23–6.

12 Gindoff PR *et al.* (1990) Efficacy of assisted reproductive technology during diagnostic and operative infertility laparoscopy. *Obstetrics and Gynecology.* **75**:299–301.

13 Mastroianni L *et al.* (1983) Intrauterine pregnancy following ovum recovery at laparotomy and subsequent in vitro fertilization. *Fertility and Sterility.* **40**:536.

14 Roh S *et al.* (1988) In vitro fertilization with concurrent pelvic reconstructive surgery. *Fertility and Sterility.* **49**:96–9.

15 Wardle PG *et al.* (1986) Endometriosis and IVF: effect of prior therapy. *Lancet.* **1**:276.

16 Damewood M and Rock J (1988) Treatment independent pregnancy with operative laparoscopy for endometriosis in an in vitro fertilization program. *Fertility and Sterility.* **50**:463–5.

21

Operative Hysteroscopy with Electricity

BRUCE McLUCAS

Introduction

The hysteroscope was introduced by Pantaleoni[1] at the end of the 19th century and popularized by Lindemann almost 25 years ago[2]. Since then it is not the instrument that has changed so much as its function, from diagnostic to therapeutic.

This is a pattern that has been seen in all areas of surgical endoscopy. For instance, Takagi invented the arthroscope in 1917 in Japan: but the instrument was little appreciated until David Dandy demonstrated the efficacy of meniscectomy via arthroscopy in 1979[3]. Within the next two years, it seemed that almost every North American orthopaedic surgeon had taken a course in arthroscopy.

Much the same phenomenon has occurred in hysteroscopy, with the renewed interest in electrosurgery. Norment and colleagues first advocated the hysteroscopic use of a diathermy current for the resection of endometrial polyps and myomata in 1957[4].

Recently a resecting loop has been devised to add to the hysteroscope for the resection of widely based endometrial polyps and submucosal fibroids. A resection of these tumours of the uterine canal under direct vision is somewhat similar to the procedure of prostatic resection, although a resectoscope used for prostatic resection cannot be used for resection in the uterine canal. The cutting loop may be removed, and the hysteroscope used for diagnosis as well. Tumours are removed with a cutting current and later the base is fulgurated.

Technological advances in telescopes, light sources and instrument design have combined to give diathermy-powered hysteroscopy many powerful applications for today's gynaecologists (Table 21.1).

The major advance in hysteroscopic surgery has been the use of the resectoscope for endometrial ablation, and that will be the major focus of this chapter. Since DeCherney and Polan first suggested the use of the cutting loop for endometrial ablation[5], several large studies and long-term results have

1925	Stern	Cutting in antegrade fashion, two-handed 0° scope
1932	McCarthy	30° scope, retrograde motion of cutting loop, insulated sheath
1939	Nesbit	One-handed working element, loop extended by spring compression, returned by expansion of spring
1946	Baumrucker	Reverse of Nesbit spring, resting position into patient space, compression return during resection
1948	Iglesias de la Torre	Simplified Nesbit motion by using leaf spring, smoothing the action
1957	Norment	First use of electrified cutting loop with hysteroscope to resect myomas
1959	Hopkins	Rod lens system
1963		Fibre illumination introduced into resectoscope
1972		Stabilized cutting loop introduced
1973	Iglesias de la Torre	Continuous flow resectoscope
	Neuwirth	Use of resectoscope for treatment of myomas

Table 21.1: Landmarks in the development of the resectoscope.

been published. These will be discussed, to give guidance to the hysteroscopist beginning ablation procedures. Informing patients of the possibilities and complications will add to the overall satisfaction of both doctor and patient.

Operative hysteroscopy with electrical current has been used for:

- endometrial ablation
- myoma resection
- dissection of intrauterine synechiae
- septum resection
- endometrial biopsy.

We will discuss each of the procedures, and examine whether they offer the clinician an advantage over other modalities with electrosurgery, whether they can be done equally well with other operative treatments, or even be performed better without electrosurgery. Complications of hysteroscopy are dealt with elsewhere in this book.

Understanding electrosurgery

Modern electrosurgery began with the development of the spark-gap generator in Boston during the 1920s. Harvey Cushing, a neurosurgeon in Boston, pioneered the use of electrosurgery using such a generator invented by William Bovie. The early spark-gap generator created a spark which would arc across ionized air to tissue. This non-contact method of using electrosurgery still exists, although the spark-gap electrosurgical units have been superseded by solid-state circuitry which amplifies and modifies the current used for electrosurgery. Spark-gap electrosurgical units are still used in operating rooms; however, they are not appropriate for modern endoscopic procedures where variable power output is important for clear tissue margins, haemostasis and for minimizing unintended tissue damage.

Electrical currents are part of the radio frequency spectrum. There is confusion about different wavelengths because of claims that have been made to promote various electrosurgical generators. Oscillation of current is usually measured in hertz or cycles per second. A waveform has a positive and negative oscillation from the neutral point of the wave. The peak voltage is the distance from a neutral point to the positive peak of the waveform. Modern electrosurgical units produce currents between 200 000 Hz (2 KHz) and 4 000 000 Hz (4 MHz). The current used in the USA for household appliances is 60 Hz. At frequencies below 200 000 Hz, muscles and nerves will be excited by the action of electrons and cause patient discomfort. At this lower level, patients may experience electrical injury and even death from depolarization of cardiac muscles.

Early spark-gap electrosurgical units generated a continuous waveform at levels around 200 000 Hz. Cells can conduct electrical currents because of their electrolyte composition. The cell membrane will depolarize when exposed to an electrical current. In neuromuscular cells, such depolarization will cause excitation. Below 100 000 Hz the cell will be alternatively depolarized and then reversed, and the patient will experience a sensation of tetanic shock. Higher-frequency current applied to tissue does of course depolarize. Patients undergoing electrosurgery now suffer no such ill-effects because of the higher frequencies generated by modern electrosurgical units. However, at the high frequencies of modern electrosurgical units, excited ions will collide with other cellular particles, thus trading the faradic effect for a thermal one.

AM band radio transmitters send signals at the same frequencies as those used by electrosurgical units; thus all electrosurgical units could be termed radio-frequency generators.

At wavelengths above 3 500 000 Hz (3.5 MHz) it is difficult to control the path of electrons. Current will scatter away from its intended area of effect and will be governed by capacitance and inductance, causing possible unintended side effects at remote parts of the body.

Many factors determine the effect of electrosurgery upon tissue:

- waveform
- power setting
- time
- size of electrode
- manipulation of electrode
- type of tissue
- eschar.

Since the type of current chosen will have a large impact upon tissue, we will consider cutting, blended and coagulating current separately. Bipolar current passing between two closely approximated electrodes has not been shown yet to have applications for hysteroscopic surgery, although it may be most effective in laparoscopic procedures[6].

Radio frequencies

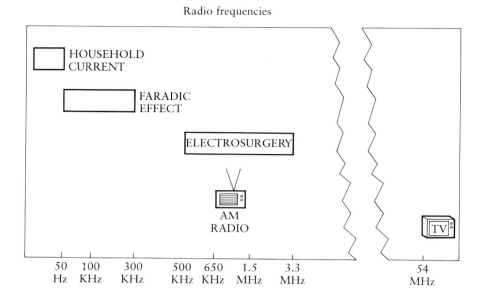

Figure 21.1: Radio-wave frequency of electrosurgery varies from 500 KHz to 3.3 MHz.

Most electrosurgical units offer surgeons a choice between 'cutting', 'blended' and 'coagulating' current.

Cutting current

The cutting current waveform can be used quite effectively to coagulate tissue if the electrode is large and in contact with tissue (the rollerball, for example):so the term 'cutting current' will be used in this chapter only because it is so named on electrosurgical units. Cutting current is produced at a frequency determined by the maker of the electrosurgical unit. The cutting current creates an arc or spark along the length of the bare wire which is held slightly above the tissue. The force which drives the current through the resistance of the tissue and the wire which the current encounters is measured in volts or ohms. The air rapidly ionizes into positive and negative electrons, allowing better transmission of the current.

Voltage is measured as the distance from the neutral point of the current to the top of the oscillating wave. The most commonly used voltage term is peak voltage. During the cutting phenomenon a spark-gap will be continuously generated.

Cutting is accomplished by the high level of heat which is produced in the arc through extreme current concentration. This high-level energy causes the cells to explode as they come into contact with the arc.

The rapid ionization of cells releases the cell's water content in the form of steam. The amount of energy necessary to drive the cutting arc during the procedure depends on the amount of resistance (generally measured in ohms) which the current must overcome. The most important factors influencing

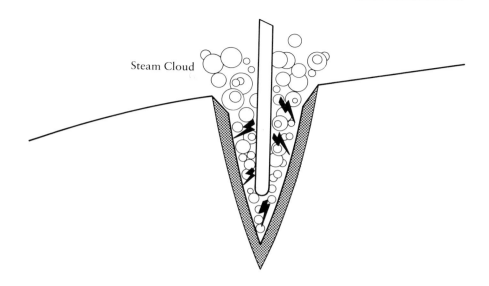

Figure 21.2: Steam is rapidly released from exploding cells when the electron energy passes through those cells.

the resistance are (1) size of wire, and (2) the cell's water content.

Thicker electrodes require higher current and cause more heat to be produced; the effect is to cause more extensive thermal damage. Stainless steel and alloys used in the production of electrodes will vary with manufacturer, and may require different settings.

The wattage chosen by the surgeon on the dial of the electrosurgical unit is not constant during the electrosurgery. This wattage is accurate at a fixed resistance determined by the maker of the unit (300 ohms). The resistance to current flow will vary not only with the factors listed above, but also according to the amount of tissue in contact with the loop. At the deepest point of the excision, the tissue resistance will be maximal; the electrosurgical unit must produce enough current to overcome this resistance and complete an excision.

If the cell's water content is high, the current can pass through the cell more easily. Bone has a much higher resistance than the uterus has (typically 300 ohms). The endometrium of a menopausal woman has less water content than that of a nulliparous woman. Similarly, the endometrium which has been scarred from previous treatment will have a lower water content. Both these circumstances will cause the surgeon to seek a higher wattage setting.

Blended current

This term is misleading, in that surgeons may believe that their electrosurgical unit can deliver a mixture of cutting and coagulating waves. Solid-state electrosurgical units generate a cutting waveform for the blended current that is intermittent; typically the wave will be interrupted 10–20% of the time.

This interruption has the same effect on the delivery of constant power as does the coagulation form. In other words, to keep a constant 30 watts of power delivered to the cervical tissue for generation of the continuous spark-gap in blended coagulation, the electrosurgical unit must compensate for the power being off for 10% of the time. If the voltage necessary to sustain the spark-gap is 1000 volts in the pure cutting current, it will be increased to 1100 volts in the blended cycle. Moreover, if the wattage is constant to the tissue, it will have to be increased by 10% to account for the off-cycle to 33 watts. We can see that the reading of '30 watts' blended current on the front of an electrosurgical unit is quite different in its tissue effects from the pure cutting setting.

Coagulating current

Terminology concerning coagulation current is not universal. The author uses a cutting current when performing endometrial ablation with the resectoscope equipped with the rollerball electrode[7]. Unlike the unmodulated sine-wave generated by the electrosurgical unit for cutting, the coagulation current is a damped waveform.

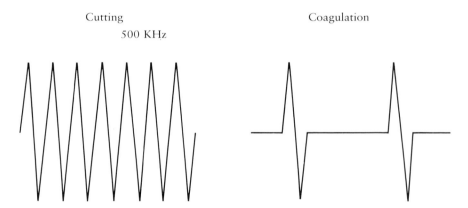

Figure 21.3: The unmodulated sine-wave is released from the electrosurgical generator at a much more rapid rate than the modulated wave associated with coagulation effect.

The waveform is created, heat is produced and then dissipates. Figure 21.3 shows the generation of a modulated wave over time and contrasts it with the cutting current. The electrosurgical unit will generate all its current at the frequency of its manufacturing specifications, mostly in the range of 0.6 MHz to 3 MHz; but the coagulation waveform will be generated in bursts of energy followed by resting periods. These bursts are rapid — between 20 000 and 50 000 Hz — but are far below the typical electrosurgical unit's capacity of 600 000 Hz. For the power delivered to the tissue to remain constant, the electrosurgical unit must compensate for the 'off-cycles' when no power reaches the tissue. During coagulation the off-periods typically account for 80–90% of the operating time, whereas the on-period is only 10%. To create the wattage to the patient similar to that delivered with non-modulated current, a much higher peak voltage accompanies each burst of power. Thus 50 watts of power to the patient in the non-modulated or cutting mode would be best described as high-frequency oscillation with low voltage of approximately 500–1000 volts necessary to drive the current. Coagulation current will require a higher voltage of 3000 volts or higher to sustain the same wattage delivered to tissue. Figure 21.4 shows the varying amplitude of voltages at different settings of 50 watts.

Rather than exploding cells, as during the cutting phenomenon, coagulation will dry the cell slowly: a process called desiccation. Desiccation may result from either the use of the non-modulated waveform when placed in contact with tissue, or with the modulated waveform crossing the air via spark-gap to the tissue (fulguration). In desiccation, the cell will be heated slowly at temperatures less than 100° F. Tissue around the blood vessels will shrink, yielding a haemostatic effect. The effects of cutting current which make it most appropriate for excision with clear margins — its ability to explode cells — would render it ineffective to deliver the high voltage necessary for cell necrosis and haemostasis.

When the cell temperature exceeds 600° C, denaturation of cell protein is produced. Further elevation of cell temperature leads to carbonization which is undesirable. The water is slowly driven out of the cells causing desiccation.

Much higher voltages are necessary to create the new coagulating waveform 20 000–50 000 times per second. These voltages can be as high as 6000 volts, but the peak voltage is usually 2000 volts. The combination of high voltage and low current in the coagulation current increases the

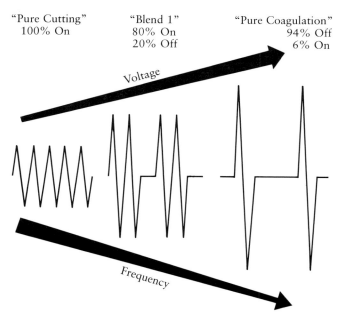

Figure 21.4: To maintain the same wattage, a modulated wave will have much higher voltage than will the unmodulated cutting wave.

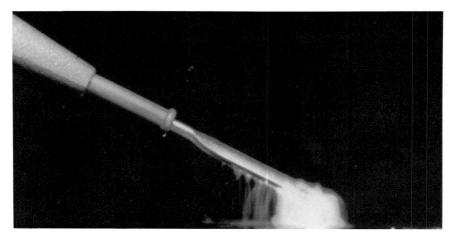

Figure 21.5: Spark jumping from the electrode to tissue using the spark gap through the air.

tendency toward sparking. Moreover, each spark carries with it a high current density. Such sparks will invariably cause tissue necrosis in the cells with which they come into contact.

Applications for endometrial ablation

The goal of ablation procedures is the destruction of endometrial tissue. Important variables to consider here are not only the quality of current but also the time of exposure. Duffy *et al.*[8] showed that exposure of tissue to 100 watts of coagulating current with four consecutive treatments of 2.5 seconds each raised temperatures of that tissue by 14° C, whereas the same applications caused temperature rises of 3.9° C in single applications. Indman and Soderstrom found that applying 50–150 watts of coagulating current via the ball-tip electrode to the endometrial cavity at the tubal ostea did not raise serosal surface temperatures more than 6° C[9]. They commented that a rise of 12° C on the serosal surface of the uterus for five seconds should be considered potentially dangerous to bowel and bladder and should be avoided[10].

For the same reason the hysteroscopic surgeon should avoid repeated exposure of the same tissue to whatever form of current is chosen. The venous system will allow cooling of the uterus with time. Duffy and colleagues[8] did show deeper destruction of tissue with the higher voltage coagulation, which should be considered when operating in areas such as the thin myometrium surrounding the ostea. A possible solution to this problem of bowel injury has been offered by Harry Reich who recommends instillation, via laparoscopy, or several litres of lactated Ringer's solution into the peritoneal cavity before ablation procedures are begun, perhaps at the time of concurrent tubal ligation[11]. This fluid will 'float' bowel off the serosal surface of the uterus.

Further, any current which might be conducted through the serosal surface will be dissipated in the electrolyte solution.

When the ball-tip electrode is held in contact with the endometrial surface for rollerball ablation, less deep tissue destruction will be generated if cutting current is chosen because of the lower voltage which accompanies this current. On balance, therefore, inexperienced hysteroscopists may elect to use this cutting current until they become familiar with the effect upon tissue.

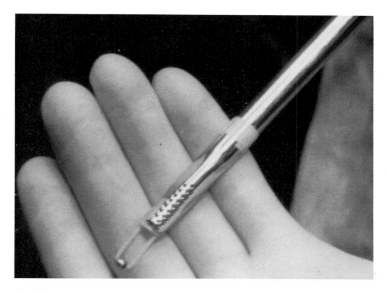

Figure 21.6: The rollerball electrode is demonstrated extending from the outer sheath of the resectoscope.

Ablation or resection

Despite increased morbidity and mortality, many European surgeons have favoured resection rather than ablation for endometrial removal[12-14]. The advantages of resection are that it is quick, it provides a tissue specimen, and no preparation is needed.

Speed is a major advantage. In resection the cutting loop is usually 8 mm wide, and thus is able to remove more tissue with each pass than the 2 or 3 mm rollerball or bar. Since fluid absorption (an important complication of hysteroscopic surgery) is known to depend upon the length of surgery, limiting the time of the procedure is important[15]. Another concern expressed about ablation is the possibility of masking endometrial cancer. With resection, the whole endometrium is submitted for pathological evaluation, and at least one case of unsuspected endometrial cancer has been detected from the resected fragments[18].

Physicians often prepare the endometrium for ablation with danazol[17] or GNRH agonists[18]. By thinning the endometrium, the hysteroscopist will have less tissue to treat, and should not only work faster, but perhaps get better results. Lefler[19] and Gimpelson and Kaigh[20] have mechanically curetted the endometrium prior to ablation procedures and reported good results. In the emergent situation, particularly in the medically unstable patient, preparation may not be possible, and surgeons should be familiar with use of the cutting loop electrode for resection in these patients.

Problems with resection

On the negative side, there is a higher rate of potentially fatal complications with the cutting loop. A recent survey of British endoscopists revealed that there have been three fatalities from the use of the cutting loop[21].

The mortality rate of approximately 0.04% is still less than the predicted 0.1% which would be expected for abdominal hysterectomy[22]. Furthermore, each of these fatalities occurred within the surgeon's first five cases. Experienced hysteroscopists serving as proctors should be sought at the onset of ablation training.

Adenomyosis

The question of iatrogenically created adenomyosis has been raised as a result of endometrial resections[23]. The theoretical mechanism for this phenomenon is that endometrial tissue under pressure of the distension medium may be driven via the transsected vessels deeply into the myometrial tissue where it may later become functional. The author has recently reviewed his patients undergoing endometrial resection and discovered nine patients who have experienced pelvic pain of dysmenorrhoea following resection and who had not complained of this preoperatively. Hormonal suppression and laparoscopy with repeat resection have been attempted in this group, but the results of retreatment are not available. Any patient complaining of dysmenorrhoea or pelvic pain in association with menorrhagia should undergo concurrent laparoscopy with the resection procedure to detect any other pathology.

Success rates

Endometrial ablation with electrosurgery is an alternative to hysterectomy for uncontrolled menorrhagia. If it is simply an adjunct, it cannot be considered a success unless performed as a measure to control bleeding, to give the patient time to donate her own autologous blood for a future procedure, or to stabilize a dangerously low haematocrit or medical condition before hysterectomy. Is endometrial ablation a definitive therapy? Table 21.2 compares hysterectomy rates following ablation in various studies. Many authors have shown that patients who initially fail to respond to treatment will do well when offered a repeat procedure (Table 21.3).

The number of patients who report amenorrhoea after ablation procedures

McLucas[7]	7/ 118	6%
Magos *et al.*[14]	16/ 234	7%
Macdonald *et al.*[21]	32/ 187	17%
Garry[25]	26/ 479	5%
Piper[37]	15/ 75	20%
Total	96/ 1 093	9%

Table 21.2: Hysterectomy rates following ablation.

McLucas[7]	3/ 118	3%
Magos *et al.*[14]	13/ 234	6%
Macdonald *et al.*[21]	18/ 187	10%
Garry[25]	13/ 479	3%
Slade[36]	35/ 220	15%
Pyper[37]	4/ 75	5%
Total	86/ 1 313	7%

Table 21.3: Rates following repeat procedures.

drops annually. The author's patients have followed trends suggested by others[14,20], becoming oligomenorrheic over time (Figure 21.7).

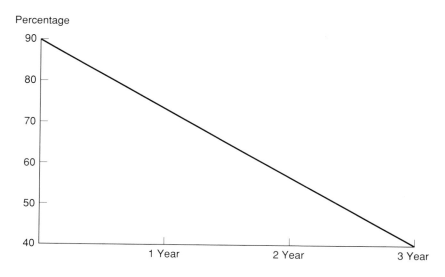

Figure 21.7: Overall amenorrhoea rates fall steadily in the years following the original procedure.

In properly selected cases, there is a 90% overall success rate of diminution in bleeding. However, attempting to measure the amount of 'normal flow' or 'light spotting' is difficult[24]. The author follows the lead of other investigators in reporting patient satisfaction as the measure of success for ablation[14].

On the face of it, the Nd:YAG laser appears to offer a higher amenorrhoea rate than that reported in resectoscope studies[25,26]. The question must be raised whether the higher cost of the laser procedure is justified.

Recurrent bleeding

Recurrent bleeding may be delayed after several years, or it may be immediate. The author has examined his treatment failures in conjunction with the radiology department, using vaginal probe ultrasound. Most of the failures, and most of the patients who continued to bleed, had functioning endometrium in the fundus[28] (Figure 21.8). This is to be expected, since the fundus and the tubal ostea are areas where the resectoscope does not function optimally in a side-to-side manner.

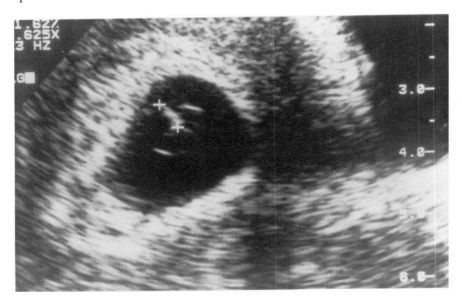

Figure 21.8: Ultrasound showing residual fundal endometrium.

When a patient experiences bleeding with or without dysmenorrhoea, she should undergo an ultrasound prior to repeat treatment. Three patients (0.2%) in the author's series have been noted to have haematometrium, and have been successfully retreated with the resectoscope under laparoscopic guidance.

Cost

Mention should be made of cost to the patient. Several studies have compared the cost of ablation with the cost of hysterectomy, and found the former to be considerably lower[28]. The overall cost to the patient may still be lower than

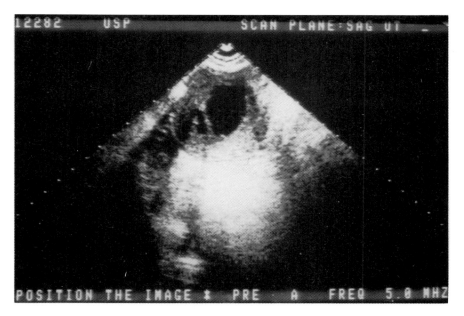

Figure 21.9: Haematometrium seen on ultrasound of the uterus.

with laparotomy, but the repeat rate of nearly 10% to achieve a 90% overall success will generate additional costs. The author recommends that patients undergo an annual ultrasound as a screening test for endometrial cancer after ablation[29]. Over a patient's lifetime, the cost of ultrasound will need to be considered as an added cost.

Other procedures

Management of uterine myomas via the hysteroscope using the polyp snare has been reported by the author[30]. Neuwirth and Amin pioneered use of the resectoscope for treatment of myomas[31]. Myomas will be covered elsewhere in this book. Surgeons are encouraged to be familiar with other non-electrical techniques for hysteroscopic myomectomy[32].

Uterine septa may be treated with the resectoscope, but March and Israel[33] recommend scissors as a safer method, as they do for the treatment of uterine synechiae. Tubal sterilization via the hysteroscope has been attempted[34], but a review showed a low success rate and serious complications, and the technique was abandoned[35].

Conclusion

Endometrial ablation and resection with electrosurgery are breakthroughs in the endoscopic technology available to the hysteroscopic surgeon. We have stressed the need for proper understanding of electrosurgery, training, and proctoring for the inexperienced surgeon. Armed with these principles, the gynaecologist will find the resectoscope to be a powerful tool and a welcome addition to his or her surgical treatment of many conditions.

References

1   Pantaleoni DC (1869) On endoscopic examination of the cavity of the womb. *Medical Press Circular*. **8**:26–7.

2   Lindemann HJ (1973) Historical aspects of hysteroscopy. *Fertility and Sterility*. **24**:230–43.

3   Dandy DJ (ed.) (1987) *Arthroscopic management of the knee*. Churchill Livingstone, Edinburgh.

4   Norment WB *et al.* (1957) Hysteroscopy. *Surgical Clinics of North America*. **37**:1377–86.

5   DeCherney A and Polan M (1983) Hysteroscopic management of interuterine lesions and intractable uterine bleeding. *Obstetrics and Gynecology*. **61**:392–7.

6   Reich H (1992) Laparoscopic hysterectomy. *Surgical Laparoscopic Endoscopy*. **2**:85–8.

7   McLucas B (1990) Endometrial ablation with the roller ball electrode. *Journal of Reproductive Medicine*. **35**:1055–8.

8   Duffy S *et al.* (1991) Studies of uterine electrosurgery. *Obstetrics and Gynecology*. **78**:213–20.

9   Indman PD and Soderstrom RM (1992) Uterine surface changes caused by electrosurgical endometrial coagulation. *Journal of Reproductive Medicine*. **37**:667–70.

10 Artz CP *et al.* (1989) *Burns: a team approach*. WB Saunders, Philadelphia. pp. 23–5.

11 Reich H (1989) New techniques in advanced laparoscopic surgery. *Baillière's Clinics of Obstetrics and Gynaecology*. **3**:655–81.

12 Hallez JP *et al.* (1987) Methodical intrauterine resection. *American Journal of Obstetrics and Gynecology*. **156**:1080–4.

13 Hamou J *et al.* (1991) *Hysteroscopy and microcolpohysteroscopy: text and atlas*. Appleton and Lange, East Norwalk.

14 Magos AL *et al.* (1991) Experience with the first 250 endometrial resections for menorrhagia. *Lancet*. **337**:1074–8.

15 Madsen PO and Naber KG (1973) The importance of pressure in the prostatic fossa and absorption of irrigating fluid during transurethral resection of the prostate. *Journal of Urology.* **109**:446–52.

16 Dwyer NA and Stirrat GM (1987) Early endometrial carcinoma: an incidental finding after endometrial resection. Case report. *British Journal of Obstetrics and Gynaecology.* **98**:733–4.

17 Goldrath MH (1990) Use of danazol in hysteroscopic surgery for menorrhagia. *Journal of Reproductive Medicine.* **35**:91–6.

18 Brooks PG *et al.* (1991) Hormonal inhibition of the endometrium for resectoscopic endometrial ablation. *American Journal of Obstetrics and Gynecology.* **164**:1601–8.

19 Lefler HT (1989) Premenstrual syndrome improvement after laser ablation of the endometrium for menorrhagia. *Journal of Reproductive Medicine.* **34**:905–6.

20 Gimpelson RJ and Kaigh J (1992) Endometrial ablation repeat procedures. *Journal of Reproductive Medicine.* **37**:431–4.

21 Macdonald R *et al.* (1992) Endometrial ablation: a safe procedure. *Gynaecological Endoscopy.* **1**:7–9.

22 Dicker RC *et al.* (1982) Complications of abdominal and vaginal hysterectomy among women of reproductive age in the United States. *American Journal of Obstetrics and Gynecology.* **144**:841–8.

23 Coltart T and Smith RNJ (1991) Letter. *Lancet.* **338**:312.

24 Hallberg L *et al.* (1966) Menstrual blood loss – a population study. *Acta Obstetrica et Gynecologica Scandinavica.* **45**:320–51.

25 Garry R (1990) Hysteroscopic alternatives to hysteroscopy. *British Journal of Obstetrics and Gynaecology.* **97**:199–207.

26 Lomano JM *et al.* (1986) Ablation of the endometrium with the neodymium:YAG laser: a multicenter study. *Colposcopy and Gynecologic Laser Surgery.* **2**:203–7.

27 Perrella RR *et al.* (1992) Sonographic findings after surgical ablation of the endometrium. *American Journal of Roentgenology.* **159**:1239–41.

28 Macdonald R (1990) Modern treatment of menorrhagia. *British Journal of Obstetrics and Gynaecology.* **97**:3–7.

29 Osmers R *et al.* (1990) Vaginosonography for early detection of endometrial carcinoma. *Lancet.* **335**:1569–71.

30 McLucas B (1992) Diathermy polyp snare: a new modality for treatment of submucous myomata. *Journal of Gynaecological Endoscopy.* **1**:107–10.

31 Neuwirth RS and Amin HK (1976) Excision of submucous fibroids with hysteroscopic control. *American Journal of Obstetrics and Gynecology.* **126**:95–9.

32 Valle RF (1990) Hysteroscopic removal of submucous leiomyomas. *Journal of Gynecological Surgery.* **6**:89–91.

33 March CM and Israel R (1987) Hysteroscopic management of recurrent abortion caused by septate uterus. *American Journal of Obstetrics and Gynecology.* **156**:834–42.

34 Quinones RG *et al.* (1973) Tubal electrocauterization under hysteroscopic control. *Contraception.* **7**:195.

35 March CM (1992) Hysteroscopy. *Journal of Reproductive Medicine.* **37**:293–312.

36 Pyper RJD (1991) A review of 80 endometrial resections for menorrhagia. *British Journal of Obstetrics and Gynaecology.* **98**:1049–54.

37 Slade RJ, Hasib Ahmed AI, Gillmer MDG (1991) Problems with endometrial resection. *Lancet.* **338**:310.

22

Laser Endometrial Ablation

JACK M. LOMANO

Historical introduction

Asherman's syndrome was first described in 1948[1]. The syndrome most commonly involves traumatic uterine synechia causing amenorrhoea, hypomenorrhoea and secondary infertility. Histological evaluation of the affected uteri show a destruction of the mucosal lining, as well as fibrous adhesions between the myometrial walls. Hysterectomy is one of the most commonly performed major operations in the USA and many hysterectomies are done for indications of excessive uterine bleeding. There is a need for a conservative method to control chronic menorrhagia.

The procedure of endometrial ablation with the Nd:YAG laser was first described by Milton Goldrath in 1981[2]. Many investigators have tried various chemicals and physical methods of destroying the endometrium. The Nd:YAG laser seems to be the most appropriate method of trauma to the uterine lining cells because of the inherent forward scatter of the laser energy as it interacts with the surface of the endometrium. There are two components to Asherman's syndrome which are necessary to produce intra-uterine synechia: there must be some form of trauma to the endometrial lining cells, in combination with the hypo-oestrogen state. Asherman's syndrome is most commonly seen following abortion or pregnancy when the genital tissues are atrophic. The source of tissue trauma in naturally occurring Asherman's syndrome is very often a vigorous D&C or a significant postpartum endometritis.

Many investigators have attempted to create an Asherman's syndrome with various chemical and physical means. However, iatrogenic tissue trauma has failed in the past to create it for two reasons: first because there have been significant complications with reflux of materials into the fallopian tubes, resulting in significant salpingitis and peritonitis, and secondly because of the tremendous capacity of the endometrium to generate itself. There must be a complete destruction of the basalis layer of the endometrium in order to have a complete Asherman's syndrome. An incomplete Asherman's syndrome results in hypomenorrhoea and scant menstrual cycles because of cyclic bleeding of small tufts of regenerated endometrial tissue.

There are approximately 750 000 hysterectomies performed annually in the USA. It is estimated that 20–30% of these hysterectomies result in some type of morbidity. This morbidity is most often minor febrile morbidity which can be treated successfully with modern antibiotic therapy. However, 600 women die annually as a complication of hysterectomy; and because of the large number of hysterectomies, the procedure consumes vast amounts of healthcare dollars. It is estimated that 30–40% of all hysterectomies are performed due to some type of abnormal uterine bleeding. Certainly if a less complex minor procedure to treat refractory menorrhagia could be found, there would be considerable reduction in morbidity, mortality and expense. The procedure of laser endometrial ablation has been developed as an alternative to hysterectomy in patients with chronic refractory menorrhagia.

What is a laser?

When energy is applied to an atom, the electrons orbiting that atom jump to a higher energy level. This unstable condition lasts a very short time, and when the electron returns to the ground state, a photon packet of energy is emitted. If the photons hit other unstable atoms, additional photons will be emitted.

Laser energy (light amplification by the stimulated emission of radiation) is collimated and parallel, which minimizes divergence of the transmitted light. Moreover, it is coherent (ie all waves are in phase) and monochromatic (ie only pure colours are emitted from the tube).

There are four major medical lasers on the market today. The carbon dioxide laser has an infrared wavelength of 10 600 nm. Its effect on biological tissue is independent of colour and it is instantly absorbed by water with minimal scattering into body tissues. The argon laser produces a visible blue–green light at a wavelength of 488–515 nm. It is easily transmitted through clear liquid as well as fibreoptic systems. Argon laser energy is absorbed by water. A relative newcomer, the potassium triphosophate crystal (KTP) laser, emits a wavelength of 532 nm in the blue–green range. Like the argon laser, it can be transmitted fibreoptically and is absorbed by water. On the other hand, the neodymium YAG laser has a solid crystal of yttrium, aluminium and garnet surrounded by neodymium. The Nd:YAG laser light is in the near infrared region with a wavelength of 1064 nm. This laser can be transmitted through clear liquids, as well as fibreoptic systems, and is an excellent coagulator because of its forward scatter. As it strikes human tissue it is selectively absorbed by any tissue with colour. This forward scatter means that the Nd:YAG laser is the most valuable laser for destroying the endometrium.

Patient selection

Patients with chronic refractory menometrorrhagia that has not responded to surgical D&C or hormone manipulation with progesterone and androgenic medical therapy become candidates for laser endometrial ablation. It is a conservative procedure designed to benefit the 30–40% of women who would otherwise undergo hysterectomy for chronic menorrhagia. The goal is to reduce the amount of menstrual flow enough to eliminate the need for a major surgical procedure. Candidates usually have a long history of dysfunctional uterine bleeding. Many will already have undergone multiple D&C procedures as well as variations of hormone regimens in order to control their heavy flow.

Other women who may benefit from laser ablation are those classified as high-risk surgical patients because of major medical problems (ie cardiac and pulmonary disorders or obesity) which require bedrest and decreased ambulation and can result in postoperative complications.

Contraindications and complications

Laser ablation is not appropriate for premalignant or neoplastic lesions of the endometrium since patients with chronic menometrorrhagia are at high risk for endometrial cancer. Candidates for this procedure must have had a benign endometrial sampling within six months prior to the procedure. It is also important that these patients are closely monitored for the development of endometrial carcinoma or endometrial hyperplasia following the ablation. Since the cervix remains open following the procedure, patients with endometrial neoplasia are likely to present menorrhagia which would prompt the physician to do an endometrial sampling to rule out neoplastic disease.

In addition, patients with recent pregnancy or active pelvic inflammatory disease should be excluded as candidates for endometrial ablation. Patients must be willing to accept sterility following the procedure, because of the postoperative intrauterine scarring and subsequent Asherman's syndrome created by the laser. To date, however, there has been no prospective study that absolutely guarantees laser endometrial ablation as a sterilizing procedure. Postoperative sampling of the endometrial cavity will show low cuboidal epithelium with surrounding fibrosis and rare endometrial glands. Even though this is not compatible with normal implantation, patients must be counselled with regard to postoperative birth control measures.

The preoperative evaluation should begin with a pelvic examination to confirm relatively normal anatomy. Patients with large myomata (which have been growing for more than 16 weeks) and patients with adnexal enlargement are not considered to be candidates for endometrial ablation. An office hysteroscopy and endometrial biopsy should be performed to rule out the presence of significant submucous myomas, endometrial hyperplasia and other pathologic conditions that would preclude ablation. If a submucous fibroid occupies more than one-half of the uterine cavity, it is best approached with an abdominal incision. Submucous fibroids occupying less than half of the volume of the uterine cavity can be approached hysteroscopically with the Nd:YAG laser (Figure 22.1). The myomas are transsected with the YAG laser using a contact method until the entire myoma is removed down to the level of its attachment to the uterine myometrium.

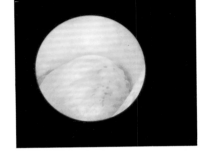

Figure 22.1: Submucous fibroids occupying less than half of the volume of the uterine cavity are approached hysteroscopically with the Nd:YAG laser.

Preoperative preparation

One of the components of Asherman's syndrome is an atrophic endometrium, and therefore most surgeons prefer to prepare the endometrium prior to proceeding with Nd:YAG laser treatment. Dr Goldrath and his colleagues have recommended danazol 400 mg twice daily for four weeks prior to the proposed surgery. This creates a thin atrophic endometrium, exposing the basal regenerative layer which the YAG laser energy must penetrate in order to assure a complete Asherman's syndrome. YAG laser energy, dispersed at 40–60 W of power, will result in a penetration of the endometrium at 4–6 mm in depth. It therefore becomes imperative that the endometrium is less than 6 mm in thickness.

GNRH agonists

Other investigators have elected to use one of the GNRH agonists in order to create the atrophic state of Asherman's syndrome. These drugs operate at the level of the pituitary gland to suppress FSH and LH activity. This results in a hypo-oestrogen state with regression of the endometrium and atrophy consistent with Asherman's syndrome. It has been found that GNRH agonists require an additional two weeks of therapy in order to obtain a suppression equivalent to danazol therapy. Intramuscular leuprorelin given at a dosage of 3.75 mg six weeks prior to surgery, and a second equivalent dosage four weeks prior to surgery, causes atrophy of the endometrium sufficient to complete laser ablation of the endometrium.

Although most patients on GNRH agonist therapy will complain of mild hot flushes, these complaints are not serious enough to warrant the discontinuation of therapy. Patients on danazol, however, have very few side-effects because the drug is only used for a four week period. Most of the androgenic side-effects of danazol commence six to eight weeks following initiation of therapy. Both of these drugs are relatively well tolerated by patients, although expense can be a significant factor for those who have limited financial resource. There is no scientific evidence that other drugs may be equally effective in producing an Asherman's syndrome. There are sporadic reports of the use of intramuscular madroxyprogesterone as well as progestin dominated birth control pills for endometrial preparation. In addition, it is possible that the atrophic component of Asherman's syndrome is not an absolute prerequisite to the destruction of the endometrium. Perhaps Nd:YAG laser energy could be applied to the endometrium during the early proliferative stage of the cycle. This could result in significant penetration of the endometrium in the basalis layer. There is a definite need for long-term prospective studies to determine the degree of uterine synechia as it relates to various types of preparation of the endometrium.

Procedure

To perform endometrial ablation, a surgeon must have a basic understanding of the mechanics and physics of the Nd:YAG laser and the surgical skills of an accomplished hysteroscopist. Proper operative equipment is vital to the success of the procedure. The system must allow for adequate uterine distension, irrigation and drainage of the operative site. The irrigation system should create optimal visualization during the surgery which will enhance the safety of the procedure. Hysteroscopy can be accomplished through a video camera or by direct vision through the lens of the operating telescope. The surgeon may select a beam splitter which will allow for direct visualization by the surgeon, while a portion of the light is transferred to a television video monitor allowing other members of the operating team to view the procedure.

Dilation of the cervix

Endometrial ablation is an outpatient surgical procedure. After induction with general anaesthesia, the patient is prepared for hysteroscopy. Regional anaesthetics can be used for those patients who do not tolerate general anaesthesia. Paracervical anaesthesia has been found to be unacceptable to most patients. The cervix is grasped with a doubletoothed tenaculum and dilated significantly to allow the hysteroscope to advance through the cervical canal. A system of overdilation of the cervix (Figure 22.2) allows the egress of the distending media to flow around the hysteroscope, over the posterior weighted retractor and finally into a plastic collecting drapery. The fluid flows into standard suction canisters which are used to record the amount of fluid that is returned from the patient. The amount of fluid that the patient has absorbed intravascularly can be estimated by subtracting the amount of fluid recovered in these canisters from the amount of fluid used to distend the uterine cavity. A gravity flow system which results in 75–100 mgHg pressure to distend the uterine cavity is preferred. The surgeon must select the larger arthroscopic tubing to obtain these pressures. Irrigation pumps add significantly to the expense of the procedure with no measurable improvement in visualization of the uterine cavity.

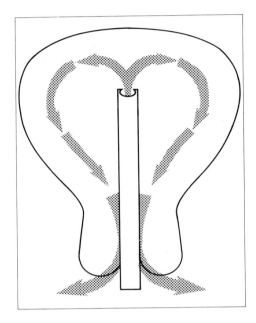

Figure 22.2: A system of over-dilation of the cervix allows the egress of the distending media to flow around the hysteroscope. The use of hysteroscopic pump systems does not require overdilation of the cervix.

Distending media

The distending media for endometrial ablation should be a balanced electrolyte solution such as normal saline or lactated ringers. Hypotonic solutions such as 5% dextrose and water can be absorbed intravenously resulting in electrolyte disturbance in the patient. High viscosity dextran solutions should not be used in operative hysteroscopy because of the potential for intravenous absorption and secondary allergic reaction or fluid overload.

Inspection and visualization

Following inspection of the uterine cavity, a 600 μm fibreoptic strand is passed through the operating channel of the hysteroscope (Figure 22.3) attached to an Nd:YAG laser with power capacity of 50–100 W in a continuous pattern. The laser energy is discharged at 40–60 W of power as the fibre is directed at the endometrial lining. Protective goggles must be worn by all personnel in the operating room in order to prevent retinal eye injury.

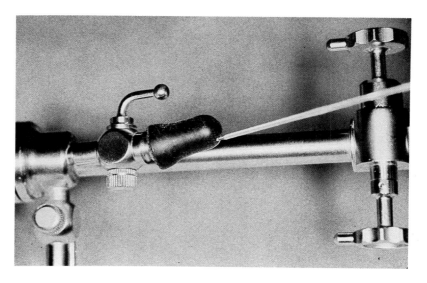

Figure 22.3: A 600 μm Nd:YAG laser fibre is passed through the operating channel of the hysteroscope. The power requirement for successful ablation ranges from 60 to 80 W in a continuous mode.

Endometrial ablation is performed under direct vision or through the video monitor. Depth perception is slightly poorer with the video system than with direct visualization through the telescope. The operating surgeon must be able to see the fibreoptic tip as well as the reflection of the helium neon beam onto the endometrium prior to firing the laser. Firing the laser while the fibreoptic tip is still in the distal end of the hysteroscope can result in significant damage to the lens system. The fibreoptic tip must never pass through the endometrium, in order to avoid damage of the uterus and intra-abdominal organs. The endometrial surface is destroyed by systematically and continuously moving the hysteroscope in a triangular pattern so that the endometrium is ablated down to the level of the internal cervical os. The ablation should begin at each cornual opening of the fallopian tubes. As the laser energy is discharged, the cornual openings will close as a direct result of tissue oedema and muscular spasm. This closure is only temporary, but does prevent the reflux of the distending media through the fallopian tubes into the peritoneal cavity. Once both the cornual areas are ablated, the surgeon should make a path connecting them and then continue the ablation along the side walls of the endometrial cavity. The success of the procedure depends on the completeness of the ablative process. It is important that the surgeon proceeds in a systematic fashion with slight overlapping of the paths of destruction as the lateral walls are ablated. To avoid a cervical stenosis with subsequent haematometrium, laser energy should not be discharged into the endocervical canal.

Bleeding

If significant bleeding is encountered during the procedure, the Nd:YAG laser energy can be discharged in a non-contact fashion to coagulate the bleeding vessel. If the YAG laser energy is insufficient to control the uterine bleeding adequately, the surgeon can put in place an intrauterine Foley catheter with a 50 cc balloon. Once the balloon is inserted into the uterine cavity and filled with normal saline, a downward traction should be placed to occlude the cervical os. The pressure of the bleeding vessel will eventually be surpassed by the distension pressure within the uterine cavity with resultant haemostasis. If the balloon becomes necessary for uncontrollable bleeding, the patient should be admitted overnight and the catheter balloon removed the following morning. The patient will have to return at a later date for the completion of the endometrial ablation.

Dragging vs Blanching

The procedure of endometrial ablation was originally described by Goldrath[2] and further documented by Lomano[3] and Loffer in 1987[4]. In the

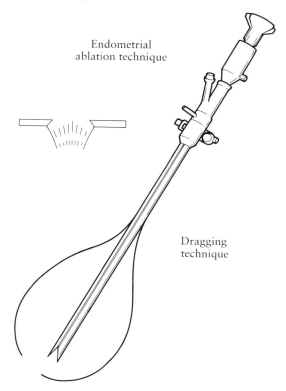

Endometrial
ablation technique

Dragging
technique

Figure 22.4: The procedure of endometrial ablation (dragging technique). Application of this technique requires complete destruction of the endometrium since small pieces of tissue may remain in between the furrows.

dragging technique (Figure 22.4), the Nd:YAG laser fibre is brought into direct contact with the endometrium while the laser energy is discharged in a continuous wave using 40–60 W of power. The surgeon moves the hysteroscope in a back-and-forth motion to create furrows of thermally destroyed endometrium. Thermal conduction of the Nd:YAG laser energy to the proteins of the endometrium results in charring of the endometrium. As the fibre cuts through endometrial blood vessels, bleeding into the endometrial cavity can obscure the visual field. In addition, the open veins and arteries can conduct the distending fluid into the vascular system of the patient, with the risk of fluid overload. Significant fluid overload in patients with a compromised cardiovascular system can lead to pulmonary oedema and congestive heart failure.

The blanching technique described by Lomano (Figure 22.5) involves withdrawing the fibre 1–5 mm from the endometrial surface prior to firing the YAG laser energy[5]. Using this technique, the surgeon employs an additional 10 W of power and proceeds with a symmetrical endometrial ablation down to the level of the internal cervical os. The blanching technique results in changing the endometrium from its normal tan or pink colour to snow-white. As the YAG energy passes through the endometrial tissue, there is coaptation of the blood vessels within the endometrium. This prevents

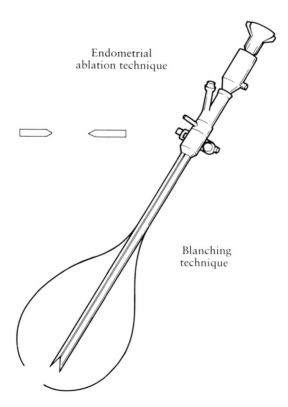

Endometrial
ablation technique

Blanching
technique

Figure 22.5: The procedure of endometrial ablation (blanching technique). The risk of fluid overload is slightly less with this technique as deep laser energy coagulates blood vessels.

bleeding into the distending media and prevents the distending media from entering into the patient's vascular system. Using the endpoints of charring in the dragging technique and the snow-white effect with the blanching technique, the surgeon maintains a consistent 4–6 mm of thermal necrosis of the endometrium.

The blanching technique prevents the problem of visual field clouding as well as fluid overload in patients with a compromised cardiovascular system. However, it is difficult to develop a right-angle approach in the lower uterine segment to accomplish the blanching technique. For this reason, the surgeon should proceed with endometrial ablation using the blanching technique in all areas of the endometrium that are accessible with direct discharge of the laser energy. In the lower uterine segment an open angle approach is not always possible, and the surgeon has access to the endometrium only with a tangential angle of the laser fibre. It is often necessary to complete the endometrial ablation in the lower uterine segment using the dragging technique originally described by Goldrath[2].

When using the dragging technique, the 600 μm fibre is in direct contact with the endometrium. This results in a much smaller spot size than when the fibre is withdrawn in the blanching technique. Because of the larger spot size, an endometrial ablation technique is accomplished in a shorter time than with the dragging technique. In the dragging technique the fibre also comes in direct contact with carbon particles, resulting in over-heating of the fibre and fracture of its terminal portion. These fractures can result in an extremely large spot size, significantly diminishing the power density. Therefore the laser must be held in contact with the tissue for a longer period of time. This problem adds to the time necessary to accomplish the dragging technique. The problem can be solved by replacing the fractured fibre with a new fibreoptic bundle. It is important to overlap the patterns of tissue destruction in both techniques (Figure 22.6).

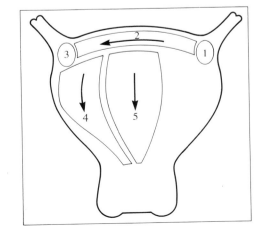

Figure 22.6: Regardless of the type of technique selected (drag vs blanch), it is important to overlap the tissue destruction to prevent residual remnants of tissue from being left at the completion of the procedure. A completely destroyed endometrium provides very satisfactory long term results.

Postoperative results

Patients are discharged on the day of surgery, with instructions to avoid strenuous activity for two or three days. There is often a watery or bloody discharge for up to six weeks following endometrial ablation. Delayed haemorrhage is an extremely rare complication. Postoperative endometritis, also a rare complication, is easily treated with second generation cephalosporin drugs. Unlike with hysterectomy, most patients are able to resume normal activities after three days and also to return to work relatively quickly, adding to the financial benefits of this procedure. Premenstrual syndrome has also been shown to improve following laser ablation[6].

Our results demonstrate a dramatic decrease in menstrual flow in patients with normal, enlarged or fibroid uteri (less than 16 weeks' gestational size)[7]. Table 22.1 demonstrates the pattern of flow prior to endometrial ablation in each of these three categories. Table 22.2 demonstrates a marked reduction in menstrual flow following Nd:YAG laser ablation. About 50% of patients undergoing laser ablation of the endometrium will become totally amenor-

	Normal uterus	Enlarged uterus	Uterine fibroids
Amenorrhoea	0	0	0
Light flow	1 (1%)	0	2 (6%)
Normal flow	2 (3%)	6 (9%)	1 (3%)
Heavy flow	33 (53%)	51 (79%)	11 (33%)
Severe flow	27 (43%)	8 (12%)	19 (58%)
Total	63	65	33

Table 22.1: Menses prior to ablation.

	Normal uterus	Enlarged uterus	Uterine fibroids
Amenorrhoea	34 (54%)	32 (49%)	16 (49%)
Light flow	9 (14%)	27 (42%)	13 (39%)
Normal flow	15 (24%)	5 (7%)	4 (12%)
Heavy flow	5 (8%)	1 (2%)	0
Severe flow	0	0	0
Total	63	65	33

Table 22.2: Menses after ablation.

rhoeic, and an additional 30–35% will have light cyclic flows, very often requiring only one or two tampons per month. Approximately 95% of patients are satisfied with the results. Only two of 161 patients had to undergo hysterectomy because of ongoing menometrorrhagia. Repeat endometrial ablation can be offered to patients with persistent bleeding.

There have been sporadic reports of gas embolization during endometrial ablation when the surgeon has incorrectly selected a 'gas fibre' as opposed to a 'bare' urological fibre. The use of a gas-cooled sapphire tip is totally inappropriate for ablation of the endometrium.

Conclusions

Endometrial ablation is a safe and effective alternative to hysterectomy in patients with chronic menorrhagia refractory to surgical and medical therapy[7]. It reduces the bleeding sufficiently to avoid major surgery in the majority of patients. Endometrial ablation may decrease the symptoms of the menstrual syndrome. The enlarged or fibroid uterus is not necessarily a contraindication to endometrial ablation and may be effective in at least temporarily controlling bleeding. The blanching technique minimizes the problems of visual field clouding and potential fluid overload. Ongoing perspective randomized studies will be required to determine the long-term effectiveness of the procedure.

References

1   Asherman JG (1948) Amenorrhea traumatica atretica. *Journal of Obstetrics and Gynaecology.* **55r:23.**

2   Goldrath MH *et al.* (1981) Laser photovaporization of the endometrium for the treatment of menorrhagia. *American Journal of Obstetrics and Gynecology.* **140:14.**

3   Lomano JM (1987) Ablation of the endometrium with the Nd:YAG laser: a multicenter study. *Colposcopy and Gyneocological Laser Surgery.* **2:4.**

4   Loffer FD (1987) Hysteroscopic endometrial ablation with the Nd:YAG laser using a non-touch technique. *Obstetrics and Gynecology.* **69:4.**

5   Lomano JM (1988) *American Journal of Obstetrics and Gynecology.* **159:152–5.**

6   Lefler H Jr (1989) Premenstrual syndrome improvement after laser ablation for menorrhea. *Journal of Reproductive Medicine.* **34:905–6.**

7   Garry R, Erian J and Grochmal SA (1991) A multi-centre collaborative study into the treatment of menorrhagia by Nd:YAG laser ablation of the endometrium. *British Journal of Obstetrics and Gynaecology.* **98:357–60.**

23

Endometrial Ablation Using SideFire Laser Fibre

ROYICE B. EVERETT

Introduction

Abnormal uterine bleeding accounts for approximately 200 000 hysterectomies in the USA each year, or approximately 20–30% of the 750 000 hysterectomies performed annually[1]. Several different methods to control abnormal uterine bleeding have been developed, because of the morbidity and the length of recovery associated with traditional hysterectomy.

Historical development

Prior to 1981, all of these modalities resulted in either unacceptable side-effects or were unsuccessful in causing significant long-term reduction in bleeding because of the significant regenerative powers of the endometrium[2]. In 1981, however, Dr Milton Goldrath reported his successful use of the Neodymium:YAG laser to accomplish endometrial ablation[3].

The Nd:YAG laser is particularly suited to this operation since it has a very deep penetrating wavelength resulting in approximately 4–6 mm of tissue coagulation. In addition to the deep destructive power of the Nd:YAG laser, the patient was pre-treated with 200 mg of danazol four times daily for two to four weeks to cause a hypo-oestrogenic state and therefore a reduction in the depth of the endometrial lining. Complications reported in this initial study include fluid overload due to extravasation of the distending media into the intravascular space.

Dragging

This report by Goldrath[3], as well as early reports by Lomano[4], described the so-called 'dragging' technique, in which the laser fibre is brought into direct contact with the endometrial lining, causing charring of the endometrium from thermal conduction of the Nd:YAG laser energy to the endometrial tissue. This technique necessarily involves cutting through endometrial blood vessels as well as opening up lymphatics as the endometrium is stripped away with a vaporization cutting mode. It was felt that this technique, which involves opening up veins and arteries as well as lymphatics to the fluid medium, could be partially responsible for the fluid overload in some patients, causing the complications of cardiovascular overload, congestive failure and pulmonary oedema.

Blanching

In 1987, Loffer[5] described a separate technique involving blanching of the endometrial lining by withdrawing the fibre 1–5 mm from the surface of the endometrium and firing the Nd:YAG laser energy directly into the tissue without the fibre coming in contact. This particular technique causes coagulation of the endometrium as well as blood vessels and lymphatics, therefore theoretically causing less potential for fluid loss. The end-point in this technique is an observed colour change from the usual pink to tan colour of the endometrial lining following hypo-oestrogenism to a snow-white fluffy cotton appearance. This technique necessarily closes blood vessels and coagulates the entire lining, as opposed to the cutting and ablation of the dragging technique. This results in less fluid loss as well as a significant increase in the amenorrhoea rate over the dragging technique[6].

Since the traditional laser fibre allowed laser energy to come out directly only in the same axis as the fibre, treatment of the sidewalls and lower uterine segment was extremely difficult; at best, it resulted in a tangential firing of the laser beam, therefore resulting in a much larger spot size and difficulty in obtaining adequate coagulation of the side walls. Therefore a method to blanch (in a non-touch technique) the entire lining of the uterus was sought. In 1987, Everett introduced the concept of a laser fibre that would deliver the energy from the fibre at a 90° angle to the fibre axis. These early attempts resulted in fibres which were either ineffective in delivering reflection of the laser beam or absorbed too much of the laser energy resulting in overheating of the tip itself.

Everett[7] used a side-firing laser device known as the Lateral-Lase Fiber on an initial group of seven patients. This fibre did improve results in a small group: six patients had slight spotting or amenorrhoea and one patient had a reduction to normal flow. However, the fibre was inadequate for long-term use and the design was abandoned. In 1990, the tip was re-engineered and redesigned as what is now known as the SideFire fibre manufactured by Microbiomed in Dallas, Texas and sold by MyriadLase of Forest Hills, Texas.

Description of the device

The solid gold tip of 99.95 + % purity shown in Figure 23.1 incorporates a flat mirror that deflects the central ray of the beam emerging from the flat end of the 600 μm diameter fibre through a 105° angle, resulting in a laterally directed beam. Gold was chosen as the material comprising the entire tip primarily because of its high infrared reflectivity of >98% for wavelengths >1 μm[8], which includes the 1.064 μm wavelength of the surgical Nd:YAG laser, its high thermal conductivity (3.15 Wcm^{-1}C)[9] and its relative inertness to body tissues and fluids (biocompatibility).

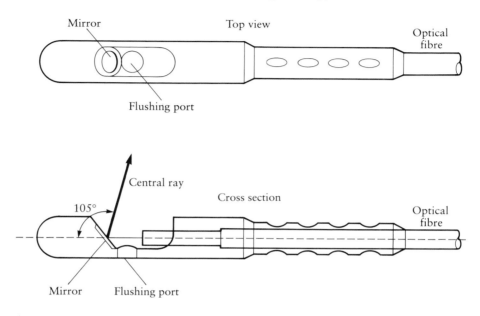

Figure 23.1: Schematic top and side views of the SideFire device.

The monolithic or singleblock design of pure gold was chosen to optimize both volume heat transfer and heat sinking to the aqueous irrigating solution normally used during laser coagulation of tissue. The lack of surface oxidation and relative resistance to build-up of a proteinaceous layer on the surface of the gold tip serves to maintain heat sinking during lasing in irrigated body cavities at Nd:YAG laser input power tested up to 80 W.

A hole connecting the lateral bottom surface of the tip and the chamber surrounding mirror and fibre end serves to direct fluid flow over the mirror and fibre end, helping to flush debris and further minimize build-up of proteinaceous material.

The device incorporates a flat-ended 600 μm diameter fused silica 3 m fibre with polymeric cladding and buffer coat. The fibre is attached to the surgical laser via an SMA 905 connector.

A holding and torquing device with the cross-section of a hexagonal cylinder can be positioned axially along the fibre length. This device allows axial translation and torsion about the fibre axis for angular positioning of the laser beam.

Optical performance

Intensity profiles measured across the beam emitted from both typical flat-ended and SideFire fibres are plotted in Figure 23.2. Profiles measured along two mutually perpendicular diameters of the flat-ended fibre pattern were averaged and plotted as shown. Mutually perpendicular profiles determined for the SideFire tip were plotted separately.

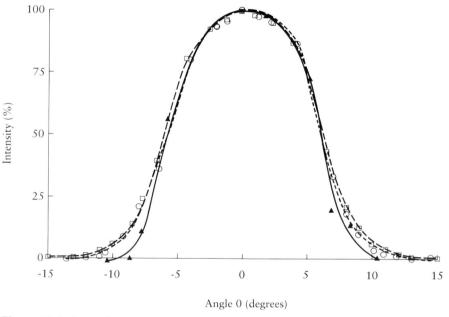

Figure 23.2: Laser beam intensity profiles determined for the bare-ended and SideFire tipped fibres. ▲, bare tip; ○, SideFire tip (R1 direction); □, SideFire tip (R2 direction).

The light-intensity pattern emitted by the flat-ended fibre distinctly shows a 7° divergence half-angle, and the essential retention of the divergence angle is shown in the intensity profiles of the SideFire pattern[10]. Integration using the flux integral 6 for flat-ended and SideFire tip data gives the angular power distribution or the fraction of total energy within the intensity profile emitted in the conical volume lying between the axial ray and the cone angle θ[11]. These profiles are shown in Figure 23.3. The 7° half-angle divergence of the bare-ended fibre and the emission into a cone of 15° half-angle containing over 95% of the energy reflected by the SideFire tip are evident.

The measurements of the power emitted by a family of six representative bare-ended and six SideFire fibres fabricated using bare-ended fibres of the same lot gave computed values of average emitted power in air and associated standard deviations of 19.4 ± 0.42 W and 18.12 ± 0.32 W, respectively, at 20 W input laser power setting. Average percentage of incident power-reflected by the gold mirror of the SideFire device is computed to be

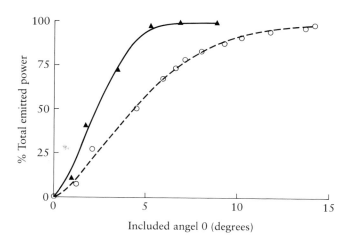

Figure 23.3: Angular distribution of relative values of the total power emitted by bare-ended and SideFire® tipped fibres. ▲, bare tip; ○, SideFire tip.

$93.4 \pm 3\%$ for the representative fibres tested. Approximately 2% of the loss arises from the small absorption by gold; the remainder we ascribe to higher angle scattering from small mirror imperfections[11].

Patient selection and preparation

The patient selection and preoperative preparation is carried out as described in detail elsewhere in this book. To summarize this process, any patient who is a candidate for hysterectomy secondary to abnormal uterine bleeding that has no other pathology or symptoms necessitating removal of the uterus itself, is a candidate for endometrial ablation. For preoperative preparation either Danocrine or Depo-Lupron (leuprolide acetate) is adequate for endometrial suppression, because of reliability of administration and reduction in side-effects. We prefer Depo-Lupron. Other medication regimens using medroxyprogesterone acetate as well as birth-control pills have been suggested; however, these alternative preparations have all resulted in a decrease in postoperative success.

Procedure

Once adequate endometrial suppression has occurred, the patient is taken to the operating room where the cervix is dilated and the hysteroscope placed under general anaesthetic. The hysteroscope should have a dual-flow system, allowing both for infusing of distending media as well as aspiration through unique ports which extend the length of the hysteroscope. This dual-flow system ensures adequate cleansing during the entire case and permits good visualization and adequate distension. Direct viewing through the scope is a possibility, although using a video monitor allows for better visualization. Once the hysteroscope is in place and the field of view is clear, the bare urologic 600 μm fibre is used, beginning in the ostial portions of the fundus at 60 W to go around the circumference of ostia. The fundus of the uterus is then ablated so that all of the tissues that are at right angles to the axis of the fibre can be treated. Once this is accomplished, the SideFire fibre is placed into the uterine cavity and the laser is advanced to 70 W. The entire side walls anterior and posterior are treated in a blanching technique with the laser reflecting at 105° to the forward axis of the fibre. This allows for total perpendicular access of the laser beam to the side walls of the endometrial cavity. Moreover, this allows for total blanching of the entire uterine cavity, therefore resulting in a greater depth of uniform penetration in the side walls as well as decreased disruption of vasculature and blood vessels and a consequent reduction in fluid loss. Everett[12], in his first 27 patients treated with the latest version of the SideFire fibre, reported a total amenorrhoea rate of 86%: ie 23 of the 27 cases have resulted in total amenorrhoea, while the other four patients have slight bleeding for three days each month. This study would tend to confirm the theoretical benefit of having the Nd:YAG energy available for right-angle delivery to all intrauterine tissue and allowing for complete destruction of the lining of the uterus. Since the fibre never comes into contact with the endometrial lining, perforation and bowel injury are not possible, and avoiding disruption of the uterine vasculature results in a decrease in fluid loss into the intravascular space. The rate of amenorrhoea is substantially higher than reported rates in patients treated either with the Nd:YAG laser alone or with the rollerball unipolar cautery technique[13–15]

Conclusions

Endometrial ablation is a safe and effective alternative to hysterectomy, regardless of the technique used or the instrumentation. However, it would appear from these early studies that use of the SideFire fibre and the technique of blanching the entire uterine cavity have resulted in significantly increased amenorrhoea rates. It is obvious that we need to follow up a much larger number of patients, and for a longer period of time, before we can draw any firm conclusions about the benefits of this technique.

References

1 National Center for Health Statistics (1987) *Hysterectomies in the States 1965–84*. Pub. No. 88–1753. US Dept of Health.

2 Droegemullen W *et al.* (1971) Cryosurgery in patients with dysfunctional bleeding. *Obstetrics and Gynecology*. **38**:256.

3 Goldrath MH *et al.* (1981) Laser photovaporization of the endometrium for the treatment of menorrhagia. *American Journal of Obstetrics and Gynecology*. **140**:14.

4 Lomano JM (1987) Ablation of the endometrium with the Nd:YAG laser: a multi-center study. *Colposcopy and Gynecology Laser Surgery*. **2**:4.

5 Loffer FD (1987) Hysteroscopic endometrium ablation using the Nd:YAG laser using a non-touch technique. *Obstetrics and Gynecology*. **69**:4.

6 Lomano JM (1988) Dragging as blanching technique for endometrial ablations with the Nd:YAG laser in the treatment of chronic menorrhagia. *American Journal of Obstetrics and Gynecology*. **159**:152.

7 Everett RB (1989) *Proceedings of the 18th annual AAGL meeting.*

8 Wolfe WL (1978) Property of optical materials. *Handbook of optics*. New York. pp.1–157.

9 Weost RC (1933) *Handbook of chemistry and physics*, 54th edn. CRC Press, Cleveland, Ohio.

10 Judy MM *et al.* (1993) Sidefiring laser-fiber technology for benign prostate hypertrophy in medical lasers and systems II. In: Karns M, Pluney CM (eds). *Proceedings of the SPIE*, 86–91.

11 Moon P (1961) *The scientific basis of illumination engineering*. Dover Publications, New York. p.607.

12 Everett RB (1994) Endometrial ablation using SideFire laser fiber. *Journal of AAGL*. **1**:253.

13 Townsend DE *et al.* (1990) Rollerball coagulation of the endometrium. *Obstetrics and Gynecology*. **76**:310.

14 Donell JF *et al.* (1992) Hysteroscopic endometrial ablation using the rollerball electrolyte. *Obstetrics and Gynecology*. **80**:329.

15 Vancaillie TG (1989) Electrocoagulation of the endometrium with the ball end resectoscope. *Obstetrics and Gynecology*. **74**:425.

24

Hysteroscopic Surgery for Menorrhagia: Long-Term Outlook and Anxieties

JOHN ERIAN and MARTIN STEEL

Introduction

Minimal access treatments for menorrhagia include transcervical (electro-surgical) resection of the endometrium (TCRE) or rollerball coagulation, hysteroscopic endometrial laser ablation (HELA) and radio-frequency abla-tion (RFA). Other modalities such as cryosurgery to the endometrium and endometrial heating have also been investigated. HELA and TCRE have been the techniques adopted most enthusiastically, and these operations are rapidly becoming widespread.

HELA was first described in 1981 by Goldrath et al., who reported 18 cases[1]; TCRE was first described in 1983 by de Cherney and Polan, who reported 11 cases[2]. Therefore, currently the maximum length of follow-up can only be around 13 years for HELA, and scarcely 11 years for TCRE. Moreover, the number of patients followed up for this length of time is very small, the majority of these operations having been performed in the last few years.

Aims of treatment

The principal application for these operations is for the treatment of menorrhagia in the pre-menopausal woman. In the majority of cases this is treating dysfunctional uterine bleeding, but there are also many cases of submucous myomata which can be successfully treated hysteroscopically. Hysteroscopic surgery is usually only applied after the failure of medical treatment, and most authors stress that patients should be counselled that the operation is performed as an alternative to hysterectomy. The aim of treatment is clearly to change the patient's menstrual pattern from an unacceptable to an acceptable level. During the procedure it is possible to attempt to destroy the entire endometrium, or to leave a small of amount of intact tissue above the cervix to allow menstruation to continue (although much lighter than before). Both techniques have been advocated by various authors, and there have also been published studies where the patient was allowed to choose between the two types of procedure. Magos et al.[3] reported 250 patients, 227 of whom had undergone a complete endometrial resection; Boto et al.[4] reported four out of 17 women who had elected for a partial resection. It seems likely, therefore, that the overwhelming majority of women wish to become amenorrhoeic, and may consider the persistence or return of even light menstruation to be a failure of treatment. When interpreting reports of successful results, it may useful to bear this in mind.

Author	Method	N	Length of follow-up (mths)	Amenorrhoea, N(%)	Improved	No better
Magos et al.[3]	E	250	3–24	≈ 25	≈ 25	≈ 10
Rankin and Steinberg[5]	E	396	4	336 (85)		60 (15)
Gannon et al.[6]	E	25	9–16	16 (64)	4 (16)	5 (20)
Garry et al.[7]	L	479	6	288 (60)	152 (39)	39 (8)
Bent and Ostergard[8]	L	42	3–24	14 (33)	20 (48)	8 (19)
Loffer[9]	L	33	3	11 (33)	20 (61)	2 (6)
Nisolle et al.[10]	L (total)	50	Not stated	17 (34)	30 (60)	3 (6)
Nisolle et al.[10]	L (partial)	100	Not stated	1 (1)	93 (93)	6 (6)
Goldrath[11]	L	321	Not stated	148 (45)	153 (48)	22 (7)
Total:	E/L	1050	3–24	493 (47)	472 (45)	85 (8)

Table 24.1: The effects on menstruation (patient satisfaction) after the procedure. E = Electrosurgery methods; L = laser ablation. Totals do not include the first two studies, where a precise breakdown of the figures is not possible.

In the short term, between six and 19% of reported patients have not been improved by the treatment (Table 24.1). Many of these patients were satisfied after a repeat hysteroscopic procedure, and the numbers requiring a hysterectomy were low. This short-term success, the minimal hospitalization and the rapid recovery to normal activities is no doubt responsible for the procedure's increasing popularity among gynaecologists and the increasing public demand.

Long-term results: published evidence

We have already noted that the maximum possible length of follow-up is currently a little more than 10 years for both HELA and TCRE. No series or even individual cases have been published involving follow-up periods as long as this. Some of the papers listed in Table 24.1 do include patients followed up for three years or more, but the data concerning this small group of patients are generally not separated from those concerning the much larger group with shorter follow-up periods, and therefore no long-term conclusions can be drawn. Rankin and Steinberg[5] presented a large series of patients followed up for four months, and contended that the success rates at eight years would be the same as those found at four months. There seems little evidence to support this, although we must concede that there is no evidence to refute this claim either. Goldrath[11] presented a series followed up for up to six years, and Loffer's series[12] had a follow-up of up to 4½ years. No differences have been suggested in those patients followed up for the longer periods of time, but again the studies include patients at varying postoperative times.

Loffer[12] stated that these data confirm that short-term follow-up success rates accurately reflect the success rates likely to be found in the long term. We feel that this is indeed likely to be the case, but cannot agree that the point has been proven. We are currently undertaking a retrospective study of all the long-term patients we have treated, and hope to be able to resolve this question. It is clear, however, that a small number of patients may return with menstrual problems after many problem-free years. The chances of this happening cannot be determined from the current literature, however, and we will need more long-term reports if we are to give patients proper information about what to expect in 10 or even 20 years' time. It is important that any patients returning because of an unexpected recurrence of or increase in menstruation are evaluated hysteroscopically and with an endometrial biopsy. This is because of the (so far theoretical) risk of an endometrial carcinoma developing insidiously after an endometrial ablation or resection (*see* below).

Anxieties in the long term

Development of endometrial carcinoma

One criticism frequently levelled at the hysteroscopic surgical management of menorrhagia is that, in creating an artificial Asherman syndrome, 'islands' of residual endometrium may remain in the fundal or cornual regions, isolated from the rest of the uterus. It has been suggested that endometrial carcinoma may develop undetected in these islands. Endometrial carcinoma accounted for over 1200 deaths in England and Wales in 1983. It frequently presents as irregular or heavy vaginal bleeding. 74% of cases present in the early stages of the disease and the prognosis in these patients is very good, the five-year survival of stage 1 being over 70%. If, after surgery, endometrial carcinoma develops in an island of endometrium which does not communicate freely with the outside, then it is possible that the diagnosis could be delayed, with serious consequences for the patient. We must therefore remain vigilant, and tell patients to report the return of vaginal bleeding, particularly if this is irregular or occurs some considerable time after the original procedure. It must also be appreciated that the very reason for the delay in presentation may make diagnosis difficult, and conventional dilatation and curettage is likely to be inadequate. We feel that a careful hysteroscopy and directed biopsy are essential methods of diagnosis.

However, anxieties are likely to prove unfounded for the following reasons.

- The frequent persistence of menstruation after surgery suggests that obstruction to flow is not a problem.

- If islands of endometrium are isolated, then a localized haematometra is likely to develop after the operation, and this would present initially as cyclical pelvic pain. The case reported by Slade *et al.* undoubtedly represents such a problem[13]. We have indeed treated such patients either by repeat hysteroscopic procedure or by hysterectomy.

- No case of a delayed presentation of carcinoma of the endometrium following hysteroscopic surgery has so far been reported.

- There are no cases in the literature of carcinoma of the endometrium being concealed by Asherman syndrome.

- Those patients who have had their endometrium completely destroyed are likely to be at a decreased incidence of endometrial carcinoma, and the overall incidence in this group is therefore likely to be reduced.

However, it is crucial that patients do not have an abnormal or malignant endometrium before the operation, and preoperative investigation is mandatory: certainly for HELA, where histological samples are not obtained, but possibly also TCRE. Rankin and Steinberg reported four out of 400 cases of TCRE showing carcinoma in the resected chippings. In two of these cases preoperative curettage was not performed, and in one the tumour was present in an endometrial polyp, which would have been available for histological analysis even after laser treatment. However, the other patient had had both hysteroscopy and biopsy, yet still had a tumour detected only by histological analysis of the chippings.

It is undoubtedly true that the risk of developing endometrial carcinoma is removed if a patient has a hysterectomy. However, if hysteroscopic surgery does not conceal these tumours and delay presentation, then it is very difficult to argue that hysterectomy is preferable on the grounds of prophylaxis alone. One possible advantage of an open operation is that the pelvic organs are directly observed, and an unsuspected pathology may be detected. Given the availability of modern diagnostic imaging, however, this is hardly sufficient justification for laparotomy; but lifelong monitoring of patients who have undergone these operations is essential in order to assess the long-term sequelae. We have already suggested that the incidence of endometrial carcinoma may be decreased due to the destruction of most, if not all, of the functioning endometrium; on the other hand it may be that the extreme heat damage and tissue destruction caused by the techniques may make carcinoma of the endometrium more likely to occur, or that uterine sarcomata could occur for similar reasons. There is no actual evidence of this, but again only long-term observation will be able to provide the necessary proof.

Hormone replacement therapy after endometrial surgery

The overwhelming majority of these procedures are performed in the pre-menopausal age group, but there is a wide age range. Our patients participating in a multi-centre study had a mean age of 39 years (range 21–54 years)[7]. This is similar to the series presented by Magos et al. (mean age 42.3, range 18–54 years). Rankin and Steinberg[5] reported a mean age of 45, with a range of 24–72 years. 15 of their patients were treated because of postmenopausal bleeding or excessive bleeding on hormone replacement therapy (HRT).

HRT is becoming increasingly common in the western world, both for the treatment of symptoms and for the putative benefits in the prevention of osteoporosis and arteriovascular disease. It is clear that over the next decade many patients who have undergone hysteroscopic surgery will seek HRT. Symptomatic relief and possible therapeutic benefit can be provided by oestrogen alone, but it is established practice to give progesterone cyclically to those with an intact uterus to prevent the development of endometrial hyperplasia and possible endometrial carcinoma. Those patients with regular menstruation or oligomenorrhoea postoperatively must be assumed to retain some intact endometrium, and should be prescribed a combined HRT preparation. There are theoretical benefits in prescribing unopposed oestrogen, however, particularly in the case of the deleterious effect on lipid metabolism of the androgen-derived progestogens. In addition, many patients experience unpleasant cyclical effects akin to premenstrual tension when taking the combined preparations. After hysterectomy, therefore, patients requiring or requesting HRT are generally prescribed unopposed oestrogen.

The question that remains unanswered is whether or not those patients who are amenorrhoeic after hysteroscopic surgery should be considered to have an intact uterus. If we could be confident that the entire endometrium had been destroyed, then we could reasonably prescribe unopposed oestrogen with impunity; but there are no published data addressing this problem.

For some time we have been looking carefully at those patients who reach the appropriate age and request HRT, or who were postmenopausal at the time of the procedure. To date we have encountered 187 such patients. Our initial treatment has been to prescribe a standard combined HRT preparation. If the patient remains amenorrhoeic after three months of therapy, then they are given appropriate counselling and placed on unopposed oestrogen (either by implant, patch or orally). After six months of such therapy, patients remaining on treatment undergo a diagnostic hysteroscopy and biopsy. If no functioning endometrium is demonstrated, then treatment with unopposed oestrogen continues. Obviously while on such therapy these patients require careful gynaecological follow-up, and the usual UK arrangements of delegating long-term management to the patient's general practitioner is not appropriate.

At present there is inadequate knowledge about how to manage HRT after hysteroscopic surgery; therefore we can only recommend that patients should be treated as if they had an intact uterus, whether they are amenorrhoeic or not. It will be many years before anyone is able to make any alternative recommendations with confidence. Meanwhile we are continuing to monitor our patients carefully to detect any long-term adverse effects.

Pregnancy after endometrial surgery

We routinely counsel our patients that the procedure will seriously impair fertility and that it is to be considered as an alternative to hysterectomy. Many authors have suggested that sterilization should be undertaken at the same time as the hysteroscopic procedure. This was often said to alleviate the problem of fluid absorption, by preventing the back flow of fluid along the fallopian tubes. This is not, however, a significant contributing factor in the aetiology of fluid overload. At the time of the procedure we ensure that the tubal ostia are coagulated by the laser, although we do inform our patients that the operation is not a method of contraception, and that pregnancy is not an absolute impossibility. We further inform patients that pregnancy may be hazardous, both to the developing fetus and possibly even to the mother herself.

To date there have been no major published series detailing the incidence of pregnancy after hysteroscopic surgery for menorrhagia, although there have been two individual case reports[14,15].

The theoretical problems with pregnancy include intrauterine growth retardation and a morbidly adherent placenta. If termination of pregnancy is chosen, there may be problems with bleeding, and it may be difficult to obtain a complete evacuation of the uterus.

One of the authors (J.E.) has personally performed around 1300 procedures using the Nd:YAG laser, and we are aware of 16 pregnancies (1.2%). As the local population is relatively stable, it is likely that this is a reasonably accurate reflection of the number of pregnancies to have resulted. Of the 16 cases:

- all had some degree of persistent menstruation
- all were made aware that if they wished termination of pregnancy then this would be available, and that indeed this may be advisable
- all patients presented before 14 weeks, so it was possible to offer a routine suction termination to those that wished it.

Thirteen of the 16 patients opted to have termination of pregnancy:

- seven had conceived between five and nine months postoperatively
- two had conceived between nine and 12 months postoperatively
- one had conceived between 12 and 18 months postoperatively
- three had conceived between 18 and 24 months postoperatively.

All of the terminations were performed under general anaesthetic by a consultant gynaecologist with crossmatched blood available. All cases proceeded uneventfully. Blood loss was not routinely measured in these cases, but in no instance was it considered to be excessive, and no patient required a blood transfusion.

Three of the patients elected to continue with the pregnancy.

Case 1: the pregnancy was complicated by mid-trimester pre-eclampsia, despite the fact that the patient was a multigravida. The pregnancy ended in an elective caesarian section at 31 weeks of gestation because of failure of fetal growth. The baby weighed 1.2 kg (less than the fifth centile) and appears neurodevelopmentally normal. Although blood loss was not excessive, it was noted that the placenta was difficult to remove at the time of the caesarian section.

Case 2: everything progressed uneventfully, except that fetal growth retardation resulted in a caesarian section at 34 weeks of gestation. Again the placenta was difficult to remove. The baby weighed 1.6 kg (again less than the fifth centile) and subsequent development also appears normal.

Case 3: as with the two cases described above, the only problem was intra-uterine growth retardation. This again resulted in caesarian section, performed because of fetal compromise at 37 weeks of gestation. On this occasion it actually proved impossible to remove the placenta, and a caesarian hysterectomy was performed. The baby weighed 2 kg (less than the 10th centile). Subsequent neonatal development again appears normal.

In all of the cases seen by ourselves the patients were not amenorrhoeic, and it may seem logical to assume that the patient is sterile if amenorrhoea results from the procedure. However, in the case reported by Mongelli and Evans, pregnancy occurred after 18 months of amenorrhoea[11]. Those patients with oligomenorrhoea (and possibly those who are amenorrhoeic) still have a small amount of functioning endometrium within the uterus. Unquestionably these patients have greatly reduced fertility (and may have been sterilized previously or at the time of the procedure), but many may retain the potential to conceive – which may occur some considerable time after the original surgery. All patients who have not been sterilized should be made aware of the possibility of pregnancy occurring even some considerable time in the future, as well as the fact that the pregnancy may be complicated and indeed hazardous.

Ovarian function after endometrial surgery

After hysterectomy with conservation of the ovaries, it is well recognized that ovarian failure can occur earlier than would otherwise have been the case had hysterectomy not been performed[16]. The conventional explanation is that it is due to interference with the ovarian blood supply. There is no doubt that hysterectomy interferes with the normal pattern of ovarian blood flow, but it is difficult to say whether there is any contributory effect due to loss of the end organ (the endometrium).

Does the ablation of the endometrium, and hence the removal of an important end organ for the ovary, influence subsequent ovarian function? It is hoped that long-term follow-up will provide the answer to this question. A very short-term (four month) analysis of the FSH and LH concentrations after TCRE has suggested that there is no immediate effect on ovarian function[4]. Only 11 patients were studied, however, and the blood levels were slightly higher than before treatment. This difference may, however, reflect a 'hangover' effect from the eight weeks of preoperative oestrogen suppression therapy.

HELA vs TCRE

Laser ablation of the endometrium has many proponents, although there are probably as many who prefer electro-diathermy resection or rollerball coagulation. Most of the debate in the literature centres on the cost of equipment, the technical ability needed to perform the operations, and the immediate complications; in our multi-centre study, however, the safety of HELA was impressive, particularly when compared to the complications of electricity later reported by others.

There are almost no comparative data on the efficiency and success rates of the two procedures: presumably because gynaecologists have rightly chosen to develop expertise in one or other of the techniques, and very few operators have developed sufficient experience to be able to produce any valid comparative figures.

The data in Table 24.1 represent different surgeons, centres, and even different countries. Despite the many differences in cases and techniques, however, there is a broad similarity in success rates and amenorrhoea rates between those studies utilizing laser surgery, and those utilizing electrosurgery.

This indicates that differences between the two techniques are likely to be minimal, at least in the short term. It is not yet possible to say whether any of the long-term effects (eg the extent of intrauterine adhesions or the possible return of menstruation) will differ between the two procedures.

It seems unlikely that major long-term differences will emerge, or that any short or long-term differences in success will be shown. At present we use the Nd:YAG laser (with a dragging, contact technique) and would recommend this, principally because of the lower operative complication rates. However, the published differences between the two techniques, particularly with regard to long-term efficacy, are so small that the best operation for any patient must be that with which her gynaecologist has had the most experience and feels most comfortable.

Conclusions

There is no doubt that the short-term results of the hysteroscopic treatment of menorrhagia are impressive. In the long term the procedure also appears effective. Although there are no precise figures available, it does seem that the majority of patients cured by the treatment are likely to remain satisfied over the years. This is certainly our personal experience, with follow-up periods of up to seven years.

Pregnancy is a risk, albeit a small one, and if pregnancy continues it is likely to be complicated. In our experience, however, termination is likely to be uncomplicated. Sterilization should be discussed with all patients as part of their preoperative counselling.

Anxieties about problems with the development of endometrial carcinoma have not so far been proven. Continued vigilance is necessary, but it seems unlikely that anything will curb the spread in popularity of these procedures. If the safety record of the procedure improves, and the long-term efficacy is proven, then these operations could become preferable to medical therapy in that group of patients who have completed their family.

References

1   Goldrath MH *et al.* (1981) Laser photovaporization of endometrium for the treatment of menorrhagia. *American Journal of Obstetrics and Gynecology.* **140**:14–19.

2   de Cherney AH and Polan ML (1983) Hysteroscopic management of intrauterine lesions and intractable uterine bleeding. *Obstetrics and Gynaecology.* **61**:392–7.

3   Magos AL *et al.* (1991) Experience with the first 250 endometrial resections for menorrhagia. *Lancet.* **337**:1074–8.

4   Boto TCA, Fowler CG and Djahanbakhch O (1989) Transcervical resection of the endometrium in women with menorrhagia. *British Medical Journal.* **298**:1518.

5   Rankin L and Steinberg LH (1992) Transcervical resection of the endometrium: a review of 400 consecutive patients. *British Journal of Obstetrics and Gynaecology.* **99**:911–14.

6   Gannon MJ *et al.* (1991) A randomised trial comparing endometrial resection and abdominal hysterectomy for the treatment of menorrhagia. *British Medical Journal.* **303**:1362–4.

7   Garry R *et al.* (1991) A multicentre collaborative study into the treatment of menorrhagia by NdYAG ablation of the endometrium. *British Journal of Obstetrics and Gynaecology.* **98**:357–62.

8   Bent AE and Ostergard DR (1990) Endometrial ablation with the Neodymium YAG laser. *Obstetrics and Gynaecology.* **75**:923–5.

9   Loffer FD (1987) Hysteroscopic endometrial ablation with the Nd:YAG laser using a non-touch technique. *Obstetrics and Gynaecology.* **69**:679–82.

10   Nisolle M *et al.* (1991) Endometrial ablation with the Nd-YAG laser in dysfunctional bleeding. *Minimally Invasive Therapy.* **1**:35–9.

11 Goldrath MH (1990) Use of Danazol in hysteroscopic surgery for menorrhagia. *Journal of Reproductive Medicine*. **35**(Suppl. 1):91–6.

12 Loffer D (1988) Laser ablation of the endometrium. *Obstetrical and Gynecological Clinics of North America*. **15**:77–89.

13 Slade RJ *et al.* (1991) Problems with endometrial resection. *Lancet*. **337**:p.1473.

14 Mongelli JM and Evans AJ (1991) Pregnancy after transcervical endometrial resection. *Lancet*. **338**:578–9.

15 Hill DJ and Maher PJ (1992) Pregnancy following endometrial ablation. *Gynaecological Endoscopy*. **1**:47–9.

16 Siddle N *et al.* (1987) The effects of hysterectomy on the age at ovarian failure: identification of a subgroup of women with premature loss of ovarian function, and literature review. *Fertility and Sterility*. **47**:94–100.

25

Complications of Operative Hysteroscopy

ANTHONY WEEKES and ERNST VOSS

Introduction

Operative hysteroscopy has revolutionized the treatment of menorrhagia, submucous fibroids and uterine septae. Patients suffering from these conditions no longer need abdominal incisions and long hospitalization. Their postoperative period is comparatively pain free and resumption of normal activity a matter of days rather than weeks. Hysteroscopy is superior to curettage in making an accurate diagnosis of pathological conditions in the uterine cavity[1] and its safety is well established. Nevertheless, like any other surgical procedure it has complications.

In a survey of members of the British Society for Gynaecological Endoscopy (BSGE), a 3% complication rate amongst 4038 cases of endometrial ablation was found[2]. In contrast, Dicker *et al.*[3] found a complication rate of 24.5% and 42.8% for vaginal and abdominal hysterectomy respectively. Sculpher *et al.*[4] in their prospective study comparing endometrial resection with abdominal hysterectomy found similar intraoperative complications (5–6%) but the hysteroscopic procedure had a 3% postoperative complications rate, compared to 38% in the hysterectomy group.

A 1991 survey of operative hysteroscopy by the American Association of Gynecologic Laparoscopists, found a complication rate of about 2.5%. This survey is the most comprehensive to date in relation to size. The number of patients reported on was 17298[5]. In 1976 operative hysteroscopies at Rush Green Hospital, the complication rate was less than 1% and there was no mortality.

Complications associated with hysteroscopy fall into four main categories:

- trauma (during instrumentation or as a result of inappropriate endometrial resection or ablation)
- haemorrhage
- related to distension media
- infection.

Trauma

Operative hysteroscopy requires the cervix to be dilated sufficiently (usually to 9 mm Hegars) to allow the passage of the operative hysteroscope. As the majority of patients are multiparous there is rarely a problem. However, in a small proportion of patients, particularly in nulliparous patients and those in their late forties, the cervix can sometimes be quite fibrous and difficult to dilate adequately. If excessive force is used, it may result in a cervical laceration which could even extend and cause bleeding from the uterine vessels. However, the latter is extremely rare. Difficult dilation of the cervix may more commonly result in the creation of a false passage or perforation of the uterus. The majority of reported cases of uterine perforation occurred during cervical dilation. The uterus may also be perforated by the operating hysteroscope particularly when the uterus is either acutely retroverted or has a small cavity.

Uterine perforation is the commonest complication of operative hysteroscopy[2,6,8]. It does not usually result in serious morbidity. However, when recognized, a laparoscopy should be performed to ensure that no damage has been done to intra-abdominal structures. If the injury is a perforation per se, and provided the rent in the uterus is not very large, it can be treated conservatively and the patient given prophylactic antibiotics. Nonetheless, if the operator is unaware of the perforation and proceeds to do an endometrial ablation or resection, serious damage may be caused to intra-abdominal structures. The authors know of several cases where this has occurred. In one patient, pieces of small bowel and a small area of sigmoid colon were resected; this patient had three major laparotomies, bowel resection,

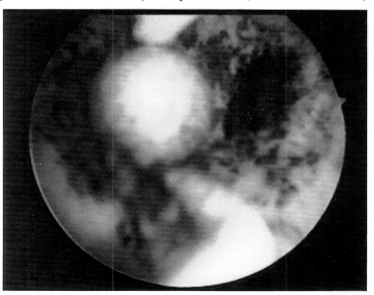

Figure 25.1: Uterine perforation with rollerball endometrial ablation.

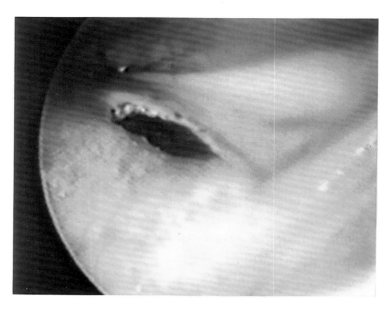

Figure 25.2: Laparoscopic view of uterine perforation in Figure 25.1.

colostomy and six weeks in hospital. In another instance of unrecognized uterine perforation, a small area of rectum was resected, a colostomy was required and prolonged hospitalization followed. Incredible as it may seem, the authors also know of a fatality associated with damage and resection of the inferior vena cava. These disasters occurred during the early 'learning curve' of a gynaecologist and serve to emphasize the necessity for preceptorships and proper training before commencing hysteroscopic surgery. The 'see one do one' philosophy is totally inappropriate. Perforation of the uterus may also occur during the operative procedure, particularly when either ablating or resecting the uterine cornua. This is not surprising as it is the thinnest part of the uterus. It is therefore imperative that extra care is taken while operating in the vicinity of the uterine cornua. A forward facing loop or the rollerball is recommended for use in this area.

Uterine perforation and its potentially serious complications can be avoided by following simple guidelines. Bimanual examination should always be performed to ascertain the position and size of the uterus. Half size dilators should be used if dilatation of the cervix proves difficult. The hysteroscope should not be introduced blindly but under direct vision and without exerting excessive force. Intrauterine operative procedures should only be performed when there is a clear view of the uterine cavity. These simple measures should help reduce the risk of uterine perforation. At Rush Green Hospital, the uterine perforation rate was 2.5 per 1000 with no associated serious morbidity. Table 25.1 shows a reported uterine perforation rate of between 0.2–1.6%. Damage to adjacent organs occurred in up to 0.22% of the cases reported.

Table 25.1: Complication rates of endometrial ablation and myomectomy: a worldwide experience.

AUTHOR	No of cases, modality	Uterine perforation	Damage to adjacent organs	Haemorrhage	Fluid over-load	Pulmonary oedema	Infection	Total complication rate	Remarks
RCOG[6]	6850 a	1.2%	0.13%	0.2%	0.4%	iu	0.4%	2.3%	UK survey conducted by RCOG
Macdonald[2]	4038 a	1.14%	0.22%	0.2%	0.4%	iu	0.97%	3%	Postal survey — UK
Erian[7]	2342 b	0.2%	0.00	0.3%	0.9%	0.4%	0.6%	2.4%	Multicentre study UK
Hill[8]	850 c	0.8%	0.00	0.8%	0.00	0.00	0.5%	2.1%	Australia
Garry[9]	859 b	0.35%	0.00	0.00	0.00	0.47%	0.47%	1.28%	Multicentre study UK and USA
Nisolle[10]	150 b	0.00	0.00	0.00	2%	0.00	iu	2%	No fluid overload since use of GnRH - a and continuous flow hysteroscopy — Belgium
Magos[11]	250 d	1.6%	0.00	0.4%	2.8%	0.00	iu	4.8%	UK
Serden[12]	216 e	0.47%	0.00	1.85%	0.47%	iu	0.92%	3.7%	USA
Goldrath[13]	335 b	0.3%	0.00	4.18%	1.49%	0.59%	1.19%	7.76%	USA

KEY:
a - diathermy, Nd:YAG and RaFEA
b - Nd:YAG
c - diathermy resection - 707 and diathermy rollerball –143
d - diathermy resection
e - myomectomy only - 90 and diathermy resection
iu - information unavailable

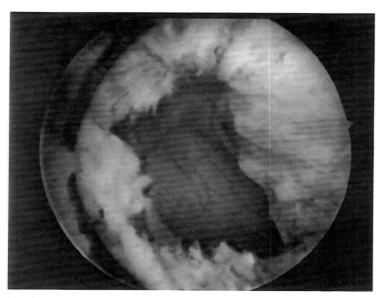

Figure 25.3: Uterine perforation with endometrial resection. Bowel visible behind perforation.

Haemorrhage

Trauma to the cervix or the uterus including perforation may cause haemorrhage. Hysteroscopic myomectomy may also be associated with quite heavy bleeding during and after the procedure. The uterine arteries may be damaged if resection or ablation of the isthmic part of the uterus is too deep.

The endometrium is extremely vascular and usually an endometrium suppressant drug is given preoperatively. There is less bleeding and a clearer view of the uterine cavity when the endometrium is prepared. The drug most commonly used, danazol, should be administered in a dose of between 400–800 mg daily for 4–6 weeks prior to surgery. Because of its known side effects (eg hot flushes, weight gain and muscle cramps), patient non-compliance may be a problem.

GnRH analogues like Prostrap, Buserelin or Zoladex (commonly used in the UK) can also be used to thin the endometrium. Brooks et al.[14] compared the effect of progestins, danazol and a GnRH analogue (leuprolide acetate) on the endometrium before endometrial resection and found that leuprolide acetate produced the most dependable suppression of the endometrium. The sample size in this study (25 women) was, however, too small to provide conclusive evidence. The relative efficacy of danazol and the GnRH analogues needs proper clinical evaluation. An advantage of GnRH analogues is that with a monthly injection patient compliance is irrelevant. There is no doubt that these drugs reduce endometrial thickness and as a result there is less bleeding.

If bleeding proves to be a problem during endometrial resection, it can be reduced by using a combination of cutting and coagulation in a blend mode. If there is excessive bleeding during laser endometrial ablation, it can be corrected by briefly increasing the intrauterine pressure. This, of course, has its dangers in relation to fluid overload and the operator should be aware of this risk. Intraoperative bleeding can make the hysteroscopic resection of submucous fibroids a very difficult operation. It usually suffices to use a blend mode and slightly higher than normal intrauterine pressure. However, as previously stated, it is not uncommon for hysteroscopic myomectomy to be followed by quite brisk bleeding; this can be controlled by the insertion of a Foley catheter with a 30 ml balloon and distension of the balloon with water. The catheter can then be removed after 4–8 hours or left in overnight. The insertion of the balloon invariably controls the bleeding and makes further operative intervention unnecessary. This catheter balloon inflation technique is also useful if there is heavy bleeding after a straightforward endometrial ablation or resection. The use of intracervical vasopressin prior to operative hysteroscopy has been claimed to reduce bleeding during operative hysteroscopy[15].

In order to minimize bleeding, the patient should be given a GnRH analogue before hysteroscopic myomectomy is attempted. A monthly injection (for two months) should reduce the size and vascularity of the fibroids by more than 30%[16]. Heavy bleeding during or following endometrial ablation or hysteroscopic myomectomy has been reported to occur in up to 4% of patients (see Table 25.1).

Distension medium

Media used to distend the uterus include:

- carbon dioxide (CO_2)
- high molecular rate dextran
- low viscosity liquids (sorbitol, glycine, dextrose and normal saline).

Each distension medium may cause specific problems. In addition, all fluid media have the potential to cause fluid overload.

Carbon dioxide

Carbon dioxide is commonly used for diagnostic hysteroscopy. Its use is limited for surgical intrauterine procedures as the view will be obscured by bubbles created by the mixture of gas, blood and mucus; there is also an increased risk of CO_2 embolism.

The safety of CO_2 in diagnostic hysteroscopy is well established. Lindemann and Gallinat[17] reported no changes in ECG, pCO_2 or pH in 40 patients during CO_2 hysteroscopy. In canine experiments, CO_2 was infused intravenously and at a rate of 200 ml/min caused only a slight increase in pulse and deepening of breathing after five minutes without a change in pH or pCO_2; at 400 ml/min toxic signs appeared and at 1000 ml/min it was lethal after one minute[18].

A laparoscopic insufflator should never be used for hysteroscopy. Modern insufflators can deliver 15 l/min or more, but even the older models that provide 1–2 l/min are extremely dangerous. However, provided the flow rate and intrauterine pressure rate are strictly controlled, the risk of significant CO_2 embolism is minimal. The flow rate should not be greater than 100 ml per minute and the maximum pressure should not be greater than 150–200 mmHg. Brundin and Thomasson[19] have suggested that heart auscultation should be mandatory during hysteroscopy procedures when CO_2 is the distension medium. CO_2 embolism can be diagnosed on auscultation of the heart by the appearance of typically metallic heart sounds. If this occurs, the procedure should be immediately abandoned. In a more recent study using ultrasound cardiography it was confirmed that precordial heart auscultation is a sufficient precautionary measure to detect cardiac gas embolism during CO_2 hysteroscopy[20]. In a series of over 2000 diagnostic hysteroscopies, the authors have not encountered a problem related to CO_2 embolism.

Liquids

The main complication with liquid distension media is excessive absorption of fluid. Fluid overload occurs between 0 and 2.8% and pulmonary oedema in less than 0.6% of cases (*see* Table 25.1).

High molecular weight dextran (Hyskon)

Dextran 70 consists of 32% dextran in 10% dextrose; because of its immiscibility with blood it gives a very good view of the uterine cavity during hysteroscopic surgery. Anaphylactic reactions to intravenous injections and intraperitoneal installation of dextran are well documented[21]. Non-cardiogenic pulmonary oedema, most probably due to the direct toxic effect on pulmonary vessels, has been reported[22,23]. Intravascular dextran may cause coagulopathy and Vercellin *et al.*[24] have reported a case of a healthy young woman who developed acute hypervolaemic pulmonary oedema and severe coagulopathy when a dilute dextran solution (10% dextran 40 in normal saline) was used for a hysteroscopic metroplasty.

Another disadvantage of this high-viscosity liquid is the caramelization on heating and adherence to instruments which can then be difficult to clean. Less serious, but still capable of causing significant morbidity, is the retention of significant quantities of dextran in the peritoneal cavity. This may cause intravascular fluid overload and ascites. As little dextran as possible should be used to minimize the risk of this complication. It has been suggested than an intravenous injection of a small quantity of dextran just prior to anaesthetizing the patient should test whether there is a risk of anaphylactic shock, but a severe reaction even to this small dose has been reported[25].

Low-viscosity liquids

Low-viscosity fluids such as glycine 1.5%, sorbitol, dextrose 5% in water and normal saline are most commonly used for operative hysteroscopy. Apart from normal saline, these liquids are low in sodium or sodium free and may thus cause hyponatraemia, as well as fluid overload and pulmonary oedema.

Glycine 1.5%, extensively used by urologists for transurethral resection (TUR) of the prostate, has been known to be associated with encephalopathy. This is thought to be due to high levels of serum glycine and its by-product ammonia[26].

It has also been suggested that glycine may be cardiotoxic[27]. To date, there have been no reports of severe TUR-type syndrome reactions associated with the use of glycine for intrauterine surgery.

Normal saline is associated with the risk of fluid overload and pulmonary oedema. This solution is favoured by a large proportion of hysteroscopists for use in laser endometrial ablation as it does not carry the risk of central nervous system toxicity. However, some hysteroscopists feel that it does not give as good a view as glycine.

In order to reduce the risk of fluid overload, several precautionary measures have been suggested. Hasham et al.[28] found that there was no fluid deficit if the mean maximum intrauterine pressure was 70 mmHg or less and, according to Lomano[29], when using the blanching technique as opposed to the dragging technique in Nd:YAG endometrial ablation, the fluid absorption was reduced from an average of 2122 ml to 246 ml.

It is essential to monitor fluid intake and output during operative hysteroscopy. Likewise, at the end of the procedure, it is just as important to find out if there is a fluid deficit. If there is a deficit of more than 1500–2000 ml, serious consideration should be given to the use of diuretics. It is essential that the patient should have a continuous urinary output measurement during and after the operation. This can only be achieved by having the use of an indwelling catheter during the procedure. Obviously, without this, any fluid balance measurement is inaccurate.

Infection

Salat-Baroux et al. reported only seven cases of pelvic infection in 4000 hysteroscopic examinations, 90% of which were done in an office setting[30]. However, in a personal series of 1976 hysteroscopies, there were ten known cases of proven infection and, apart from two, these were not of serious consequence. One patient developed a septicaemia due to beta-haemolytic streptococcus; in the other, pseudomonas was grown from the blood culture. The two cases mentioned both developed very high temperatures, rigors and sweating within a few hours of the operation. There is a case to be made for the use of prophylactic antibiotics if the procedure is unduly prolonged or the patient has had pelvic inflammatory disease in the past. However, before this becomes standard clinical practice, it should be properly evaluated. Another pre-emptive measure would be to take high vaginal swabs from all patients before operative hysteroscopic procedures. This may be particularly relevant if there is vaginal discharge or any other reason to suggest pelvic infection. It has been reported that hysteroscopy may cause a flare up of pelvic inflammatory disease.

Injuries due to electrical or laser energy

Injuries may result from the use of electricity, particularly with regard to its thermal effect. More interestingly, long-term thermal injuries to the uterine wall may result in scarring and the formation of intrauterine synechiae. It is quite possible that this scarring and adhesion formation may be responsible for the cyclical pain which some amenorrhoeic patients or patients with even scanty periods get months after endometrial resection.

Injuries due to the use of laser energy are unlikely in the uterine cavity, except perhaps at the uterine cornua where the uterus is thinnest and caution should be employed in ablating this area. Obviously, if there is a uterine perforation which is unrecognized and the laser or diathermy is activated outside of the uterus, this can then result in damage to adjacent structures[31,32].

Endometrial carcinoma

Romano *et al.*[33] reported a case in which endometrial carcinoma was diagnosed on hysteroscopy and, at laparotomy, cytology from peritoneal washings were found to be positive for carcinoma. They suggested that the dissemination of malignant cells during hysteroscopy was very likely and quoted Beyth[34] and Nagel *et al.*[35] who demonstrated that reflux of endometrial tissue may occur during irrigation of the uterine cavity for operative hysteroscopy. In our view, the possibility of spread of endometrial carcinoma as a result of hysteroscopy seems unlikely but there is a need for more extensive evaluation.

There is a possibility, in the longer term, of carcinoma developing in buried endometrium or in residual or regrown endometrium shut off by adhesions from the cervix. If this were to occur, bleeding may be a very late symptom and by the time the patient presents, the neoplasm may be advanced. This is unlikely after laser endometrial ablation, as the uterine cavity is usually a tubular open non-adhesive cavity. However, after endometrial resection, it is not uncommon to see intrauterine adhesions. In some instances, the adhesions may totally partition part of the uterine cavity from its access to the cervical canal. Whether this proves to be a real worry or a theoretical possibility can only be established by long-term follow-up of patients who have had endometrial resection.

Poor outcome

If endometrial ablation, resection or hysteroscopic myomectomy fails to relieve the patient of her symptoms, then this can be considered to be a significant complication. It is now generally believed that the majority of failures (apart from those in the early learning curve of the hysteroscopist's experience) are associated with adenomyosis. In our institution, a preliminary study of 248 endometrial resections and ablations showed that amongst the failures, adenomyosis was present in 46% of those patients who needed a hysterectomy.

Conclusions

Complications associated with hysteroscopy are infrequent (*see* Table 25.1) and are proportionally less than those associated with either diagnostic curettage or hysterectomy for benign conditions. It is essential that the gynaecologist undertaking these minimally invasive procedures should be properly trained and should follow the basic principles outlined in this chapter. (Particularly with reference to the risks inherent in the use of the instruments and distension media.) Perhaps the most important advice to the aspiring hysteroscopist is that he or she should never operate unless there is a clear view of the uterine cavity.

References

1   Gimpelson RJ and Rappold HO (1988) A comparative study between panoramic hysteroscopy with directed biopsies and dilatation and curettage. *American Journal of Obstetrics and Gynecology*. 158:489–92.

2   Macdonald R, Phipps J and Singer A (1992) Endometrial ablation: a safe procedure. *Gynaecological Endoscopy*. 1:7–9.

3   Dicker RC *et al.* (1982) Complications of abdominal and vaginal hysterectomy among women of reproductive age in the United States. *American Journal of Obstetrics and Gynecology*. 144:841–8.

4   Sculpher MJ *et al.* (1993) An economic evaluation of transcervical endometrial resection versus abdominal hysterectomy for the treatment of menorrhagia. *British Journal of Obstetrics and Gynaecology*. 100:244–52.

5 Hulka JF, Peterson HB, Phillips JM, Surrey MW (1993) Operative hysteroscopy. American Association of Gynecologic Laparoscopists 1991 Membership survey . *Journal of Reproductive Medicine*. **38**:572–3.

6 Royal College of Obstetricians and Gynaecologists (1991) *Endometrical ablation survey.*

7 Erian J, Weekes ARL and McMillan L (1993) *Hysteroscopic endometrial ablation: present and future techniques.* Presented at the World Congress in Reproductive Endocrinology, Bali.

8 Hill D *et al.* (1992) Complications of operative hysteroscopy. *Gynaecological Endoscopy*. **1**:185–9.

9 Garry R, Erian J and Grochmal SA (1991) A multicentre collaborative study into the treatment of menorrhagia by Nd-YAG laser ablation of the endometrium. *British Journal of Obstetrics and Gynaecology*. **98**:357–62.

10 Nisolle M *et al.* (1991) Endometrial ablation with the Nd-YAG laser in dysfunctional bleeding. *Minimally Invasive Therapy*. **1**:35–9.

11 Magos AL, Baumann R, Lockwood GM and Turnbull AC (1991) Experience with the first 250 endometrial resections for menorrhagia. *Lancet*. **337r:1074–8.**

12 Serden SP and Brooks PG (1991) Treatment of abnormal uterine bleeding with the gynecologic resectoscope. *Journal of Reproductive Medicine*. **36**:697–9.

13 Goldrath MH (1990) Use of danazol in hysteroscopic surgery for menorrhagia. *Journal of Reproductive Medicine*. **35**:91–6.

14 Brooks PG, Serden SP and Davos I (1991) Hormonal inhibition of the endometrium for resectoscopic endometrial ablation. *American Journal of Obstetrics and Gynecology*. **164**:1601–8.

15 Lefler HT, Sullivan GH and Hulka JF (1991) Modified endometrial ablation: electrocoagulation with vasopressin and suction curettage preparation. *Obstetricsand Gynecology*. **77**:949–53.

16 Donnez J *et al.* (1990) Neodymium:YAG laser hysteroscopy in large submucous fibroids. *Fertility and Sterility*. **54**:999–1003.

17 Lindemann HJ and Gallinat A (1976) Physikalische und physiologische Grundlagen der CO_2-Hysteroskopie *Geburtshilfe und Frauenheilkunde*. **36**:729.

18 Lindemann HJ (1980) *Atlas der Hysteroskopie.* Gustav Fischer, Stuttgart.

19 Brundin J and Thomasson K (1989) Cardiac gas embolism during carbon dioxide hysteroscopy: risk and management. *European Journal of Obstetrics, Gynecology and Reproductive Biology*. **33**:241–5.

20 Rythen-Alder E *et al.* (1992) Detection of carbon dioxide embolism during hysteroscopy. *Gynaecological Endoscopy*. **1**:207–10.

21 Borten M, Seibert CP and Taymor ML (1983) Recurrent anaphylactic reaction to intraperitoneal dextran 75 used for prevention of postsurgical adhesions. *Obstetrics and Gynecology*. **61**:755.

22 Zbella EA, Moise J and Carson SA (1985) Noncardiogenic pulmonary edema secondary to intrauterine installation of 32% dextran 70. *Fertility and Sterility*. **43**:479–80.

23 Leake JF, Murphy AA and Zacur HA (1985) Non-cardiogenic pulmonary edema: a complication of operative hysteroscopy. *Fertility and Sterility*. **48**:497–9.

24 Vercellini P, Rossi R, Pagnoni B and Fedele L (1992) Hypervolemic pulmonary edema and severe coagulopathy after intrauterine dextran installation. *Obstetrics and Gynecology*. **79**:838–9.

25 Berstein RL, Rosenberg AD, Iada EY and Jaffe FF (1987) A severe reaction to dextran hapten inhibitin. *Anesthesiology*. **67**:567–9.

26 Roesh RP *et al*. (1983) Ammonia toxicity resulting from glycine absorption during a transurethral resection of the prostate. *Anesthesiology*. **58**:577–9.

27 Coppinger SWV and Hudd C (1989) Risk factor for myocardial infarction in transurethral resection of prostate. Letter, *Lancet*. **2**:859.

28 Hasham F, Garry R, Koleri MS and Mooney P (1992) Fluid absorption during laser ablation of the endometrium in the treatment of menorrhagia. *British Journal of Anaesthesia*. **68**:11–14.

29 Lomano JM (1988) Dragging technique versus blanching technique for endometrial ablation with the Nd:YAG laser in the treatment of chronic menorrhagia. *American Journal of Obstetrics and Gynecology*. **159**:152–5.

30 Salat-Baroux J *et al*. (1984) Complications from microhysteroscopy. In: Siegler AN and Lindemann HJ (eds). *Hysteroscopy: principles and practice*. JB Lippincott, Philadelphia.

31 Kivnick S and Kanter MH (1992) Bowel injury from rollerball ablation of the endometrium. *Obstetrics and Gynecology*. **79**:833–5.

32 Perry CP, Daniell JF and Gimpelson RJ (1990) Bowel injury from Nd:YAG endometrial ablation. *Journal of Gynecological Surgery*. **6**:199–203.

33 Romano S, Shimoni Y, Muralee D and Shalev E (1992) Retrograde seeding of endometrial carcinoma during hysteroscopy. *Gynecologic Oncology*. **44**:116–18.

34 Beyth Y *et al*. (1975) Retrograde seeding of endometrium, sequela of tubal flushing. *Fertility and Sterility*. **26**:1094.

35 Nagel TC *et al*. (1984) Tubal reflux of endometrial tissue during hysteroscopy. In: Siegler AN and Lindemann HJ (eds). *Hysteroscopy: principles and practice*. JB Lippincott, Philadelphia.

Part V: The Future of Endoscopic Surgery

The Future of Endoscopic Surgery

26

The Future of Endoscopic Surgery
STEPHEN A GROCHMAL

Introduction

The location is a medical centre somewhere on the East Coast of the USA. You are accompanying the operating surgeon from the physician waiting area to the operating suite. You enter a control room, an area similar to that used in interventional neuroradiology procedures. In front of you is a large glass window, and in the distance you can see a sophisticated operating table on a cylindrical pedicle rising from the floor in the dimly lit room.

As you stare through the glass, the patient is wheeled into the operating room with the anaesthesiologist and ancillary personnel. With the patient prepared on the table and under intravenous sedation, a robotic multi-articulated unit descends from the ceiling and hovers over the patient (Figure 26.1). While under intravenous sedation, the Verres needle is inserted under direct visualization by one of the robotic arms, which the operating surgeon is controlling from the surgical control booth. As the needle is guided into the abdominal cavity, all the layers of the abdominal wall can be clearly seen

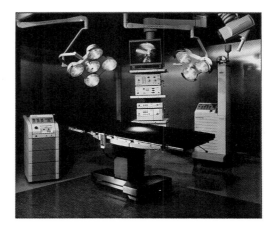

Figure 26.1: Operating room of the future with suspended electronic columns, pneumatic remote control table and laser delivery pedestals.

through its tip and accurate placement in the peritoneal cavity is confirmed. Once rapid full insufflation has been achieved, the patient is remotely manoeuvred into the Trendelenburg position.

A secondary robotic arm removes the Verres needle from the abdomen, and a large 15 mm trocar is inserted through the umbilicus by the assistant surgeon at the other side of the table. Once the trocar is in place, a large 14 mm operating three-dimensional electronic video laparoscope is placed down through the umbilical cannula and attached to one of the robotic arms (Figure 26.2). The operating surgeon in the control booth now confirms a video image on his operating screen; this three-dimensional image is as clear as in conventional open surgery. The video image from the monitor is also remotely displayed to other areas of the hospital including a classroom of second-year medical students across the street, and the pathology department who will ultimately receive the specimen (Figure 26.3). As the operating surgeon remotely manipulates the robotic arm of the electronic video laparoscope (Figure 26.4), secondary and tertiary puncture sites are made

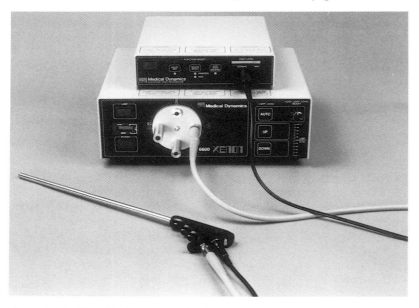

Figure 26.2: The 3D electronic video laparoscope uses two high resolution CCD imaging chips positioned at the distal tip of the scope with each CCD having its own 3-element lens system. The images from the two CCDs are processed separately and fed into special image processing circuitry housed inside an IBM compatible computer. The left and right images are then presented sequentially on the monitor at twice the normal (60 Hz) rate to eliminate flickering. As the left and right images are switched on and off, an infrared emitter which is synchronously driven, switches each lens of the liquid shutter eyeglasses on and off. For example, when the left image is displayed on the monitor the left lens on the eyeglass opens while the right lens remains closed, the reverse is true when the right image is displayed. By using the two CCDs side by side, the user sees an image from two different perspectives which closely simulates human stereoscopic vision which gives objects a realistic amount of depth that cannot be seen with a 2D image. This results in a more accurate, lifelike image and significantly aids in the manipulation of surgical instruments.

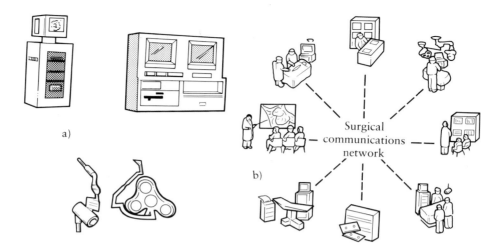

Figure 26.3: a Video cameras (hidden in the lights of the operating room, or suspended from the ceiling) collect images from the operating room environment as well as from the video recorders and video endoscopic tower. **b** Video images collected by suspended cameras (as shown in A) can be transmitted via integrated networks to classrooms, consultants' archives and other areas of the institution, and also via satellite to teleconferences worldwide.

by additional robotic arms. The assistant surgeon puts in the proper instruments and attaches them to the robotic arms which can be manipulated from the control booth.

This patient has been diagnosed as being an unruptured ectopic pregnancy. Since there is no evidence of any pelvic haemorrhage, a robotic laparolift arm is swung into place and an elevator trocar is substituted for the original 15 mm trocar as the pneumoperitoneum is slowly replaced by mechanical lift (Figure 26.5). Using laser energy via the operating channel of the electronic video laparoscope, the operating surgeon begins the initial tubal incision from the control booth by moving a joystick. This laser energy from an Nd:YAG laser is delivered from a small launch port in the wall of the operating room and transmitted overhead via an umbilical cable. The operating theatre personnel make adjustments to the laser energy with a small hand-held remote control unit. The laser itself is located at some distance from the operating theatre in a specially designed room, from which it supplies laser energy to other operating rooms throughout the building via long semi-rigid fibre cables.

The assistant surgeon, wearing a pair of 3D glasses, adjusts the monitor which hangs from the ceiling track so that it can slide back and forth. From the control booth, the operating surgeon advances 3 mm pneumatic grasping forceps into the right fallopian tube using the robotic arm, and the products of conception are extracted and passed to the nurse. There is slight oozing from the edges of the incision. The robotic arm uses Nd:YAG non-contact energy to coagulate the borders of the serosa. Copious lavage is then performed using a high-flow, high pressure irrigation aspirating system originating from one of the ceiling towers.

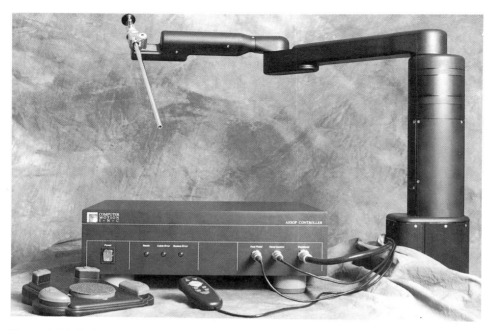

Figure 26.4: Robotic-assisted technology with the AESOP (automated endoscopic system for optimal positioning) allows complete remote control of laparoscope or secondary trocar sites. The aim is manoeuvred interactively with an intuitive foot control. Previously viewed video sites can be returned to and repeated at a button-touch throughout the endoscopic procedure. The system may also be controlled by a simple hand-held control unit. (Photo courtesy of Computer Motion Inc, California, USA.)

A specialized tissue glue is then inserted through the 3 mm cannula and directed over the incision site on the fallopian tube. An anti-adhesive material is passed down through the operating channel of the laparoscope, using the robotic arm, and is spread over the tubal surface. The robotic lift system is removed after the trocars and cannulae have been removed from the articulating robotic arm system which is then retracted back into the ceiling receptacles.

Finally you discover that a video image of the surgical procedure has been transmitted to St Mary's Regional Hospital Centre in London via satellite where consultant gynaecologists with several registered surgeons in training have been observing the surgical procedure. You failed to notice that the operating surgeon was wearing an ear-piece and a small microphone under his mask which allowed him to converse directly with the consultant gynaecologists in London, the medical students in the classroom and the pathologist in the laboratory. Furthermore, the entire procedure was performed under intravenous sedation.

If this sounds 'far out', actually it isn't. All of this technology presently exists and will be the standard by the millennium for minimally invasive surgical procedures.

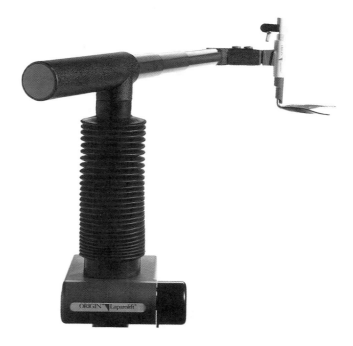

Figure 26.5: Laparolift robotic arm.

Instrumentation

Of all the problems with endoscopic surgery, the most limiting is the unavailability of proper operative instrumentation. This is true for all the surgical specialties now beginning to use the endoscopic minimal access approach. As instrumentation develops and technology improves, so does the outcome and the chances of the procedure being performed completely endoscopically. These sections of the chapter are difficult to write because by the time the book is printed, many of those developments and improvements in instrumentation which are presently on the drawing board will be in use by endoscopic surgeons.

Tissue morcellation

Most procedures currently being performed are limited by the difficulties of extracting tissue from the abdominal cavity. This inability to extract tissue has been caused by the limitations of the mechanical instruments that are used at present to remove pathological specimens through an endoscopic puncture. Whether in general surgery, gynaecology or urology, the difficulty of removing large tumours or tissue masses has always been perplexing and is still unresolved. The virtuous endoscopic surgeon would prefer to remove, morcellate, vaporize or vibrate these tissue masses completely endoscopically.

Currently the only method of morcellating tissue is the Semm hand-operated morcellator with the recently developed 'cookie-cutter-like' tissue extraction tubes which are introduced through 15–50 mm or larger ports to grind away large fragments of tissue specimen (Figure 26.6). Unfortunately, although this system is effective, it is difficult to manoeuvre and operate, often leaving the operating surgeon with an acute tendonitis and a sore hand from the twisting motion required. The best improvement would be the mechanization or electrification of this hand-operated system. Already in limited use is a shaver or automated morcellator system which is used by urologists in endoscopic nephrectomy. With this system, the specimen is placed into a Kevlar impermeable bag and brought up through one of the endoscopic ports; a grinder-like sleeve is then placed down through the port to morcellate and remove the entire kidney. Unfortunately, the specimen is removed in fragments and resembles a purée which could be perplexing to the pathologist to evaluate. These early prototypes are still under development and trial, and organizations such as the FDA (in the USA) have held up their arrival in the market place.

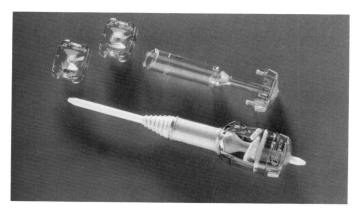

Figure 26.6: 33 mm transparent disposable trocar with alternative reduction sleeves utilized for tissue extraction.

This idea of an automated system is probably in the neophyte stage and will lead to a specific instrument being developed for this purpose. Imagine a Nicad battery handle which can be recharged within the operating room and to which a series of motorized instruments could be attached. In this case the main instrument would be the tissue morcellator, but this could perhaps be interchanged with electric scissors or pneumatic graspers. This would decrease cost as well as increase efficiency, leading to shortened operating room time.

Hand-held instrumentation

There are a number of companies developing hand-held instruments, but none of them appear to be taking consideration of the surgeon's comfort and ease of use. These instruments could be improved with ergonomically designed thumb and finger grips. Nor has any company addressed the need for a hand-held instrument which can grasp large amounts of tissue within its jaws. The difficulty of maintaining the capture of the tissue within the grasp of the jaws may lead to miniaturized pneumatic systems being devised to maintain constant pressure on the tissue specimen. One innovative approach has been the development of reusable instruments which allow a ratchet, for example, to be interchanged with a spring-loaded handle, according to the preference of the operating surgeon. This can be done within the sterile environment of the operating field.

Along the same lines, the problem with reusable scissors is that they become dull quickly during endoscopic procedures. To solve this, a reusable instrument and hand shaft with a rotatable collar but with a disposable replaceable scissor tip or shaft has been developed. These scissors are designed in various configurations to facilitate tissue incision endoscopically (Figure 26.7). The enhancement of the rotatable collar and handle which can easily be manoeuvred by one finger of the operating surgeon's hand, will make the approach of the scissors in any direction more comfortable.

(a)

(b)

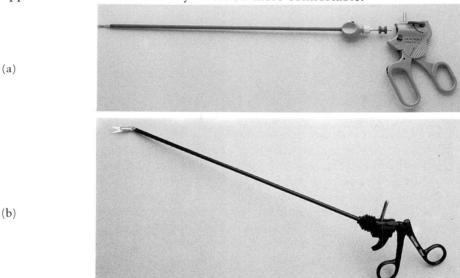

Figure 26.7: a Semi-disposable replacement shaft, with scissor tip, easily detaches from rotatable reusable handle. **b** A bendable lateral handle movement may be achieved, including horizontal displacement of the instrument tip.

Instrument diameters will increase to perhaps 20 or 30 mm as needed. They may be made of titanium, to withstand increased stress, and with operating channels to pass smaller secondary instrumentation. Just as instruments become larger, so they will also be made smaller to allow improved microtechniques in the future.

Laser applications

Lasers are used in many areas of medicine, from surgery to photodynamic therapy. Nearly all the medical specialties have come to accept the laser as a key instrument in the surgical arena. As surgery in the year 2000 will be largely non-invasive, nearly every operating surgeon will use lasers rather than scalpels in their surgical technique, and nearly all medical schools will be using lasers rather than scalpels in their classrooms.

Medical uses for diode lasers include the diode-pumped Nd:YAG lasers which, although not firmly established in clinical applications, do show promise. Many believe that diodes will replace ion lasers by the end of the decade, perhaps sooner, especially in the ophthalmological arena. They are said to be significantly less expensive than ion lasers since they do not require tube replacement.

The growing interest in minimal access treatment for benign and malignant conditions has also led to the introduction of the Nd:YAG laser via the endoscopic approach. Recent developments in design configurations of fibre delivery systems has led to the development of a side-fire laser fibre. This fibre allows approximately 93% of the laser energy to exit from the side of the fibre as it reflects off a 24 carat gold tip at the distal end of the fibre delivery system. Apart from applications in urology which appear to be promising at present, this system could also find its way into intrauterine surgery. Improved outcome for long-term amenorrhoea may be demonstrated if the clinical trials show that this application for endometrial ablation supersedes or improves the clinical outcome of patients treated with conventional fibre technology, either in a contact or non-contact mode. Presently a side fire energy is applied in a non-contact method.

To make lasers more useful as well as more effective, many manufacturers have been developing tunable devices which can operate at multiple wavelengths. One particular company has developed a tunable system that can operate at wavelengths equivalent to Alexandrite, Nd:YAG, Tm:YAG, Ho:YAG, Er:YSGG and Er:YAG lasers. The unit can deliver as many as three different wavelengths through separate fibres or simultaneously through one fibre. The ability to combine and mix various wavelengths, pulses and energy levels may well facilitate the exploration of new laser tissue interactions.

As manufacturers develop new technology, it is hoped that they will bring improvements in the life-expectancy and maintenance levels of these systems. In the future, one laser system might replace several single-purpose devices within the hospital or surgical unit. For now, however, such systems promise to be expensive until the economic scale, competition and agency approval have the effect of bringing down their prices.

Electronic visualization

In use today are the 'chip on a stick' laparoscopes, which have a small chip at the distal end of the telescope. Single-chip technology with individual pixel enhancement approaches the resolution and quality of standard three-chip systems. As chips decrease steadily in size, we will see electronic video hysteroscopes as well. By 1996, chips will be available as small as 4 mm.

Small colour cameras and monitors, measuring less than 5 cm in length and under 2.5 cm in both width and height are already available (Figure 26.8a). The micro-monitor (LCD) displays a 2 cm diagonal video image at 240 TV lines of horizontal resolution (Figure 26.8b).

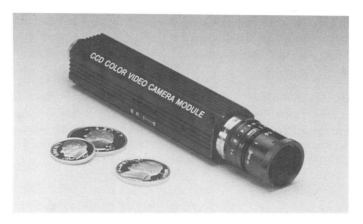

Figure 26.8a: Sony's miniature XC-777 colour camera module, with 1/3″ sensor format, is currently the smallest colour camera module available, measuring less than one inch in diameter and offering 470 TV lines of resolution (photo courtesy of Sony, Inc, Corporate Communication Dept.)

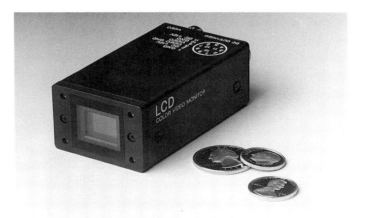

Figure 26.8b: The XC-MO7 colour LCD monitor provides OEMs with a high quality image in an ultra-small, 0.7-inch display. The XC-MO7 provides 240 TV lines of horizontal resolution and a contrast ratio of 120:1 for an exceptionally clear picture under a variety of lighting conditions. Perhaps this type of LCD display will find itself located on the proximal end of laparoscopes and hysteroscopes for a timely integrated video system optical scope! (photo courtesy of Sony, Inc, Corporate Communications Dept.)

Digitized super-cool CCD cameras and 3D systems will make endoscopic procedures appear clearer than in real life ('super real') and virtual reality training simulators will use imaging-based telepresence systems to train our future surgeons.

Widely used data-input devices known as digitizing tablets have recently found new uses when interfaced with computers to convert colour images, text and graphics into accurate digital information which can then be entered into the computer for storage or analysis. This video enhancement will allow increased accuracy for guiding instruments, needles and energy sources to their tissue targets endoscopically via remote control. Optical fibre technology has also progressed to such a point that single strands of fibre optics can now provide acceptable image on a monitor. Instead of having to insert the Verres needle blindly, visually guided needles or curettes with fibre bundles placed distally will allow in utero manipulation under video surveillance.

Hi-8 video recorder technology will allow more than 500 lines of resolution by the use of newly formatted and developed metal videotapes. A new format, W-VHS, will also appear. It captures 16:9 aspect ratio video on W-VHS format metal powder-coated tapes from soon-to-be-released with HDTV (NTSV) signals. W-VHS can also play back conventional VHS and S-VHS video signals in a normal 4:3 aspect ratio. The system can put nine hours of NTSC video on a three-hour tape plus a double track 'time-compression' recording allowing two separate NTSC video signals on the same tape recorded at the same time (Figure 26.9). Devices created by the imagination of electronic engineers will in turn stimulate the imagination of physicians to reach new levels in endoscopic procedures.

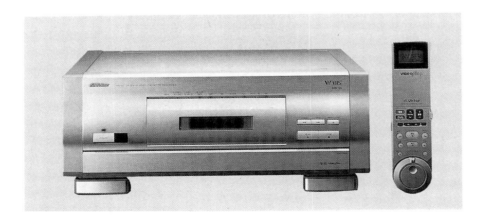

Figure 26.9: W-VHS recorder captures images from 1125-interlaced HDTV and NTSC signals – the first recorder of its kind to accomplish this (photo courtesy of JVC Professional Products.)

Future developments

As more and more surgical procedures are able to be done with minimal access techniques, the need for small ancillary hand-held accessories will become even more apparent. In the foreseeable future, development of an improved generation of retractors and retainers which can be introduced endoscopically through a trocar site will appear. These retractors will be deflectable as well as rotatable and will articulate at various angles in order to help the endoscopic surgeon isolate a particular surgical field within the endoscopic picture.

Improvements in automated stapling devices — mechanized, hand-operated or gas powered — are currently under development and some are already in use. The endoscopic stapling devices will make a laparoscopic total hysteroscopy, for example, quicker and easier, and cause minimal trauma to the surrounding vital structures such as the ureters, bowel and bladder. However, suture material will still find a place in the surgeon's armamentarium.

One of the most frustrating manoeuvres in endoscopic surgery is intracorporeal knot tying. This technique, which needs to be practised diligently, is sometimes awkward for tissue approximation. Despite the use of 3D enhancement on the video screen, endoscopic manoeuvring can still be perplexing for most endoscopic surgeons. Therefore the use of a suture clip, which can be used to secure or establish a knot-like presence once the tissue has been approximated with the needle, will make the intracorporeal approach easier. The previously developed absorbable clip appliers are the first step in allowing the endoscopic surgeon to use a true 'through and through approach' with suture material.

Additional equipment will be developed as the need arises. A good example of this is the development of the optical catheter for the Verres needle. Long seen as the last blind entry approach in endoscopic surgery, the insertion of the Verres needle can be hazardous and dangerous to the patient. As mentioned earlier, an optical fibre placed down through the sheath of the Verres needle itself can be used to enter the abdominal wall layer by layer under direct video visualization, thus avoiding major viscera below the peritoneal surface. This concept could find its way into amniocentesis, and neonatal, fetal and paediatric endoscopy, as well as neurosurgery, general surgery, gynaecology and urology.

Index